BORN TO WALK

Also by Mark Sisson with Brad Kearns

The Primal Blueprint
The Primal Blueprint 21-Day Total Body Transformation
The Primal Blueprint 90-Day Journal
The Primal Connection
Primal Endurance
The Keto Reset Diet
Keto for Life
Two Meals a Day

BORN TO WALK

The Broken Promises of the Running Boom
and How to Slow Down and Get Healthy—
One Step at a Time

MARK SISSON
WITH BRAD KEARNS
***New York Times* bestselling authors**

PRIMAL
BLUEPRINT
PUBLISHING

Library of Congress Control Number: 2024922260
Sisson, Mark, 1953– ; with Kearns, Brad, 1965–

hardcover ISBN: 978-1-7362944-1-3
ebook ISBN: 978-1-7362944-2-0

Design and layout: Caroline De Vita
Illustrations: Caroline De Vita
Cover design: Caroline De Vita
Editor: Barbara Clark
Proofreading and indexing: Tim Tate
Endnotes: Ben Gambuzza

Published by Primal Blueprint Publishing, P.O. Box 4393, Stateline, NV 89449.
For information on quantity discounts, please email hello@bradventures.com.

It is only ideas gained from walking that have any worth.
—Friedrich Nietzsche, *Twilight of the Idols*, 1889

CONTENTS

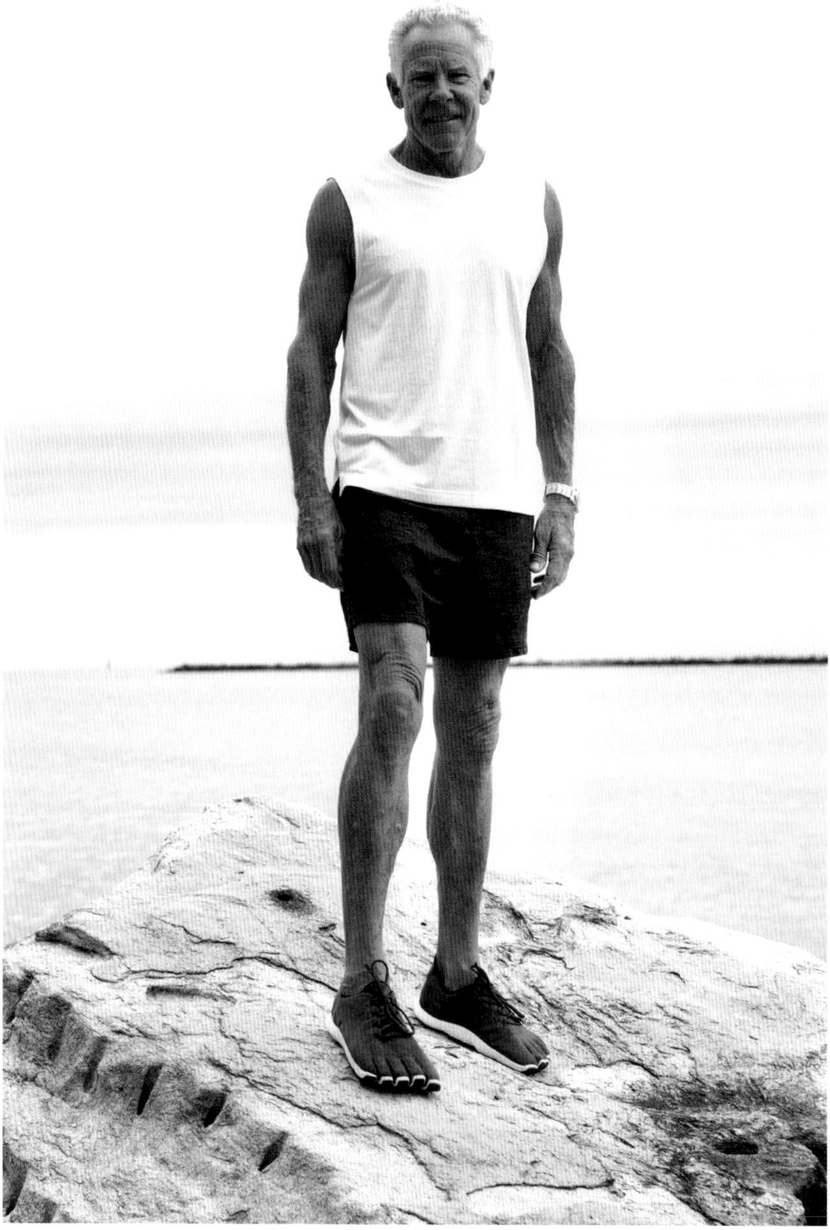

PREFACE
The Running Boom is Over—Don't Shoot the Messenger

The overly stressful way in which the vast majority of runners train today means that the race to the finish line is concurrently a race to an early death.

BEFORE WE DIVE INTO THIS BOOK, I want to offer you a brief philosophical overview to give you some context about what might appear to be an antirunning stance. It is my main thesis here that walking is the quintessential human movement pattern and that we all should do more of it, regardless of how fit we are. It is hardwired into our genes that we should walk extensively every day. In other words, we are born to walk. We are also born to lift heavy things and sprint once in a while. These are basic evolutionary adaptations that we, as bipedal creatures, made. And yes, of course, we are also born to run from an evolutionary biology perspective—but here's the kicker: we were not born to run long distances frequently, certainly not metronomically, at a pace of eight or nine or twelve minutes per mile, day in and day out, especially with the poor form and elevated heart rates typical of almost all recreational runners. This is antithetical to the pursuit of a long, healthy, happy, energetic life.

The flawed and often highly destructive born-to-run notion came about from an avalanche of hype, deception, misinformation, and fabrication that have fueled half a century of what we have come to call the running boom. If your hackles get raised now and then as you read, please remember that I'm one of you: I've been there and done that. Endurance training and racing were the essence of my existence for a couple of decades. I have many treasured memories and lifelong friendships from my days as an elite marathon and ironman triathlon competitor. I also have a keen appreciation for being out in nature daily and challenging my body to perform. As you can probably understand, a day just doesn't feel right unless I've been able to get outdoors into fresh air, open space, and beautiful scenery and put in some form of physical exercise.

In fact, I still consider myself a runner. I am a huge fan of elite racing, and I still advise many competitive runners. However, I have not run a mile in more than thirty years. At seventy-one, I have a VO2 max (see page 176) in the ninety-fifth percentile for my age group, just as I did when I finished fifth at the USA Marathon Championships at the age of twenty-seven and was running more than one hundred miles per week. Oh—but today I have twenty pounds more lean muscle mass and essentially the same body fat. This results from an enjoyable, stress-balanced, longevity-promoting regimen of walking extensively every day, sprinting once in a while, lifting weights consistently, and playing in a variety of ways.

So don't worry: I'm not categorically against running. If you absolutely love endurance running and are proficient at it, with a minimal history of injury and burnout, keep on keepin' on. I also encourage you to walk more in concert with your devotion to endurance running. But I contend that runners who are truly thriving are literally one-in-fifty success stories. They're naturally lean, athletic, energetic, and resistant to injury. They're able to execute a perfect midfoot strike every time. But unfortunately, research and anecdotal evidence confirm that the vast majority of devoted runners are chronically injured, carry excess body fat (especially health-destructive visceral fat, a.k.a. belly fat), and suffer from assorted other mental, hormonal, and cardiovascular health issues, including general overtraining syndrome.

I don't know about you, but I've had enough of the flawed, dated, and destructive approach that has been the norm in the endurance community for decades, to our great collective detriment. The vast majority of runners would be much better served (fitter, leaner, healthier, and happier) by running far less and, instead, walking more every day. There is no health benefit available from running that you can't get in a similar or better (and less injury-prone) form from a host of other activities.

My goal is to spare you some of the repeated suffering and setbacks that too many endurance enthusiasts accept as part of the game. I respectfully request that you maintain an open mind and a willingness to think critically about the information I'm presenting you. I'm going to call bullshit on harmful marketing hype from the fitness industry, the running-shoe industry, and endurance training culture, and it's not going to be pretty. I'm going to expose the worst-kept secrets of the fitness industry and running boom, including the following:

- running is not an effective way to shed excess body fat;
- runners get injured at an embarrassingly high rate;
- running shoes do not prevent injury—rather, they are the driving cause of injury; and
- hormonal burnout, mental health struggles, and cardiovascular disease are commonplace among accomplished runners.

I'm even going to call bullshit on some popular assertions about human running prowess that originated with evolutionary biologists—not because the life's work of leading scientists is flawed but because we are missing the big picture. Modern humans immersed in a life of comfort, convenience, and cushioned shoes are trying to run when they're better off walking in virtually every way.

Now that I've entered my eighth decade, I have the benefit of hindsight and accumulated knowledge. I can say with certainty that the running boom is laden with hugely destructive unintended consequences that we need to acknowledge and immediately take action to avoid if we want to live our longest, healthiest, and happiest possible lives. This is not just my opinion and personal experience: the emerging field of research surrounding what's known as the excess endurance exercise hypothesis reveals that in many, if not most, cases, the more miles you run per week and the more years you spend doing it, the more hollowed-out, hunched-over, weak, hormone-diminished, and diseased you become. If this progression sounds familiar, it's because it is the essence of the aging process. Here's a sound bite: the overly stressful way in which the vast majority of runners train today means that the race to the finish line is concurrently a race to an early death. It's time to expose the truth: it's more accurate and sensible to acknowledge that modern humans are not born to run. They are born to walk—and walk extensively—every single day.

Introduction
Born To Run? Not Really

Walking is the quintessential form of human locomotion. Running 10ks and marathons, lifting heavy weights, making pars on the golf course, and shooting three-pointers on the court are great athletic achievements, but walking lands in an even loftier category as a foundation of healthy living—right up there with sleep and nutritious food. Humans are genetically hardwired to engage in near constant low-level movement throughout the day, because this promotes optimal cognitive, hormonal, metabolic, and immune function. This is how our ancestors lived for two million years—hunting, gathering, foraging, wandering, scouting, and migrating all day every day.

In recent years, this central tenet of evolutionary biology has been cleverly co-opted to make us believe that humans are "born to run." The bestselling 2009 book of the same name by Christopher McDougall was credited with reinvigorating the running boom as well as helping drive the minimalist running-shoe fad. Alas, the maxim has been misinterpreted, misappropriated, and exploited for fitness industry profit. During my youth, I bought into the born-to-run philosophy big-time. After some initial long-distance running success in middle school and high school (great for guys like me who were too small to make the football or basketball team), the sport became my passion, my avocation—my life. I even deferred plans for medical school to move across the country so I could train for a marathon and eventually qualify for the United States Olympic Team Trials. At my peak, I ran more than one hundred miles a week for nearly a decade.

My endurance career, which also included a fourth-place finish in the Hawaii Ironman World Championship triathlon, was a valuable personal growth experience, but it destroyed my body and inflicted long-term damage to my psyche in many ways.

It's true that humans possess numerous highly evolved genetic attributes that enable them to perform feats of endurance superior to those of any other animal on earth. Our upright stature, long limbs, narrow pelvis, and slender frames, in contrast to the physiognomy of our ape cousins, allow incredibly graceful bipedal locomotion. We have efficient thermoregulatory mechanisms that adapt to prolonged exercise in the heat. Our springlike ligaments and tendons in the toes, arches, Achilles, and calves are designed for optimal impact absorption and harnessing of kinetic energy for forward propulsion. Unlike our ape cousins, we possess a large and powerful gluteus maximus that is designed particularly for running. We have short toes, which greatly improve the mechanical efficiency of the foot in comparison to long-toed animals. We even have a nuchal ligament, which connects the base of the skull to the spine and prevents excessive head bobbing while running.

In fact, the fittest humans can outlast cheetahs and antelopes and even fare well against horses, especially when temperatures are warm or hot. The 2000 documentary *The Great Dance: A Hunter's Story* captures a persistence hunt—humans' most ancient and elementary form of hunting—on film for the first time. In the film, San hunters in the 110-degree heat of the Kalahari Desert track a kudu antelope for four hours, driving it to its ultimate demise by exhaustion. The endurance running hypothesis advanced by many evolutionary anthropologists asserts that persistence hunting is a key reason that humans ascended to the top of the food chain. Compare and contrast our graceful locomotion with the plodding, waddling, easily overheated great apes for further evidence of our evolutionary endurance superiority.

But these scientific insights, combined with a hefty dose of modern fitness-industry marketing hype, have led us to celebrate the idea that humans are natural runners—that training for marathons is one of our birthrights. For the past fifty-plus years, we have laced up our cushioned shoes and headed off down roads and trails searching for the promises of the runner's high, a trim physique, and protection against the diseases caused by a sedentary lifestyle. We've been buoyed by culture-shaping ad campaigns from Nike (before the epic "Just do it" campaign launched, in 1988, Nike fueled the running boom with 1977's "There is no finish line"), and dreamy quotations from scientific experts, elite athletes, and journalists alike.

Consider Dr. Louis Liebenberg, an evolutionary biologist on the faculty at Harvard: "By exploring our past, we are rediscovering new limits to our endurance that we were never fully aware of." There's also elite ultrarunner and Appalachian Trail record setter Scott Jurek, who said, "I do feel a connection to some ancient, Neolithic, warrior spirit in these races…That connection to our primal self is drawing people to ultrarunning." And Christopher McDougall offers: "If you don't think you were born to run, you're not only denying history. You're denying who you are."

As I explain in detail in this book, we've taken valid evolutionary biology assertions about the survival attributes humans honed through two million years of life-or-death selection pressures and run with them—in the wrong direction. The aggressive marketing of the born-to-run fantasy has frequently compromised the collective health and well-being of earnest runners.

Humans are not born to run long distances any more than we're born to swim, sumo-wrestle, or race motorcycles. It's as simple as this: endurance running—anything beyond a mile or two—is too physically stressful for most enthusiasts. Attempting a 5k or 10k run (never mind a marathon), even at a modest jogging pace, will cause most people to quickly transition from burning predominantly fat to burning predominantly glucose. This results in a stressful, exhausting, depleting workout. It is not an effective way to become fit or healthy.

In addition, recreational runners are injured with stunning regularity. A 2021 review of twenty-four studies involving thousands of runners by researchers in the UK and France revealed an annual injury rate of between 37 and 56 percent. *Runner's World* reports 46 percent. A newsletter published by the Yale School of Medicine reports 50 percent. The Wake Forest University School of Medicine's Center for Injury Biomechanics says that 79 percent of runners get an overuse injury every year. The American College of Sports Medicine reports that 25 percent of all runners are sidelined by injury at any given time. Most of these statistics are worse than those coming out of the NFL, where 31 percent of players are injured annually, 4 percent at any given time.

Most people (except highly conditioned and genetically gifted front-of-the-pack athletes) lack the baseline metabolic, musculoskeletal, and cardiovascular health to attempt an activity as strenuous as running. Mind you, I'm not talking about training for marathons or ultras: I'm talking about trying to run nonstop for as little as ten or fifteen minutes. After only a few minutes of running, your heart rate can easily drift outside of the comfortable aerobic zone, prompting increased stress-hormone production, elevated glucose burning, lingering muscular soreness and fatigue, and prolonged recovery time. A pattern of such medium-to-difficult workouts—as recommended by popular books, magazine articles, coaches, personal trainers, expert-guided group running programs, and one's peers—can lead to exhaustion, depletion, brain fog, difficulty dropping excess body fat, and an assortment of genetically programmed survival compensations that will make you generally less active in daily life.

We've breezily tried to emulate mythical figures, great champions, and modern-day social media influencers, foolishly ignoring the profound genetic differences and practical limitations that separate the select few humans who really are born to run (or have painstakingly become adapted to run over years and decades) from the rest of us. "Born to run" is a cute aphorism and compelling marketing hook, but it's a big fat ruse and has f*ck-all to do with how you can get healthy, happy, and fit in hectic, high-stress modern life. We need to come down off our runner's high, slow to a walking pace, start thinking clearly, and apply a more sensible and genetically optimal strategy in pursuit of the all-important cardiovascular health that prevents disease and promotes longevity.

* * *

The running boom began in the late 1960s and early 1970s in the United States. Early kindling came from Bill Bowerman's 1967 book,

Jogging, and Dr. Kenneth Cooper's 1968 book, *Aerobics*. The boom reached a tipping point when Frank Shorter won the marathon at the 1972 Olympic Games in Munich. Then the "shoe dogs" in Oregon—Nike cofounders Phil Knight, the company's longtime CEO, and Bill Bowerman, author and University of Oregon track coach—invented the heavily cushioned waffle-sole shoe in 1972, which allowed the masses to take off jogging down the roads and trails of America and pushed the Nike enterprise off into the stratosphere.

Soon the early adopters whom passing motorists considered crazy had scientific validation of their runner's high. In the early 1970s, three different research teams independently discovered that human brains have special receptors for morphinelike pain-killing and mood-elevating chemicals called endorphins that are released by the pituitary gland in response to strenuous exercise and that these chemicals have potentially addictive properties. As the thinking went, why wallow in the neighborhood watering hole when you can get high and healthy at the same time? Running-boom momentum was further bolstered when Jim Fixx wrote the 1977 sensation *The Complete Book of Running*, then jogged across our television screens with his turn in the iconic American Express "Don't leave home without it" series of commercials. In 2009, *Born to Run* captivated runners with a fanciful tale about the mysterious Tarahumara peoples in Mexico's isolated Copper Canyon and their amazing feats of endurance.

Don't get me wrong: the running boom and other aspects of modern fitness culture sure beat couch-potato culture and the patterns of inactivity, atrophy, lifestyle-related disease, and accelerated aging that have become today's norm. The incredible physical feats of today's endurance stars are amusing, entertaining, and awe-inspiring: legendary Kenyan Eliud Kipchoge, the greatest long distance runner ever, a two-time Olympic marathon champion who broke the unfathomable two-hour marathon barrier in 2019; American Courtney Dauwalter, widely recognized as the most dominant ultramarathon racer in the world; American author and ultrarunning showman Dean Karnazes, who ran fifty marathons in each of fifty states in fifty days; and even the zany characters featured in McDougall's book, including Barefoot Ted McDonald and Caballo Blanco, a.k.a. Micah True. Caballo, became a folk hero for his zany, off-the-grid ultramarathon adventurer lifestyle, including a prodigious training output (170 miles a week) and a habit of kickin' it with the Tarahumara every winter in primitive accommodations. His legacy was tarnished after he was found dead in 2012, at the height of his book-driven popularity, in the remote Gila National Forest of New Mexico. After not returning from a planned twelve-mile training run, a massive multiagency search and rescue effort over two hundred thousand acres ensued. True's body was finally recovered and retrieved on horseback. An autopsy revealed that he was the victim of a "Pheidippides cardiomyopathy" heart condition, causing death during exertion.

I hereby declare an end to the running boom. Humans are born to walk, not run.

As a lifelong athlete and coach, I have tremendous respect for people pushing the boundaries of human endurance. It's beautiful to take inspiration from them and fuel the pursuit of daunting and scary personal performance goals. Even David Goggins, the former Navy SEAL and bestselling author of *Can't Hurt Me*, who has been lionized for executing some ridiculously extreme and ill-advised endurance feats, has helped many people get off the couch, overcome self-limiting beliefs and behavior patterns, push beyond their comfort zones, and cross distant finish lines.

But because of the disastrous unintended consequences of running and the tremendous upside of a walking-centric lifestyle, I hereby declare an end to the running boom. Humans are born to walk, not run. I will stand my ground against any evolutionary biologist who refutes this contention. It's clear that Homo sapiens has the genetic capability to perform amazing endurance running feats driven by the fight-or-flight instinct, but that does not mean we should be replicating those feats on a regular basis.

As we marvel at our genetic capacity for endurance, we must also acknowledge that nearly all modern humans have completely squandered these gifts in the incessant pursuit of convenience and luxury. Raise your hand if you've tracked any antelopes for hours in one-hundred-degree temperatures recently, and you may be excused from class to go train for your next half-marathon. Otherwise, let's reflect on the fact that our amazing locomotive talents have been buried under collective tons of excess body fat, weak and atrophied musculature and connective tissue, diminished aerobic capacity (use it or lose it!), dysfunctional feet resulting from a lifetime of wearing elevated, restrictive shoes, and distracted, hyperconnected brains primed for sedentary instant gratification.

***

In part 1 of this book, you'll learn about the deception, false pretenses, flawed assumptions, and misguided good intentions that buoyed the running boom but led to decades of frustration and disappointment among devoted runners. For example, endurance training does not help you lose excess body fat; elevated, cushioned shoes don't prevent injury but rather cause injury; and the prevailing approach to endurance training—what I call chronic cardio—leads to depletion, exhaustion, recurring overuse injuries, suppressed immune, hormonal, and metabolic function, and even mild-to-serious heart problems among the fittest runners. I'll explain that the type A mindset that is so common among devoted fitness enthusiasts often causes them to become their own worst enemy, and I'll argue that the struggle-and-suffer ethos that pervades modern fitness culture and marketing messaging is missing the point.

The daunting physical challenges that push you beyond the comforts and predictability of modern life can bring you tremendous satisfaction, but your approach must promote health and psychological well-being instead of compromising it. We commonly talk about exercise addiction with levity and even celebration, but it's nothing to make light of. Yes, it's a step above addiction to destructive behaviors or substances, but it can still be harmful. It may require a mindset adjustment—slow down, enjoy the scenery, and detox from the runner's high—but the payoff will be enormous. You'll have more energy and vitality, more success dropping excess body fat, and vastly lower your risk of recurring injuries and burnout.

In part 2, I'll show that slowing down, walking, and building an aerobic conditioning base is the secret to health, longevity, and achieving all manner of fitness goals. I'll present a plan of action that will get you taking the first steps toward a healthy, happy, energetic, and long life with walking as a centerpiece of your daily routine. I'll explain that walking is not an à la carte fitness indulgence like hot yoga, spin class, and Pilates but rather an obligatory daily behavior critical to healthy cognitive, hormonal, endocrine, and metabolic function. Then we'll get to my current obsession with footwear and how to carefully and steadily transition from destructive "brace and encase" modern shoes to a barefoot-inspired lifestyle. And although walking and other forms of low-level aerobic activity are foundational to a healthful, active lifestyle, I'll also show you how to incorporate other activities that promote full-body fitness and broad-based athletic competency into your regimen.

PART I

THE UNINTENDED CONSEQUENCES OF THE RUNNING BOOM

CHAPTER 1
Opening The Floodgates In One Fell Swoosh

Since the 1970s, runners have gone from being a peculiar and marginalized group to a prominent element of the mainstream fitness scene. Readers of a certain age might remember the days when seeing someone jogging down the street was a cause for concern. ("What is he running from? What did he steal?") Today, we have mass-participation events in nearly every community, ranging from Thanksgiving turkey trots to big-city marathons with more than fifty thousand participants. This is by and large a good thing, as is any other fitness movement that gets people off the couch and into action.

After all, the biggest public health problem we face in the world today is the virtual pandemic of lifestyle-related diseases driven by lack of activity and overconsumption of nutrient-deficient processed food—what experts are calling energy toxicity. We burn too little energy and store too much of it, simple as that. Any dent we can make in this overarching problem is a huge win. What I aim to do with *Born to Walk* is refine our approach to cardiovascular endurance exercise so that it's less destructive, more fun, and for effective for disease prevention and promoting longevity. I'm starting a walking boom!

The Pholly of Pheidippides

Until recent decades, no human ever ran a long distance for recreational purposes—not in prehistoric times, not in the ancient world or in the Middle Ages, not in the days of the American Wild West, and not during the Industrial Revolution. Our ancestors ran for their lives or their livelihoods—no other reason. Today's popular term for a low-key community running event, "fun run," was an oxymoron throughout human history . . . until the running boom.

If you've been around the running scene, you've surely been regaled with the legend of Pheidippides, the legendary Greek *hemerodromos* (meaning "daylong runner," or professional courier). As the tale goes, in the fifth century BCE Pheidippides ran the twenty-five miles from Marathon to Athens to report the news of a Greek victory over the mighty Persian army in the Battle of Marathon. Pheidippides reached the Acropolis, then announced to the gathered archons (magistrates): "Nike! Nike! Nenikekiam" (Victory! Victory! Rejoice, we conquer), then dropped dead on the spot. This dramatic and inspirational tale has become entrenched in running lore and served as the inspiration for the modern-day marathon race. The only problem? It's not true.

Historians have gone to great pains to separate fact from fiction in the life of Pheidippides (530–490 BCE), and it's now widely agreed that his fateful Marathon-to-Athens run never happened. The myth originated from an 1879 poem titled "Pheidippides," for which author Robert Browning gleaned information from unreliable ancient texts that were written decades or centuries after Pheidippides's death. He then further embellished that information using poetic license. Alas, Browning's fanciful poem inspired the French linguist Michel Bréal to propose that the first Olympic Games, held in Athens in 1896, should include a twenty-five-mile marathon. Today's familiar 26.2-mile distance was introduced at the 1908 London games, supposedly so the race could start at Windsor Castle and finish inside the Olympic stadium, and was finally standardized in 1921.

Actually, Pheidippides's endurance exploits were far more amazing than the legend suggests. This man wasn't some mythical (and obviously poorly trained) schlub who kicked the bucket after running a mere marathon. Scholars now confirm that Pheidippides ran an astonishing 306 miles in four days to convey critical military intelligence between the Athenians and the Spartans—potential allies in the Battle of Marathon, which historians contend is a pivotal event in European history. He ran the 153 miles between the two cities, going virtually nonstop for thirty-six hours over an arduous route, to request the Spartans' help against the Persians. Upon learning that the Spartans were celebrating a religious holiday and couldn't depart immediately, Pheidippides realized that he needed to return to Athens and convey the news urgently. He took a short catnap, then ran back to inform his leaders in time for them to make strategic adjustments.

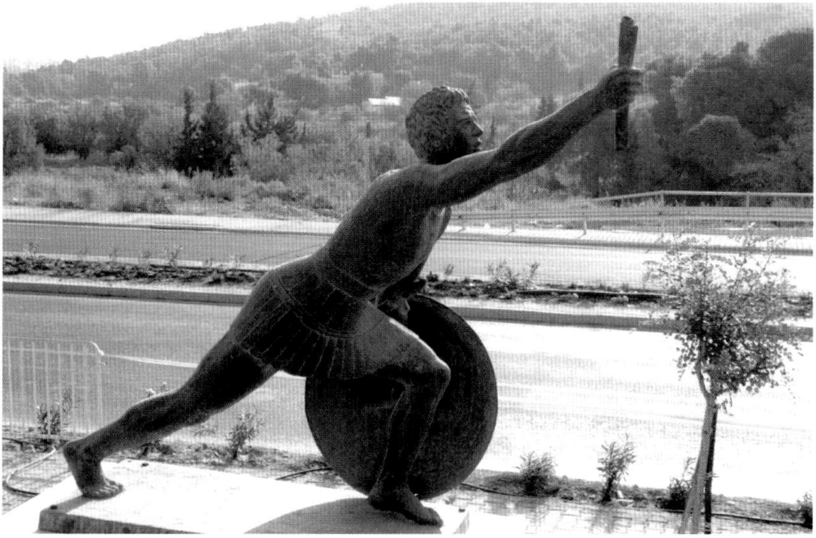

Pheidippides was way more heroic than most people think. He actually ran 306 miles in four days.

In Dean Karnazes's book *The Road to Sparta*, he details the accurate research about Pheidippides's exploits and chronicles his reenactment of Pheidippides's ancient journey. In 2014, Karnazes and other intrepid ultramarathoners participated in an organized event called the Spartathlon—a race covering the 153 miles from Athens to Sparta. For authenticity, Karnazes fueled his effort only with BCE-inspired fare—figs, olives, cured meats, and honey–sesame seed paste. Karnazes writes: "The Battle of Marathon is one of history's earliest recorded military clashes, and the valiant drama of a single lone runner stands enduringly as one of the greatest physical accomplishments ever." Considering that Pheidippides battled hot weather and extremely difficult, hilly terrain, wore rudimentary footwear and consumed only basic nutrition, and had to navigate by the stars, this was indeed a superhuman performance, even by today's standards.

Karnazes, a highly accomplished and highly trained ultramarathoner equipped with modern footwear and navigational aids, finished the Spartathlon in just under thirty-five hours, meeting his goal of matching Pheidippides's time. Pheidippides was surely pushed to his limits during the 306-mile jaunt: in fact he famously had what we might today describe as a heat- and fatigue-induced hallucination when he reached the top of Mount Parthenion (elevation, according to Karnazes, 3,608 vertical feet) on his return trip to Athens. There he encountered the intimidating god Pan, who had the face of a human and the horns of a goat. Pan complained that he wasn't being properly revered by the Athenians, even though he served as a strong ally for them during wartime. Pan told Pheidippides that Athens should build a temple to honor him. So after Pheidippides reported the mystical encounter, the Athenians established a sacred precinct of Pan beneath the Acropolis and held annual sacrifices and torch races in his honor.

***

Here are some key takeaways for those studying at home: first, the basis for the modern-day marathon distance of 26.2 miles is historically inaccurate. Sorry: I know this revisionist history puts a damper on the fantasy of today's marathoner, who channels the spirit of Pheidippides and collapses at the finish line to the accolades of family and friends. But if we truly want to honor Pheidippides, the marathon distance should be 306 miles!

Second, Pheidippides was not running for sport, nor was he running for a book deal. He was a soldier following military orders in wartime—a life-or-death mission. A well-trained *hemerodromos* could outrun a horse over the mountainous Greek terrain (in fact, a rough translation of the name Pheidippides is "spare the horse"), thus achieving a critical tactical advantage when dealing with the advancement of opposing cavalry.

Third, *hemerodromoi* were a special breed—perhaps one-in-a-thousand or one-in-ten-thousand specimens among the ranks of ordinary soldiers. *Hemerodromoi* were revered as statesmen for their unique ability to convey sensitive military and political information in a timely manner. When going about their duties en route, they were given something like diplomatic immunity as well as aid and support. They were carefully selected for their endurance prowess and trained with military rigor. The role was often passed down from father to son, an indication of the importance of genetic advantages in endurance running.

Today, when aspirants plunk down $295 to enter the New York City Marathon, they are no more honoring their ancestral past or connecting to an ancient warrior spirit than they would be if they were to swim the English Channel. And I am certainly not denying human history or denying who we are as a species when I assert that running a marathon, like swimming the Channel, is an incredibly extreme, arduous, potentially health-destructive, and unnatural endeavor.

Modern endurance running started as a pub game in England after the Industrial Revolution, when cross-country paper chases became popular. A trail marked by shredded paper was laid down through the woods by so-called hares, and then the course was raced by "hounds." Today's nickname for cross-country runners—harriers—comes from this tradition. Those races offered an opportunity, beyond darts and other indoor activities, to show off one's athletic prowess and perhaps win a beer and bragging rights. The races were run on natural surfaces such as grass, dirt footpaths, and walking trails—certainly not paved roads. Leather shoes were more than adequate for all those surfaces.

Later, cross-country racing became a schoolboy sport around the world, but again, these races were held on golf courses or woodsy trails in natural settings. There was no need for cushioned shoes. Also in the 1800s, some runners started to compete on tracks at longer distances (5k and 10k), but the tracks were made of dirt or cinder—very forgiving to the foot. Athletes could wear spikes and land on the midfoot to enable running at high speed. Like *hemerodromoi*, those who pursued running were naturally slender and inclined for endurance, just as rugby and football players are naturally large and powerful and basketball and volleyball players are tall. There were no joggers in the early days, only racers—just as there are no casual football or rugby athletes.

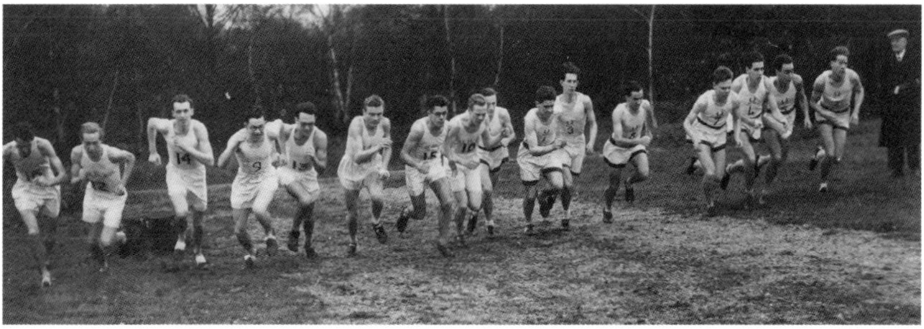

Notice any common physical attributes among the harriers? They are all very slender. The man wearing the number 9 is Olympic gold medal steeplechaser Chris Brasher, and the athlete farthest to the right is the first sub-four-minute miler, Sir Roger Bannister.

Competition at a distance as long as the marathon didn't emerge until the 1896 Olympic Games. Though the Boston Marathon, the world's oldest, is an annual event dating back to 1897, mass-participation marathons didn't really flourish until the 1970s. Boston had fewer than three hundred entrants each year all the way up to 1964 and fewer than three thousand entrants all the way up to 1977. That's not a "century-old tradition of marathon running," as some have called it: it's a century-old cultural oddity—like the century-old tradition of three-legged races at the county fair.

THE MARATHON ORDEAL OF FEMALE MARATHONERS

Incredibly, women weren't allowed to run the Boston Marathon until 1971, and they weren't allowed to run an Olympic marathon until the 1984 games in Los Angeles. This was because the Amateur Athletic Union and Olympics officials across the globe were worried that training for and running a grueling marathon would defeminize women. Medical and sports authorities in the 1960s went on record to say that such strenuous exercise might cause the uterus to fall out of place and result in infertility. They also expressed the concern that hair might sprout on a woman's chest or back from the rigors of such manly training.

Much earlier, stuffy Olympics organizers hit the brakes on women's endurance competition after the 1928 games in Amsterdam, when a bunch of women collapsed after running the longest event on the docket, the 800 meters. The International Olympic Committee resisted adding distance events for females for decades, then reintroduced them slowly. The women's 800 meters didn't return to the Olympics until 1960. The women's 1,500 meters was introduced in 1972, and then the women's 3,000 meters and marathon were added in 1984.

In concert with the social justice movements of the era, trailblazers Roberta Gibb and Kathrine Switzer forced the issue of female participation in the Boston Marathon in the mid-1960s. In 1966, Gibb jumped out of the bushes to "bandit" the race (i.e., run without an official entry number) and finished with a fantastic time of 3:21—which would have been good for 126th place overall. Gibb finished unofficially again in '67 and '68.

In 1967, Switzer registered for a race number as K. V. Switzer and set out on the course with her female features concealed and boyfriend Tom Miller at her side as a bodyguard in case of potential trouble. Miller was indeed called into action a few miles into the run when race official Jock Semple jumped off the press bus, grabbed Switzer from behind, and tried to remove her from the course. Semple also knocked Switzer's coach and training partner, Arnie Briggs, to the ground as Briggs tried to protect her. Miller then executed a clean body check that sent Semple flying; the dramatic image found its way into newspapers around the country and ultimately became iconic within the women's athletic movement. Switzer went on to become the first official female finisher, but the AAU and Boston organizers responded by banning females from competing until 1972.

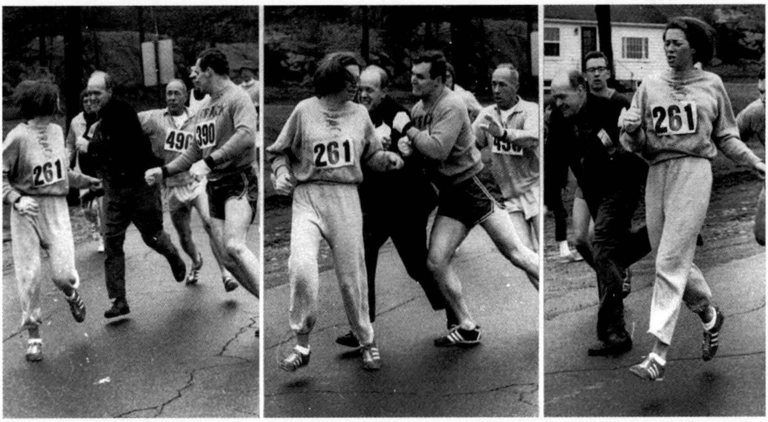

Runner Kathrine Switzer attacked by race official Jock Semple while running in the 1967 Boston Marathon.

* * *

In the days preceding the running boom, there were no joggers, only runners. These people were universally lean, highly trained, competitive, had strong baseline athletic ability, and exhibited excellent technique, especially with the all-important midfoot landing. They were iconoclasts: runners had to deal with rudimentary shoes, be comfortable in solo countercultural pursuits, and have a willingness to endure physical suffering at a level unmatched by any other mass participation sport. Running a 2:59 marathon entails prolonged suffering—try running a single mile in under seven minutes if you don't believe me.

What's more, the population as a whole was much lighter in the early days of the running boom. Someone who was considered out of shape then was vastly better positioned to start jogging than today's XL-size couch potato. The level of obesity in America, and globally, has more than tripled since the 1960s. In 1974, only 15 percent of people in the United States were considered obese. In 2024, that figure has risen to 43 percent, and fully 70 percent of Americans are considered overweight.

It's likely that a good percentage of pioneering runners were keeping the flame alive after competing in their school days, just as I was. And there were surely some people who jumped into distance racing, took to it immediately, and came to believe that they were born to run. These runners possessed a natural talent not only for efficient oxygen consumption during strenuous exercise but also for avoiding injury—thanks in no small part to the fact that virtually every serious runner fell into the featherweight category. Consider that Frank Shorter raced at five foot ten and 134 pounds. *One thirty-four!* The marathon GOAT Eliud Kipchoge ran his 1:59 at five foot six and 115 pounds. The 1996 Atlanta Olympic Games marathon gold medalist, Josia Thugwane of South Africa, was only five foot two and ninety-nine pounds. Ethiopian-born Dutchwoman Sifan Hassan, one of the greatest and certainly the most versatile distance runner in history, with world-class performances and loads of championship medals at distances ranging from 800 meters to marathon, races at five foot seven and 108 pounds. (In the 2021 Olympic Games, she won gold medals in the 5,000 and 10,000 meters and bronze in the 1,500 meters. In the 2024 Olympic Games, she won gold in the marathon and bronzes in both the 5,000 and 10,000 meters). I laugh at photos of an emaciated version of myself running the 1975 Boston Marathon at five foot ten and 142 pounds—carrying twenty-five pounds less muscle mass than I do today at age seventy-one. Imagine: at the time, I was considered too muscular to seriously contend with the world's top marathoners.

It's essential to realize that the running boom has been popularized by highly adapted mini humans. Like our ancestors *Homo floresiensis* (nicknamed the Hobbit, standing around three feet six inches tall and known to have lived some fifty thousand years ago), *Homo marathoniensis* is a small creature. But unlike *Homo floresiensis,* it is present in the population at a level of only one in fifty. No joke: of the fourteen million people who have completed a marathon in the United States since 1975, only 280,000 (2 percent) have finished in under three hours. Before the running community cleansed itself with political correctness, the rule was that if you broke three hours for a marathon, you could call yourself a runner. If you couldn't break three, you were a jogger.

In 2023, the average marathon time among 1.1 million finishers worldwide was around 4:30—shuffling along at ten minutes and eighteen seconds per mile. Finishing 26.2 miles at all is still a grand accomplishment, but mere finishing is about perseverance rather than suffering for a fast time. By comparison, consider the 1979 Nike–Oregon Track Club Marathon, in which 351 of the 689 finishers broke three hours—51 percent of the field! Today's viral Instagram marathon poser-influencer at the front of the pack ("@sub3_is_me"!) would have been *midpack* in '79. I ran a respectable 2:21 at the Nike OTC—good for a victory in most marathons today—and finished in forty-eighth place. Today's *average* finish time of 4:30? Bringing up the rear in '79—669th out of 689 finishers in Eugene.

At one extreme of the elite athlete's physique, we have ninety-nine-pound Josia Thugwane winning Olympic gold, and at the other extreme we have the legendary sumo champion Akebono—a.k.a. Chad Rowan, the first non-Japanese-born person to reach the top rank of yokozuna—who wrestled at six foot eight and 514 pounds (admittedly much bigger than the average elite sumo wrestler, who stands six feet tall and weighs only 337 pounds). Athletic champions are indeed born with the unique genetic attributes that give them the potential to become world-class—whether a eleven-pound newborn in Japan destined for sumo or a Kalenjin child in the Great Rift Valley of East Africa destined for long-distance running.

For the rest of us, only one thing is certain: we are all born to walk.

Nike! Nike! I Sóla Váfla (Victory, Victory, the Waffle Sole)

In the early days of the running boom, there were no support groups for novices, and the average fitness-conscious person wouldn't dare run around the neighborhood for five kilometers without stopping, let alone attempt a marathon. The general sentiment was, "That's crazy!" Old-time runners wore what today would be described as a minimalist shoe. In my teens, I actually started long-distance running in classic Converse Chuck Taylors. My first pair of proper running shoes were Onitsuka Tiger Marathons, and they weren't much different from bare feet: they had a very thin rubber sole, zero arch support, and zero elevation of the heel. These shoes compelled you execute an ideal midfoot landing. If you didn't, the consequence was the dreaded heel strike, a painful landing, and too much impact trauma to run more than a few minutes.

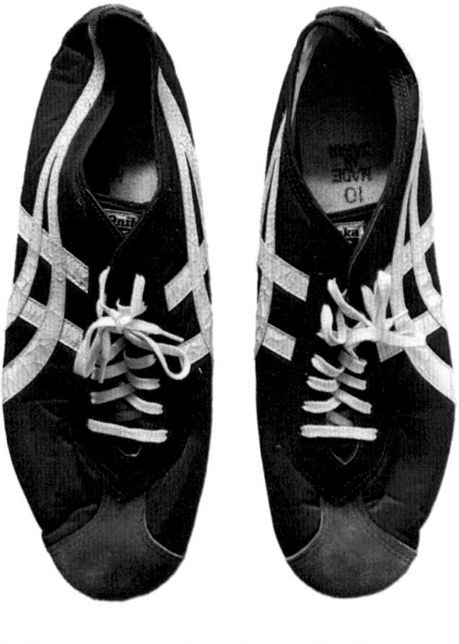

Rudimentary running shoes, like these Onitsuka Tiger Marathons, were an entry barrier to the sport. You had to be highly athletic, resilient, and exhibit excellent form in order to run in them without injury.

In the mid-1960s, none other than the Nike cofounder and longtime company CEO, Phil Knight, started to import shoes from the Onitsuka company in Japan and sell them to serious runners in the United States. These bare-bones Tiger Marathon shoes acted as a built-in governor: running correctly at respectable speeds in flimsy shoes puts a lot of demand on your arches, Achilles tendons, and calves. If you push things too hard, you will get immediate feedback in the form of soreness and inflammation at your weakest link. It was not uncommon for me to wake up the day after a hard twenty-mile run with some kind of physical issue: a supertight left Achilles, a burning second right metatarsal, or knotted calf muscles. I would have to back off for a couple of days, then things would clear.

Minimalist running shoes also acted as a governor because they limited the number of people who dared to lace them up and attempt to jog or run even a short distance at a decent speed. If one was overweight, unfit, or even fit but lacking connective-tissue resiliency (e.g., a competitive swimmer trying out running), it was not going to be smooth sailing, especially on pavement.

In the late 1960s and early 1970s, the running boom started to take shape, and the iconoclastic University of Oregon track-and-field coach Bill Bowerman was a central figure within it. Bowerman coached forty-four all-Americans and nineteen US Olympians, including the late running hero Steve Prefontaine. His runners were NCAA champions in 1971, and he coached the US Olympic team runners in '72. One could argue that he kindled the boom with his 1967 book, *Jogging*—which leveraged his dynasty-level success at Oregon. But even before Bowerman, there was the legendary distance coach Arthur Lydiard, from the active, fit, outdoorsy nation of New Zealand. Lydiard-coached runners Peter Snell, Murray Halberg, Rod Dixon, Dick Quax, and John Walker won Olympic medals and broke world records starting at the 1960 Olympics in Rome, and their winning streak continued throughout the 1960s and 1970s.

Lydiard was the first coach to recognize the importance of overdistance aerobic training to build a base for competitive success at short events. The Lydiard mantra, "Train, don't strain," ushered in a new era of sophisticated endurance training methods. Prior to 1960, long-distance runners mostly ran arduous interval workouts around a track. The idea of accumulating road, trail, or sand-dune miles to prepare for races lasting as little as a couple of minutes on the track was practically unheard of before Lydiard.

But things changed quickly when the black-clad Kiwis started crushing the global competition. After winning 800-meter gold in Rome, Snell shattered the world record in 1962 with a time of 1:44:30. This remains a world-class mark today and would have qualified him for every single Olympics final through 2021—and would have been good for a few gold medals. While the Lydiard principles are still popular today among elite performers, the train-don't-strain philosophy has been widely disregarded by most recreational runners (more on that in chapter 4).

Bill Bowerman visited New Zealand in 1961 and was profoundly influenced not only by Lydiard himself but also by the fact that running and physical fitness were central elements of Kiwi culture. When he returned home, he established jogging clinics for ordinary citizens in Eugene and eventually published his popular book. Dig the bullet points on the back cover of *Jogging*.

- It is free
- It is easy
- It is relaxing
- It can be done alone or in groups
- It is fun
- It is good for the heart and lungs—the organs which may determine your life span

In 1968, Dr. Kenneth Cooper of the soon-to-be-famous Cooper Institute, in Dallas, published his magnum opus, titled *Aerobics* (some thirty million copies sold to date), promoting comfortably paced aerobic activity as a way to prevent disease and increase longevity. Then Frank Shorter put the hammer down on the field in Munich by winning Olympic marathon gold in 1972. It was the first marathon gold for an American since 1908. Nothing like a gold medal to get Americans interested in a sport.

Bowerman's novel ideas about balancing training load with sufficient recovery time, along with his holistic strategies for personal and competitive excellence, made him a John Wooden for distance runners. Bowerman was also an inveterate tinkerer. He was obsessed with shoe weight, postulating—quite accurately, performance physiology labs would later confirm—that shaving a few ounces off a racing shoe would save loads of time over long distances. "Shave one ounce off a track spike and you move fifty-five fewer pounds over the course of a mile race!" he crowed way back in the 1960s. Bowerman was known to handcraft and custom-fit track spikes for his dominant Oregon Ducks distance runners.

If you go deep into Nike lore—detailed in books such as *Shoe Dog*, *Swoosh*, and *Bowerman and the Men of Oregon*—you'll learn that Bowerman is the father of the modern-day cushioned running shoe, which has enabled the masses to participate in running for better or for worse. One of Bowerman's runners was the supremely talented but often injured Kenny Moore. Moore took fourth place in the 1972 Olympic marathon behind Shorter and went on to become a preeminent running author (he wrote the aforementioned *Bowerman and the Men of Oregon*) and screenwriter until his death, in 2022. Moore's fragility—including a metatarsal stress fracture that served as the last straw for Bowerman, who vowed never again to tolerate an inferior training shoe—was a strong impetus for the coach to develop the first extra-cushioned, elevated-heel, arch-supporting running shoe. He designed it, and Onitsuka manufactured it as the Onitsuka Tiger Cortez. After Knight and Bowerman had falling-out with their Japanese partners, Blue Ribbon Sports was renamed Nike, and they started manufacturing their own shoes—thus the Tiger Cortez became known as the Nike Cortez.

The efforts of Nike representatives who attended local track meets and sold cutting-edge footwear out of the trunks of their cars were wildly successful. Unlike today's fledgling fitness and fashion brands, which grow via paid influencer spots and search-term advertising, Nike grew via an authentic grassroots approach: it made the most innovative shoes for the best runners in the world. Years later, Phil Knight had the brilliant insight that just making the best shoes was not enough, and he oversaw the creation of the iconic Nike advertising campaigns and athlete-ambassador relationships that transformed both the footwear industry and modern advertising culture.

At the '72 Olympic marathon, four of the top seven runners were wearing Nike shoes. Steve Prefontaine was even hired in the prime of his career to be Nike's "international public relations manager." Yes, during the "shamateurism" years, prior to the fully professional Olympics movement, which matured in the 1990s, athletes couldn't get paid for endorsing products: they had to do actual work. In 1975, Prefontaine sent some Nikes to a runner on the East Coast named Bill Rodgers, who wore them to win the 1975 Boston Marathon in an American-record time of 2:09:55—kicking off a legendary marathon career that included four Boston and four New York City Marathon victories.

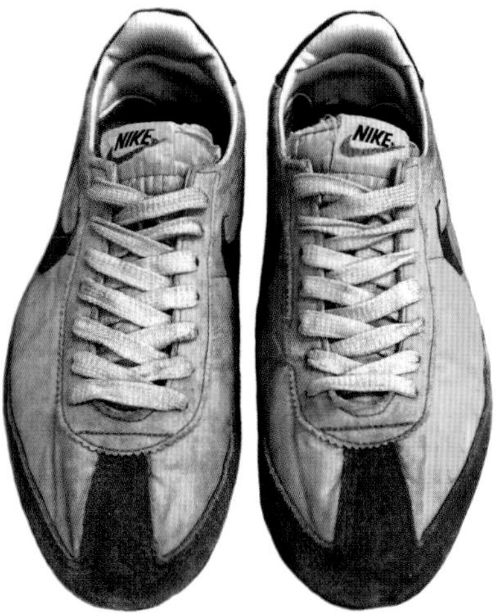

A pair of these Oregon Ducks–colored Oregon Waffle shoes worn by Steve Prefontaine in 1975 sold for $163,800 at a 2022 Sotheby's auction.

Besides Nike's fortuitous and incredibly prescient grassroots marketing efforts, the cultural zeitgeist was working in the company's favor. Recall that the 1970s came to be known as the Me Decade—a collective turn away from the tumultuous social and political upheavals of the 1960s and a pivot toward the self. Fitness and self-help crazes abounded—meditation retreats, aerobics classes, and, of course, jogging. In the 1986 book *Breakthroughs*, chronicling sixteen innovative companies, authors John M. Ketteringham and P. Ranganath Nayak wrote about Nike: "With the sudden emergence of that fitness movement, a scruffy, idiosyncratic, anti-Establishment shoe company was in the position to be the touchstone for a generation."

Bowerman and Nike's signature running shoe would soon evolve from the Cortez to a new model with a distinctive black rubber sole containing protruding nubs—it was named the Nike Waffle Trainer. Indeed, Bowerman fabricated the gridlike waffled sole by pouring liquid urethane into an ordinary waffle iron to create a molded rubber tread, then glued it to the bottom of a typical canvas upper and added a tongue and laces to form a shoe. The protruding rubber nubs from the sole provided excellent grip on a variety of surfaces and added a bit of rebound spring.

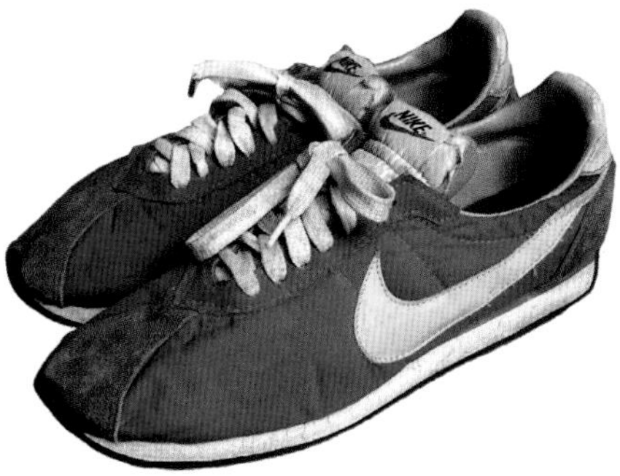

The Nike Waffle Trainer shoe was released in 1974.

Bowerman believed that an elevated heel would take a bit of strain off the Achilles tendon and that a generally more cushioned and supportive shoe would allow his elite runners to train hard without getting injured. This made for lots of NCAA titles and Olympic medals, but the elevated heel has also led to decades of injury problems and dysfunction among heavier, less well adapted ordinary runners who lack certain genetic gifts. I remember putting on a pair of Waffle Trainers for the first time and feeling like I could fly! They were sleek, lightweight, grippy, and springy. They felt great for cranking out five-minute miles, and they felt great to the thousands of novices who were running around the block for the first time. A *Time* magazine piece described them: the shoes were "grabbed by the army of weekend jocks suffering from bruised feet."

Nike had successfully eliminated the primary obstacle holding back the running boom—the obligation to pound the pavement while wearing woefully inadequate Onitsuka Tiger Marathons. With the release of the Waffle Trainers, any novice who coughed up $24.95 could start plodding down the road with poor technique and not experience any immediate penalty. That would come later, a result of excessive and inappropriately dispersed impact trauma. Give the masses cushioned shoes and promote them with brilliant advertising campaigns, and you can transform American (and eventually global) culture, bringing running to the forefront.

* * *

Running is a simple and pure activity that can be done almost anywhere. For those reasons, it can help us overcome the fears, inhibitions, and logistical challenges that keep us from moving. Just lace up some swooshed shoes and take off down most any road or trail. No worries about measuring up to a formidable opponent on the tennis court or in a pickup basketball group. No qualms about venturing into an intimidating gym environment to mix it up with the bros—just head out the door. Just do it, because there is no finish line . . .

In a short period of time, Nike-wearing heroes became household names. I remember being in awe when I saw a multistory banner on the side of a building depicting Joan Benoit Samuelson, the American legend who won the first-ever women's Olympic marathon in 1984 in Los Angeles.

The running boom thrived for decades. It had a bit of a lull for a while, then it rebounded, and now, in the third decade of the twenty-first century, huge numbers of recreational event participants and shoe sales are being recorded. I'm calling the running boom a big fat destructive lie because it lures millions of people into an overly stressful endeavor under false pretenses. You can find some perky bodies and smiling faces on the roads and trails, but the sport is also tainted by casualties—overweight, injured, exhausted, frustrated, and discouraged enthusiasts socialized to believe that fatigue, injury, and burnout are par for the course.

CHAPTER 2
The Broken Promise of Weight Loss

THE MOST EGREGIOUS BROKEN PROMISE of the running boom is also the most obvious: endurance running does not help you lose excess body fat. Full stop. It's likely that the most common goal of recreational joggers is to drop excess body fat, but their workouts are too strenuous and exhausting to be effective in that way. Yes, you burn calories logging the miles, but a pattern of workouts that are slightly to significantly too stressful prompts an increase in appetite, especially for quick-energy carbs, which you deplete during sugar-burning workouts.

Endurance running also leads to a reduction in general everyday movement and a reduction in resting metabolic rate. Perhaps most important, it prompts your hormones to signal the body that it needs to shed lean muscle mass and hoard body fat. These observations led scientists to develop what's called the compensation theory of exercise. In essence, when you push your body too hard with exhausting, depleting workouts, it engages in an assortment of hardwired compensations to conserve energy. And by conserve energy, I mean preserving stored body fat as well as signaling the body to become consciously and subconsciously lazy in everyday life.

Compensation for the Victims

Glenn Gaesser, professor of exercise physiology at Arizona State University and author of *Big Fat Lies: The Truth About Your Weight and Your Health*, studies the ways in which exercise and diet affect obesity, fitness, and health. He is a leading proponent of the idea that exercise, although it doesn't directly support weight loss, delivers comprehensive health and longevity benefits: "It looks like exercise makes fat more fit," Dr. Gaesser said. There are more than two hundred meta-studies and individual studies supporting this assertion. It also confirms my longtime contention that 80 percent of your body composition is determined by diet: the other 20 percent is influenced by sleep, stress management, and sensible exercise. However, I'd argue that the idea that exercise is ineffective for fat loss applies mostly to people who are not fit enough to be running or participating challenging group classes such as CrossFit and Peloton—their stressful workouts further immerse them into a carbohydrate-dependency cycle.

Someone with an effective fitness regimen builds *metabolic flexibility*—the capacity to burn a variety of fuel sources, especially stored body fat, based on demand. This person's well-planned workouts help stabilize appetite and energy levels, so he can eat sensibly and reach and maintain ideal body weight effortlessly. The effort is still 80 percent about diet, but fit people naturally make good decisions and control their food intake because they have constant access to internal sources of energy—namely, stored body fat.

To appreciate the compensation theory, consider your behavior in the hours and days after completing an extreme endurance challenge. I'll wager there's lots of sitting around and eating involved. It's a long-standing tradition in the endurance community to demolish a brunch buffet after proudly completing a community 10k or half-marathon—not to mention the obligatory carbo-loading the day before.

The idea that endurance exercise doesn't meaningfully contribute to fat reduction can be validated by looking at the body composition of folks on the starting lines of marathon and ironman triathlon races around the world. Participants must adhere to an incredibly time-consuming and rigorous training program, so you'd think they would be universally lean and mean. Unfortunately, this is not the case—something that's obviously not being broadcast by those with vested interests in the movement. On the first page of my 2016 book, *Primal Endurance*, I called this strange phenomenon the "elephant in the room" of the endurance community.

Tim Noakes, the eminent South African exercise physiologist (his research has been cited an astonishing sixteen thousand times), author of the most comprehensive endurance training and physiology book of all time—the 944-page *Lore of Running*, published in 1985—and modern-day low-carb-diet advocate, offers the most infamous example of the idea that runnin' don't get ya skinny. Noakes was an accomplished endurance runner for decades, having finished more than seventy marathons and ultramarathons—notably, he is a seven-time finisher of the legendary Comrades Marathon, a fifty-five-mile ultramarathon that takes place in Durban. This is the world's oldest and largest ultramarathon, having started in 1921: there were nearly twenty-five thousand participants in 2019. Noakes's research on substrate utilization during exercise, detailed in *Lore of Running*, helped popularize the practice of carbo-loading.

Unfortunately, when Noakes reached age sixty, he discovered that he was not able to outrun the metabolic disease that his father contracted at a similar age and eventually succumbed to. When Noakes was diagnosed as prediabetic, he tipped the scales at 225 pounds, even though he was still highly devoted to endurance running. So he decided to experiment with a low-carb diet, famously inspired by an unsolicited email advertisement that first landed in his spam folder. Noakes's personal keto folly was a dramatic step to take, because he was essentially refuting a good chunk of his life's work in the process. As another prominent low-carb author and advocate, Gary Taubes, observed: "[Noakes] was a marathoner who became obese and diabetic. He was angry."

Upon ditching the grain-based meals and sugary energy drinks favored by his running brethren, Noakes lost loads of weight in short order. He ultimately lost nearly fifty pounds, reversed his disease risk factors, and gleefully shared his story with his peers in academia and the general population, especially in his native South Africa. Unfortunately, his enthusiasm for this radical "new" diet—in his best-selling 2013 book, *The Real Meal Revolution*, he emphasized that he was simply advocating the high-fat, low-carbohydrate Banting diet, which originated in London in the 1860s—didn't sit well with his stuffy peers, and he became embroiled in controversy. Much of this was fueled by Noakes's aggressive and irreverent communication style: one viral video shows him theatrically tearing out the pages of the diet chapter of his own book to emphasize how radically he had renounced the so-called carbohydrate-glycogen model of endurance performance. This posits that a high-carbohydrate diet will stock the liver and muscles with glycogen, the stored form of dietary carbohydrate, which will then serve as the primary fuel for endurance efforts.

Noakes came under global scrutiny when he was forced to stand trial in South Africa for medical ethics violations relating to his frequent tweeting of antiestablishment dietary advice, though he was acquitted of the charges in 2017 and again in 2018. At a keynote presentation early in his low-carb journey, amid heated criticism from the audience for his refutation of conventional nutritional wisdom, Noakes was compelled to stand in front of the audience, gesture to his new physique, shrug his shoulders, and exclaim, "What can I say? Trust me."

Despite Noakes's high-profile success story, and despite respected research from other leaders in the field of low-carb endurance performance, including Dr. Stephen Phinney and Dr. Jeff Volek, coauthors of *The Art and Science of Low Carbohydrate Performance*, the running community does not appear to be solving the girth problem anytime soon. (Dr. Volek was chair of the highly regarded 2015 University of Connecticut FASTER study—Fat-Adapted Substrate Oxidation in Trained Elite Runners—which essentially refuted the foundation of the carbohydrate-glycogen model.) An article on the Asics website titled "How to Lose Belly Fat by Running" offers this sage advice: "A simple way to tweak your running to lose belly fat is to head away from the roads and onto the trails. Although your pace is likely to be slower, trail running provides more of a total body workout to help you tighten up those problem areas." If you're getting a visual right now of a large earnest jogger jiggling down a rocky slope in hopes of oscillating fat off his body, you can see why I'm so exasperated.

"They" say you can't outrun a bad diet, but you also can't outrun the adverse effects that your running habit has on your dietary habits. Here's what typically happens when an earnest fitness enthusiast starts out on the roads and trails toward a weight-loss destination.

First, initial weight-loss success is enjoyed, thanks to a combination of (1) a reduction in (inactivity-driven) systemic cellular inflammation; (2) a reduction in glycogen storage and consequent water retention; (3) some loss of lean muscle tissue, especially if running is paired with calorie restriction; and (4) some shedding of excess body fat. Realize that each gram of glycogen in your body binds with three to four grams of water. That's around five pounds when you are fully stocked with around five hundred grams of liver and muscle glycogen, so anyone who starts to put in some training hours can quickly drop several pounds.

They say you can't outrun a bad diet, but you also can't outrun the adverse effects that your running habit has on your dietary habits.

But after you get active and drop that first ten or more pounds, your body starts to recalibrate. First, the glycogen-water weight can come right back on after a few big meals and/or recovery days. This is why you might return home from a weeklong cruise having gained five to ten pounds, by the way. Also, the more energy you burn with your new hobby, the more the aforementioned genetically hardwired compensation mechanisms kick in.

Furthermore, when you improve your fitness, you become more calorically efficient during workouts. So that six-mile run requires fewer calories than it did when you were just starting out. Yes, this is a good thing! What's not a good thing is when newly efficient exercisers continue to indulge in the extra portions and sweets and treats they feel they've earned. Over time, many well-intentioned runners who faithfully log consistent weekly miles will drift back to their metabolic set points.

The compensation theory is the reason you don't lose an easy twenty-four or forty-eight pounds of excess body fat per year by running twenty-four or forty-eight miles a week—even though such massive weight loss would be predicted by comparing carefully tracked exercise expenditure against carefully tracked caloric intake. Unfortunately, the calories in–calories out model of weight loss is oversimplified and inapplicable to most living, breathing human beings. In many cases, one's body-composition set point can even drift higher amid a dogged devotion to weekly mileage. This is the result of what I call the Ben & Jerry's effect (morning run = evening pint) and the fact that one becomes lazier as the day wears on, both consciously ("I ran this morning, so I deserve to relax; I'll rake the leaves another day") and subconsciously (moving more slowly, feeling less peppy, and conveniently forgetting or otherwise not getting around to raking the leaves).

This also happens to so-called charity runners, who comprise an estimated 20 to 25 percent of all marathoners. These mostly novice folks enroll in organized group training programs led by expert coaches in their hometowns, agree to raise money for charity, and prepare for an exciting destination race that's typically affiliated with the charity. Charity group-training programs are offered for marathons, half-marathons, ironman triathlons, century (one-hundred-mile) bike rides, and other events. Members of these groups—the Leukemia & Lymphoma Society's Team in Training program is the world's largest—are able to bypass stringent qualifying standards and sold-out registrations and gain entry into prestigious events such as the Boston Marathon. Charity marathon-training programs typically kick off six months before the event, and participants are subjected to guided workouts of quickly escalating degrees of difficulty to prepare them—on an inappropriately tight timeline—for the big day. This crash course can result in a brutal escalation of fatigue, peer pressure, and anxiety about the rapidly approaching event. Among the Team in Training benefits listed to entice participants is that "coaches [are] present at the race to ensure everyone finishes." How about that for pressure?

The first step in escaping from the sugar-burning, sugar-chomping, fat-loss-frustration loop is to stop running and start walking. The compensation effect doesn't kick in after a long walk—in fact you get a boost in energy and fat burning and a natural stabilization of appetite. Then your still-energetic self can perform the short-duration, high-intensity workouts that don't drain glycogen or prompt hunger spikes, as a medium-to-difficult hourlong run does. Instead, high-intensity strength and sprint workouts get you ripped. You experience a boost in metabolism for up to seventy-two hours afterward via a process called excess post-exercise oxygen consumption (EPOC; see page 218) and send your body powerful signals to build or maintain lean muscle mass and shed excess body fat.

Sadly, we continue to obsess over self-quantification devices that calculate our calorie burn and count our calorie consumption, but it's largely to no avail. Humans are not machines with gas gauges: we are dynamic organisms with many nuanced variables that influence our rates of energy expenditure and storage. Perhaps we buy into this garbage because we're bombarded with marketing messages. Or perhaps we wish to quantify everything in order to guarantee success, or maybe we just want to indulge our control-freak tendencies. Regardless, it's time to do away with this flawed mentality—and ditch the ridiculous and often highly inaccurate technology that tells us how many calories we've eaten and burned.

The Slippery Slope of Visceral Fat

Dr. Philip Maffetone is one of the world's leading experts on endurance training. He's been a coach to many world champions in distance running and triathlon and is the author of many bestselling books, including *The Big Book of Endurance Training and Racing*. He and Arthur Lydiard are the widely acknowledged fathers of aerobic-based endurance training. For some forty years, Dr. Maffetone has been promoting the groundbreaking idea that fitness is not the same as health and that you can actually trash your health in pursuit of extreme fitness goals. In Dr. Maffetone's 2017 book, *The Overfat Pandemic*, he asserts that 76 percent of the global population (some 5.5 billion people) are what he calls overfat. This term describes having excess subcutaneous and/or visceral fat that causes a measurable impairment of health.

Experts such as Dr. Maffetone, Dr. Ronesh Sinha (host of the *Meta Health* podcast and author of *The South Asian Health Solution*), researchers at the Cleveland Clinic, and many others contend that you can quickly determine if you are overfat by calculating your waist-to-height ratio—you want your waist circumference to be less than half of your height. For example, a five-foot-nine, 175-pound male with a thirty-five-inch waist is certainly not in the overweight or obese category and probably looks reasonably fit in street clothes. But alas, half of sixty-nine inches is only 34.5, so this man qualifies as overfat. Researchers call him TOFI—thin on the outside, fat on the inside. The overfat ranks include a significant number of people considered to be of normal body weight but who carry excess amounts of the extremely health-destructive visceral fat, a condition called normal-weight abdominal obesity. Yep, it's a stringent standard to be taller than double your waist circumference, and billions of people are flunking—couch potatoes and die-hard runners alike.

Visceral fat—also known as belly fat, hidden fat, intra-abdominal fat, visceral adipose tissue, and beer belly—is a distinct type of fat that accumulates around the abdominal organs as well as the heart. Visceral fat is metabolically active: it secretes hormones and other substances directly into the bloodstream. Consequently, like the thyroid and adrenal glands, it is classified as a separate endocrine organ—except this organ is unwanted and wreaks havoc on healthy metabolic and endocrine function. Visceral fat is far more destructive to health than the largely harmless subcutaneous fat, which typically accumulates on the hips, thighs, and rear end. Subcutaneous fat is soft and squishy because it's just below the skin, while visceral fat is firm because it gathers deep within the abdomen in the spaces surrounding the organs. Men have a greater predisposition to store visceral fat than women, because they tend to accumulate less subcutaneous fat. Men also have a larger omentum—a protective flap of tissue that surrounds the intestines and is another favored spot for accumulation of particularly firm visceral fat.

Visceral fat is far more destructive to health than the largely harmless subcutaneous fat, which typically accumulates on the hips, thighs, and rear end.

Your body is actually trying to protect you from metabolic damage by storing excess energy as subcutaneous fat. Only when the delicate hormonal systems that regulate energy utilization and storage capacity are overwhelmed or dysregulated will you start to accumulate visceral fat. This means that people with a genetic predisposition for skinniness can actually fare worse from adverse lifestyle practices than those with an endomorphic body type, who have a greater capacity for "adipose expansion." When one is unable to efficiently transport fat from the bloodstream into storage depots, triglycerides (fats circulating in the blood) rise to unsafe levels. Then fat begins to deposit in the liver, leading to nonalcoholic fatty liver disease, or NAFLD, and settles around skeletal muscles, the heart, and abdominal organs. This condition is called lipotoxicity.

Visceral fat accounts for around 10 percent of the body's total fat content, but it is perhaps the single most important and outwardly visible indicator of overall health disturbance and disease risk. If you have even a moderate spare tire, you are not healthy—even if you can break four hours (or three hours!) in a marathon, finish a century ride, crush a CrossFit workout with the young guns, or score double digits in an adult basketball league game. Visceral fat secretes large amounts of substances known to interfere with normal glucose and fatty-acid metabolism, including inflammatory cytokine proteins such as interleukin-6, TNF-alpha, and MCP-1 and adipokines such as leptin, adiponectin, resistin, and retinol-binding protein 4. Visceral fat suppresses sex hormone levels and drives systemic inflammation, oxidative stress, mitochondrial dysfunction, and broad-scale hormonal and metabolic dysregulation. Visceral fat can interfere with leptin signaling between the brain's appetite center and the digestive system, leading to overeating and fat storage instead of fat burning.

Extensive research from around the world, including the United Kingdom, India, and California, reveals that visceral fat increases the risk of insulin resistance, type 2 diabetes, metabolic syndrome, heart disease, breast cancer, colon cancer, and dementia. One UK study revealed that women double their risk of heart disease over a twenty-year-period when they carry excess visceral fat. Each additional two inches of waist circumference raised the risk by 10 percent. Research from India revealed a three- to fourfold increase in breast cancer risk in those with excess visceral fat. A thirty-six-year study in California found that those with abdominal obesity in midlife were three times more likely to develop dementia decades later. Risks for other conditions such as poor lung function, migraine headaches, and asthma are elevated when visceral fat is present. A study of 350,000 European males and females revealed that those with large waists had double the risk of dying prematurely.

When you accumulate a bit of visceral fat, its inflammatory, hormone-altering properties beget the accumulation of more visceral fat and systemic inflammation over the ensuing years and decades. For example, visceral fat contains an enzyme called aromatase, which converts, or aromatizes, testosterone into estrogen. This can happen when testosterone creams or injections are prescribed for dudes with low T and large bellies. There are no free lunches when you are metabolically deranged—sorry. Visceral fat also inhibits the release of human growth hormone by the pituitary gland, promoting fat storage and loss of muscle mass. Compromised sex-hormone status, both in males and females, diminishes energy, vitality, libido, cognitive performance, motivation, and athletic performance and recovery. This slippery slope of gradual visceral fat accumulation is so commonplace that we have come to consider expanding waistlines part of the normal aging process. Alas, spare tires are indications of metabolic and hormonal damage from adverse lifestyle practices, not part of chronological aging. Losing abdominal muscle strength and mass with aging is also a factor, because the intestines and organs tend to spill outward to contribute to that beer-belly look.

Unfortunately, the vast majority today's runners and fitness enthusiasts carry spare tires and fail to meet the proper waist-to-height ratio. Even highly accomplished veterans sporting physiques that are borderline emaciated can be classified as overfat. Spare tires linger on fit specimens for variety of reasons, most of which come down to inflammatory lifestyle practices. Perhaps the main culprit is consuming nutrient-deficient processed foods that contain refined grains, sugars, and industrial seed oils, which drive insulin resistance and systemic inflammation. This includes most of the performance powders, bars, and gels peddled to endurance athletes for use during exercise. The cumulative load of hectic, high-stress modern life—chronic cardio, poor sleeping habits, emotional stress, environmental endocrine disrupters, and so on—can also drive visceral fat accumulation because you overtax delicate fight-or-flight mechanisms designed for occasional short-duration use only.

Fattened by Fight or Flight

Your endocrine system makes no distinction among stress inputs—interacting with an unreasonable boss, missing an airplane flight, delivering an important presentation, arguing with a mean boyfriend, or running six miles at a strenuous "tempo" pace. The fight-or-flight response is designed for brief peak-performance efforts, or what the primitive part of your brain, the amygdala, perceives as life-or-death situations. The concept that running is a great release from the stress of the workplace or the responsibilities of home life can be valid from a purely psychological perspective, but physiologically, the stress response is triggered regardless of whether the stimulus is positive or negative. Striving to achieve a consistent output of weekly mileage at a heart rate slightly or significantly above your fat max heart rate (the intensity at which the maximum number of fat calories are burned per minute; I'll cover fat max in detail in chapter 6) is effectively piling more stress on top of an already stressful life. This then piles more visceral fat onto the bit you started to accumulate after your twenties.

Following is a quick overview of the ways in which chronic stress makes you fat.

- Excessive fight-or-flight stimulation prompts chronic overproduction of **cortisol**, the preeminent stress hormone. Cortisol gets a bad rap these days, but it's important to clarify that the *chronic overproduction* of cortisol is the problem. Healthy cortisol production is what gets us alert and energized in the morning and able to execute all manner of physical and mental peak-performance tasks. Chronic overproduction is like liquidating your assets (see page 38).
- One of cortisol's roles is to promote **gluconeogenesis**—the conversion of amino acids, including lean muscle tissue, into glucose for use as quick fuel. In fight-or-flight circumstances, fat burning is put on hold in favor of stripping muscle and turning it into glucose. This is a desirable emergency fuel source, but too much gluconeogenesis screws up your metabolism.

- When you are making lots of glucose—and eating lots of processed carbs, because cortisol spikes one's appetite for quick energy—you chronically overproduce **insulin**, a condition known as hyperinsulinemia. Hyperinsulinemia prevents you from mobilizing stored body fat for energy, making you reliant upon dietary calories to get through the day. You'll know this is happening if you feel hangry when you skip a meal.
- **Hyperinsulinemia** also promotes visceral fat accumulation and prompts systemic inflammation and oxidative damage—the latter two being widely acknowledged as the true root causes of heart disease. Public health and medical experts contend that hyperinsulinemia is the number one health problem in the world today, because it is a driving cause of obesity, type 2 diabetes, cardiovascular disease, and cancer.

Chronic cardio is stressful and inflammatory: you can be fit and fast and still sport a spare tire. Mind you, I'm not talking about elite endurance athletes, who all have low body fat and zero visceral fat because of their incredibly high energy expenditure in training. However, the supremely fit are often unhealthy in other ways. The chronic stress of their arduous training regimens causes immune suppression, recurring musculoskeletal injuries, and even cardiovascular disease driven by repeated scarring and inflammation of the heart. I'll discuss the excessive endurance exercise hypothesis at length in chapter 4.

LIQUIDATING YOUR ASSETS VIA TOO MUCH FIGHT-OR-FLIGHT STIMULATION

In addition to the accumulation of visceral fat, there is other damage associated with being a stresshead, because immune and digestive function are suppressed every time you trigger fight-or-flight. When you lace up your shoes and take off down the trail, start in with another argument, or are called on for your presentation, you trigger the peak-performance protocol: elevated heart rate, blood pressure, body temperature, respiration, focus, and mental acuity. Meanwhile, digesting food and fighting off an airborne virus are put on the back burner. Remember, the amygdala judges your conference-room presentation and your interval workout as if they were the same thing. Dr. Tommy Wood, assistant professor of pediatrics and neuroscience at the University of Washington and former head of Physicians for Ancestral Health, calls our modern abuse of fight-or-flight "liquidating your assets."

Chronic suppression of digestive and immune function is why so many endurance athletes suffer from frequent minor illnesses and complain of chronic digestive disturbances, a key early indicator of overtraining. For example, a survey published in *Medicine & Science in Sports & Exercise* revealed that 31 percent of the participants in the Hawaii Ironman World Championship complained of significant gastrointestinal distress during the event. These are the best-trained and fastest triathletes in every age group from all over the world, each meeting rigorous qualifying standards simply to get to the starting line, yet one-third of them are making unscheduled pit stops for leaky pipes, cramps, bloating, vomiting, and more. Crazy!

I averaged six colds a year during my decade of marathon training. I was the fittest guy any of my friends knew but possibly the least healthy. Imagine—dealing with *sixty* colds during your twenties, your biological prime! I was a finely tuned elite athlete obsessed with eating the best food, getting perfect sleep, and following the best recovery protocols, but the abuse I inflicted upon my body was similar to what a hard-partying globe-trotting rock star does to himself—and we both rocked a lot of Lycra.

Chronic cardio may seem badass—runners still judge their peers according to their weekly mileage, as if they were forming a caste system—but it's antithetical to a lean, athletic physique. When you engage in specialized athletic training, you send powerful genetic signals to your body, telling it to adapt to the stress you place upon it. Just as a bodybuilder pumps iron and chugs protein shakes all day to signal his body to produce muscle, a serious runner flips the genetic switches and asks his body for increased oxygen utilization and blood volume in the heart (hey, I thought I would throw some good things in) *as well as* decreased muscle mass and bone density. That's right: weekly mileage causes you to become less muscular and more brittle, because a lighter chassis goes faster.

Over time, this running-driven loss of muscle mass reduces your metabolic rate, but your pattern of exceeding your fat max heart rate and drifting into the glycolytic (glucose-burning) zone routinely prompts an increase in appetite that encourages you to overeat. The appetite center in your brain, ultrasensitive and highly calibrated for survival, is saying, "Better stuff my face in case this fool tries to do the same thing again tomorrow."

You will particularly crave quick-energy processed carbohydrates in a desperate attempt to recover from a chronically stressful training program on top of a hectic, fight-or-flight lifestyle. An overstressed body is fueled by glucose, whereas a stress-balanced, active, energetic body builds metabolic efficiency and prefers fat for fuel, both at rest and during comfortable low-level movement, such as walking and structured cardio sessions conducted at or below fat max heart rate.

The chronic abuse of delicate fight-or-flight mechanisms also suppresses testosterone and human growth hormone. The effects of poor sex hormone status extend far beyond the oft-highlighted low libido: it also causes visceral fat storage, muscle loss, and increased risk of the most common lifestyle-related conditions, such as heart disease, metabolic disease, cognitive disease, and assorted cancers.

High-Intensity Interval Training, Burnout, and Carbohydrate Dependency

Antiaging fitness strategies should be focused on preserving hormone status, bone density, lean muscle mass, explosive power, balance, and mobility. Of course, they should also support cardiovascular fitness, which most runners do fine with—unless they overstress the heart muscle and compromise overall cardiovascular health in the process. There is absolutely nothing more important to a long, healthy, happy, energetic life than nailing these various fitness objectives. Dr. Peter Attia, author of the 2023 book *Outlive: The Art and Science of Longevity*, explains, "Exercise not only delays actual death but also prevents both cognitive and physical decline better than any other intervention. It is the single most potent tool we have in the health-span-enhancing toolkit—and that includes nutrition, sleep, and meds." Interestingly, Attia used to believe that diet was the best intervention until emerging research convinced him and others that exercise was king.

It's important to realize that the massive vitality and longevity benefits of exercise can only be enjoyed through a sensible and strategic approach that honors our genetic expectations for health. This is why I created my Primal Blueprint blend of low-level cardio, resistance training, sprinting, and play, which avoids overly stressful exercise patterns that lead to injury, burnout, and accelerated aging. The primal-inspired approach to fitness is simple, sustainable, time-efficient, low-key, and low-tech.

Virtually any able-bodied citizen, even one burdened by morbid obesity and near-zero fitness activity, can get started by putting one foot in front of the other and going for a walk around the block. And a gentle, enjoyable walk around the block can be vastly better for health and longevity that forcing an unfit person to exercise to the point of exhaustion, as seen in the infamous *The Biggest Loser* television series. In addition, resistance exercise can be scaled even to unfit elderly subjects. In fact, elderly subjects generate the quickest strength-improvement rate of any age group. It's hard for a muscle bro to increase his strength by 10 percent in one year, but Grandma can double her strength in eight weeks. Even all-out sprints can be executed by novices performing low- or no-impact activities.

Unfortunately, the fitness industry has brainwashed people to regard strenuous high-intensity interval training (HIIT) workouts as the ultimate exercise protocol for fitness and weight loss. People who want to get fit have been conditioned by powerful marketing forces to join a gym, join a running group, hire a trainer, or purchase a cardio machine for home use—and to let the suffering begin. In general, they are doing their jogging, stair climbing, elliptical training, and group classes—boot camp, barre, Bodypump, boxing, kickboxing, Curves, F45, Orangetheory, spin, step, and Zumba—at effort levels that are slightly to significantly too stressful. The same goes for home-based workouts—Peloton, P90X, lululemon Studio, Tonal, and guided sessions using YouTube or a smartphone app. A HIIT workout can be highly effective in theory, but in practice it is widely misused: people not only perform too many intervals that last too long, with too little rest between them—thanks to peer pressure and a lack of individual instruction in group settings—but also perform these workouts too frequently.

An HIIT workout can be highly effective in theory, but in practice it is widely misappropriated.

In many cases, we seem to be trying to counter the adverse effects of a sedentary lifestyle by engaging in what I call blended workouts—those that target a variety of energy systems and muscle groups in a single session. As one website promises, "F45 Training merges . . . high-intensity interval training (HIIT), circuit training, and functional training in order to provide you with the results you're looking for—all in just under an hour." Keep in mind that there is nothing inherently bad about these protocols: exercise physiology research validates the rapid fitness improvements experienced when doing HIIT correctly. Workouts of this nature give you an aerobic conditioning effect, because your heart rate is elevated for the entire class; a strength-training effect, because you're challenging muscle groups with resistance exercises; and high-intensity stimulation, because your heart rate spikes and muscles burn during short, explosive efforts. Furthermore, someone who is movement-deficient and fitness-deficient will benefit hugely from doing any form of exercise—even if it's unsustainable over the long term.

But the big problem with chronic cardio, HIIT, and blended workouts is that, for a lot of people, they are too difficult, performed too frequently, and are crammed into an overly stressful lifestyle. Blended workouts can also increase injury risk: complex movements are not a good idea when the muscles and central nervous system are fatigued. For example, CrossFit classes often integrate Olympic lifts such as the snatch and the clean and jerk, which require explosive power and precise technique. If the participant has already completed several sets of rope climbs, box jumps, and laps around the block, and is then asked to quickly move a weighted bar through space, even a slight technique imperfection can cause acute injury to an already overloaded or misaligned joint or muscle.

If you are in a pattern of cranking out challenging blended workouts, or pounding the pavement to the tune of thirty miles a week at beyond your fat max heart rate, then zipping through a productive day of multitasking and running around town, then sinking into the couch and polishing off a full pint of Ben & Jerry's in the evening, you have departed from your ideal mode of existence as a fat-burning beast and have become dependent upon dietary carbohydrates as your primary source of energy.

THE CARBOHYDRATE-DEPENDENCY ROLLER COASTER

Are you stuck in a carbohydrate dependency cycle? Monitor your energy level, mood, appetite, and cognitive function at the twelve-, twenty-four-, and thirty-six-hour marks after a challenging workout. You may feel alert and energetic for several hours following a lively morning session, but if you experience significant lulls later on, or experience any of the following symptoms, you may be on the roller coaster of carbohydrate dependency.

- **Fragility:** Frequent overuse injuries; minor respiratory infections; digestive disturbances
- **Low fuel efficiency:** Declining energy in the latter stages of a workout; craving sugar immediately afterward
- **Crankiness:** Decline in energy and cognitive function if you skip a meal
- **Afternoon blues:** Periods of brain fog or diminished cognitive function, especially in the afternoon
- **Cravings and Bingeing:** Episodes of appetite spikes and overeating, especially in the aftermath of challenging workouts or in the evening hours

It's telling that a chronic exercise pattern consisting of steady-state cardio, frequent HIIT sessions, and/or "kinda hard" blended workouts will leave you too tired to engage in the most longevity-promoting fitness practices. These include walking and other forms general everyday movement; taking frequent breaks from periods of stillness; performing regular brief, intense strength workouts featuring full-body exercises with explosiveness and precise technique—and quitting before you feel drained and depleted; finding time for spontaneous, unstructured outdoor play; and performing occasional, very brief all-out sprints.

Particularly when it comes to getting stress hormones and inflammation under control and reducing visceral and subcutaneous fat, slowing your cardio down to a walk is a critical first step to success. Then sprinkle in a couple of strength-training sessions and one short sprint session a week (a duration of thirty minutes for these sessions is plenty), and you can quickly experience breakthroughs in body composition, energy, mood, and cognitive function. You can also minimize your disease risk factors and improve your longevity prospects (see chapter 9 for a complete plan). You can do all this in less time, with less suffering, than would be possible if you followed a typical pattern of chronic cardio and/or blended workouts.

How to Get Rid of Belly Fat

For a variety of reasons that are extremely important for die-hard chronic cardio enthusiasts to understand, you cannot easily burn off a spare tire simply by logging more weekly mileage. Even when you increase your calorie burning and mind your portion sizes, belly fat can linger because of deeply rooted hormone dysregulation.

The good news is that once you make the necessary lifestyle changes, belly fat can come off quickly and efficiently. Since belly fat, unlike subcutaneous fat, is metabolically active—the very property that makes it harmful—your body can efficiently excrete it through breath and urine more quickly than it can excrete subcutaneous fat. Belly fat can seem stubborn only because your approach is flawed, but subcutaneous fat is stubborn and clings to those problem areas because it's less metabolically active. Following are the most effective ways to reduce belly fat quickly.

Eliminate Processed Foods

Consuming heavily processed, nutrient-deficient, chemical-laden foods prompts your digestive tract to release lipopolysaccharide (LPL) into the bloodstream. LPL is an endotoxin, or an internally manufactured toxin, that promotes systemic inflammation and interferes with your ability to burn energy. Refined industrial seed oils such as canola, corn, soybean, sunflower, and safflower oils are arguably the single worst things you can consume in the modern food supply. They trigger endotoxins; severely hamper fat metabolism; promote oxidative stress, inflammation, and insulin resistance; and cause an immediate and prolonged disturbance in healthy arterial function. Dr. Cate Shanahan, who often warns consumers of the dangers of industrial seed oils, contends that their toxic properties make them "literally no different from consuming radiation in a bottle."

Dr. Robert Lustig, pediatric endocrinologist at the University of California–San Francisco, widely regarded as one of the world's leading antisugar crusaders, argues persuasively in his book *Metabolical* that if you simply eliminate processed foods, you won't get fat, won't get diabetes, and won't get metabolic disease. That's a bold contention upon which Lustig stakes his esteemed reputation and life's work. Practically, you must agree that this makes perfect sense. Do you really think that obesity and metabolic dysfunction are the results of eating too many eggs, salmon, steaks, salads, and fresh fruit? When you consume exclusively wholesome, nutrient-dense foods, your magnificently fine-tuned appetite and satiety mechanisms guide you to consume the optimal amount of energy to truly thrive.

Eliminate or Greatly Reduce Alcohol Consumption

They don't call it a beer belly for nothing! Alcohol calories are known as the "first to burn." Because alcohol is a poison, it must be metabolized immediately after it enters the bloodstream. This causes the burning of all the other calories to be put on hold—removed from the bloodstream and stored as fat.

Note that this is different from the popular but inaccurate notion that alcohol gets "converted" into fat. Actually, these nutrient-devoid, nonsatiating liquid calories prompt you to consume excess food calories, and *those* calories are converted into fat. For example, when you drink a daiquiri or margarita, the alcohol calories get burned immediately while the sugar in the mixers gets removed from the bloodstream and sent to storage. Then, once the alcohol is processed by the liver, which takes around an hour, you typically get the munchies because your bloodstream has become devoid of energy.

When the liver becomes overwhelmed with too much energy and/or toxins to process, it can accumulate fatty deposits—the aforementioned NAFLD. Since your liver is the control tower for all manner of energy and micronutrient processing and distribution, an overwhelmed, poorly functioning liver promotes all manner of disease and dysfunction. This includes the suppression of sex hormones and the accumulation of visceral fat.

Consume Nutrient-Dense Foods

If you ditch processed foods and then kick-start an extreme calorie-restriction program, or if you think you can shed visceral fat through starvation, you will activate compensation mechanisms. Chronic stress-hormone production to make the sugar you ain't getting from your diet, as well as chronic inflammation, can ultimately keep your tummy at square one.

Instead, strive to consume an animal-based diet from the best sources (grass-fed beef, pasture-raised chickens and their eggs, wild-caught fish, and heritage-breed pork) along with sufficient natural, nutritious, easy-to-digest carbohydrates from your favorite well-prepared plants, fresh produce, and fermented foods. Eat at a leisurely pace in a pleasant, low-stress environment to the point of satiety and refrain from crash diets and extremes. Get metabolically fit first, then worry about dropping excess fat.

Slow Down!

If you are enmeshed in chronic cardio or an otherwise overly stressful exercise routine, slow down and reduce your total weekly workout energy expenditure. Losing visceral fat is about managing the preeminent stress hormone, cortisol. If your overall life-stress score is too high, you promote systemic inflammation, appetite dysregulation, and the accumulation of more visceral fat. Instead of being a sugar-chomping, fat-storing, inflamed, and exhausted endurance junkie, mix things up with a sensible, ancestral-inspired program that covers a broad base of fitness objectives. You'll have more energy for everyday life and increase your overall fitness competency.

When it comes to your beloved endurance goals, you may astonish yourself with performances that are as good or better than they were when you were cranking out big mileage and hanging on by a thread. This happened to me when I retired from elite marathon and triathlon racing and transitioned to a busy career as a personal trainer and young father in my midthirties. I'd get plenty of low-level cardio activity daily by hiking, jogging, and cycling with my clients—at a pace vastly slower than my training pace as a recently retired elite athlete—steering safely clear of chronic cardio. When little blips of free time opened up in my schedule, I would go and blast some short, high-intensity hill sprints or commence an all-out assault on the VersaClimber (my favorite cardio machine ever, by the way). For fun on the weekends, I would jump into races in which the professional endurance athletes I coached were competing. With extremely minimal structured endurance sessions, lots of nonstrenuous "going through the motions" with my clients, and some occasional explosive blasts, I shocked myself at age thirty-eight by performing at several major international competitions only slightly behind where I had been in my prime, right on the heels of the world's best multisport athletes.

My results helped my clients embrace my counterintuitive ideas about slowing down and paying more attention to low-level aerobic conditioning. Besides the thrill of crushing my chronic cardio–immersed competitors and coming in just behind the pros, I was free to live my life without being obsessed with training and feeling continually nagged by aches, pains, and minor illnesses. Instead of remaining skinny because of my high-mileage regimen, I naturally added lots of longevity-boosting and aesthetically appealing lean muscle mass while my body fat stayed in the single digits. Slowing down works!

Go Hard

Comfortably paced cardio fine-tunes your fat-burning abilities, but it's not going to result in miracle fat reduction because the metabolic demands of a comfortable aerobic workout are not a shock to the body. Your body has strong homeostatic drives to remain at a genetically influenced metabolic set point. If you want to shed that last ten or twenty pounds, you need to aggressively force your body to burn more fat. This is where high-intensity resistance training and sprinting come in. Resistance exercise prompts the body to build and maintain lean muscle mass, which helps increase your metabolic rate. With your fat-burning capabilities optimized from extensive low-level movement, your strength sessions help you burn fat around the clock—without the rebound effects of increased appetite and everyday laziness prompted by chronic cardio.

Sprinting is a tremendous trigger for fat reduction because the penalty for carrying excess body fat when sprinting is severe. This is especially the case for high-impact sprinting on flat ground, but low- or no-impact sprints also help your body become leaner and more powerful.

Fat loss is just one of the ways in which sprinting delivers by far the best return on investment of any workout. Even doing a single sprint workout once every seven to ten days, consisting of four to eight sprints of ten to twenty seconds each, with extensive rest between efforts, can improve fitness and body composition better than miles and miles on the road (details in chapter 9). You get appropriate fight-or-flight stimulation followed by a quick return to homeostasis without the compensation factors such as fatigue and increased appetite kicking in. You also reduce perceived exertion and improve efficiency at all lower levels of intensity.

Remember: it's not about the calorie burn during workouts but rather about the hormonal signaling prompted by your overall exercise program—ideally a mix of frequent low-level movement, regular high-intensity resistance workouts, and occasional all-out sprints.

Prioritize Sleep and Downtime

Even mild sleep deprivation can make your metabolic and endocrine hormones go haywire and send you into a tailspin of inflammation and chronic stress-hormone production. We pay plenty of lip service to the importance of sleep, but execution can easily fall by the wayside when we are lured into evenings filled with artificial light and digital stimulation.

Resolve to make your evenings quiet, mellow, and as minimally lit as possible. Use UV-blocking orange lenses, orange lightbulbs, or candlelight instead of harsh, bright lighting. Create a relaxing wind-down ritual in which you end screen time early, walk the dog around the block, and take a relaxing bath before some easy reading and lights-out. Create a sleep sanctuary that is completely dark, cool, uncluttered, simple, and restful. This means using blackout curtains, covering up the small illuminations emanating from electronic devices, keeping the room at sixty-eight degrees Fahrenheit or below—a cooling mattress is helpful if you wake up feeling warm at night—and having absolutely no screens, desks, or paperwork stacks in your bedroom.

Sleep hygiene is paramount, but you also have the obligation of creating downtime during the day. Resolve to get good at Mister Rogers–style transitions between the workday and leisure time. Learn to power down or at least put down your mobile device and engage with nature or real humans.

Manage Stress

Chronic overproduction of stress hormones causes inflammation, which in turn contributes to the accumulation of belly fat, so learning to disengage the fight-or-flight mechanisms that get you through your hectic days, and learning to trigger calming parasympathetic nervous system function, will improve your metabolic and hormonal functioning. We want to figure out ways to trigger that activity on demand (i.e., "unwind") instead of being locked in chronic sympathetic nervous system dominance. Probably the most simple and reliable way to do this is by walking: getting fresh air, being in open space, receiving direct sunlight, and engaging in gentle locomotion will quickly transition your mind and body into a calm state of being. Meditation is another excellent way to trigger parasympathetic nervous system activity, as are formal movement practices such as yoga and tai chi and self-care routines such as massage and acupuncture. It also helps to soak in a sauna, hot tub, or bubble bath.

It's imperative to discover your own personal sweet spot, one where you have enough stimulation to keep you energized, engaged, and purposeful but not enough to make you feel frazzled. You don't want to feel bored and aimless, and you don't want to feel worn out. The late Dr. Hans Selye, the father of modern stress research, called this sweet spot of optimal stimulation eustress (as opposed to distress). We also have to be wary of cultural forces that get us sucked into exhausting patterns. Power down to avoid hyperconnectivity. Nurture gratitude. Practice mindfulness exercises to counter the pressures of consumerism and FOMO.

CHAPTER 3
The Broken Promise of Cushioned Shoes

Nike turbocharged the running boom by making a promise that its shoes would help you excel and avoid injury. The promise certainly emanated from heartfelt good intentions of Phil Knight, Bill Bowerman, and the other pioneers as well as whatever rudimentary research was available at the time and the anecdotal evidence of top athletes winning major races in Nikes. Alas, the promise has been egregiously broken over and over for millions of earnest runners over the course of the past half century. Modern running shoes are a decided departure from our human genetic expectations for health—right up there with processed foods and artificial light after dark.

When we don modern footwear, we are interfering with the extremely precise and delicate interactions between our feet and legs, interactions that have been honed by 2.5 million years of human evolution. The dangers of messing with our species-appropriate locomotion techniques manifest themselves in many ways, including chronic foot pain and both chronic and acute foot injuries. Shoe manufacturers promise that their wares prevent injury. But in truth, running shoes not only don't prevent injury; they are the driving cause of overuse injuries.

The Research Reveals . . . Nothing

A 1997 study in the *British Journal of Sports Medicine* reported that shoe manufacturers are engaging in "deceptive advertising . . . that may represent a public health hazard" because there is not a single shred of scientific evidence that shoes can lessen impact forces and prevent injury. The study suggested that expensive high-tech running shoes caused 123 percent more injuries than less expensive shoes with less cushioning and none of the rigid support material for the arches, sole, or heel cup known as motion-control technology.

A 2022 Chinese study found that running shoes with the typical ten to fifteen millimeters of "vertical drop"—the elevation of the heel above the midfoot and toes—caused a 15 percent increase in patellofemoral joint stress (stress on the joint where the kneecap meets the femur) compared to shoes with five millimeters of vertical drop or less, a feature common to all "minimalist" shoe models. In addition, the researchers found that elevated running shoes contribute significantly to the extremely common condition called runner's knee, a.k.a. chondromalacia. They explained that elevated shoes promote a heel-strike gait, which increases knee extension to the point of causing pain and injury. Following is a classic example of running-shoe hype, deception, and outright falsehoods from the shoe manufacturer Saucony.

> Our technology ensures enhanced stability for a more productive workout that's less likely to result in injury. No matter the terrain, our men's stability running shoes for overpronation help to decrease muscle tightness and prevent your foot, shin, and knee from twisting while you run by steadying your stride.

Steve Magness, former elite high school miler, exercise physiologist, coach of numerous top professional runners, author of *Do Hard Things* and *Peak Performance*, and publisher of the popular blog *The Science of Running*, offers a heavily scientifically referenced article on his blog titled "Why Running Shoes Do Not Work." Magness explains that the entire premise of elevated, cushioned running shoes is deeply flawed. "Running shoes are built upon two central premises, impact forces and pronation. Their goals are simple, limit impact forces and prevent overprontation. This has led to a classification system based on cushioning, stability, and motion control. The problem is that this system may not have any ground to stand on." Hmm. "It's a significant mindset jump if you think about it," Magness observes in a huge understatement.

Magness cites three studies concluding that lower-extremity alignment—the degree of pronation, or how much the arch flattens and the foot caves in during the running gait—doesn't influence injury rate and another study finding that motion-control shoes do not alter pronation or change the kinematics of the tibia or calcaneus (the large bone in the heel)—your foot pronates anyway!

Shoes ruin your proprioception, or kinesthetic awareness.

If shoes don't lessen impact forces, why do we feel so comfortable floating down the street in super-cushioned shoes? The main reason is because shoes ruin your proprioception, or kinesthetic awareness—your sense of the positioning, force, movement patterns, and weight distribution of your limbs and trunk moving through space. In cushioned shoes, you essentially deactivate the sensory nerves on the bottom of your feet, one of the most nerve-dense areas of the body—hence acupressure's focus on the soles—and disconnect your feet and ankles from their important role in initiating and stabilizing the complex neuromuscular activity going on in other parts of your body.

Jay Dicharry, physical therapist, biomechanical expert, and author of *Running Rewired*, offers a thoughtful summary of the problems associated with cushioned shoes: "The foot no longer gets the proprioceptive cues that it gets unshod. The foot naturally accommodates to surfaces rapidly, but a midsole [the cushioned material in a shoe between the tread and the "upper" that you slide your feet into] can impair the foot's ability to react to the ground. This can mute or alter feedback the body gets while running." It's kinda like getting Novocain for a tooth extraction. You feel fine during the dental procedure (akin to pounding the pavement on your run) because you're numb (wearing cushioned shoes). After the meds wear off, you're hit with the pain and inflammation caused by pliers yanking a tooth out of your gums; this is akin to getting an overuse injury.

Cushioned shoes make each of your jarring, inefficient foot strikes feel comfortable, while your toes, arches, Achilles tendons, shins, calves, knees, hamstrings, quads, hip flexors, and lower back get traumatized by inappropriate impact loads and shearing forces. Over time, you experience

- atrophy of the arch and important stabilizer muscles of the foot,
- atrophy and loss of mobility in the critically important big toe as well as the other toes,
- weakening and shortening of the calf muscles and Achilles tendons,
- a strength imbalance between the hamstrings and quadriceps, and
- a misshaping of the primary structural components of the foot—small bones, cartilage, and tendons.

As a result, you'll likely experience chronic aches, pains, injuries, poor movement mechanics, and referred pain and dysfunction throughout the lower extremities and even into your lower back. Amid all this atrophy and dysfunction, it's common to make technique compensations that further ingrain inefficiencies and injuries—especially if you neglect complementary mobility and strengthening exercises or if you rush back to the roads too soon after you're injured.

True, the first cushioned Nike also shoes compromised proprioception for Kenny Moore, Bill Rodgers, and other elite runners launching the brand and the boom—including me. But we were executing midfoot landings under featherweight frames. The shoes took a bit of the edge off the musculoskeletal torture of our one-hundred-mile weeks, especially when we were running at quick paces, so we could dance on the razor-thin edge between peak performance and overuse injury. Today, elite runners are still obligated to exist on that tightrope between injury and victory, and they can all be seen training and racing on the latest, greatest high-tech shoes. Shoe endorsement deals are also typically their primary source of income. Alas, overuse injuries are still common even among the most genetically gifted and highly conditioned runners on the planet, who have huge financial incentives to stay healthy. Meanwhile, half of recreational runners are still injured every year—even after enjoying the benefits of decades of running-shoe-industry research, substantial advancements in materials technology, insights derived from sophisticated biofeedback devices, and vastly improved training strategies. Christopher McDougall, author of *Born to Run*, remarked in an interview:

> Running shoes are based on a kind of cult idea—that our feet are flawed and we need shoes to correct those flaws. The shoe companies are in the business of selling shoes. But there's no evidence from running shoe manufacturers that they're right. There's no scientific data that running shoes reduce injury.

McDougall goes on to say in the book, "Blaming the running injury epidemic on big, bad Nike seems too easy—but that's okay, because it's largely their fault." I've spoken to numerous elite runners and coaches about this conundrum of "needing" cushioned shoes to train optimally, knowing that they are not great for overall foot health. My ideal scenario—heads-up to all Olympic runners reading this book—would be to train in the shoes that work best for you (and pay you the biggest fee) but to spend all possible remaining waking moments either barefoot or in a barefoot-style minimalist shoe. This strategy will strengthen feet, helping mitigate the negative effects of training hard in cushioned shoes and potentially improving your performance when wearing the necessary shoes.

This suggestion also applies to elite basketball players, tennis players, golfers, cleated soccer players, and football players. But it is even more urgent for recreational runners, who have much less aerobic fitness, foot strength, and overall musculoskeletal resiliency compared to an elite athlete. Running is vastly more stressful for a recreational runner than it is for an elite runner—even when the former is jogging slowly and the latter is cruising along for a couple of hours at six-minute miles. Not only do recreational runners need to up their barefoot game, they also need to slow down and focus on full-body fitness, as I'll explain in chapter 9.

The Design Flaws of Modern Shoes

What we must do right away is acknowledge that shoes do not lessen impact trauma, control pronation, improve foot functionality, or optimize explosiveness, endurance, balance, or any other performance attribute. They protect our feet from the trauma associated with playing sports, performing labor, avoiding obstacles and debris, avoiding heat and cold, and so forth. Shoes can be accurately described as a necessary evil—it's now undisputed that they directly cause atrophy and dysfunction in the feet and throughout the lower extremities.

Long-term shoe use makes us increasingly reliant upon high-tech shoes, expensive orthotics, arch supports, braces, cushions, and perhaps even medications and surgical procedures to keep us moving. Much as prescription drugs alleviate symptoms without addressing the cause and consequently make you more reliant upon them to settle your stomach or ease your back pain, running shoes beget further reliance on running shoes. This is a classic example of what I call digging a hole to install a ladder to wash the basement windows.

Following are the most health-destructive properties of modern footwear.

An Elevated Heel

A typical dress shoe, running shoe, or sneaker will have ten to thirty millimeters of vertical drop. Katy Bowman, MS—founder of the Nutritious Movement organization, author of popular books such as *Move Your DNA*, *Rethink Your Position*, and *Don't Just Sit There*, and one of the world's leading experts on barefoot functionality—proposes that an elevated heel is the single most destructive aspect of modern footwear: "Just placing a little wedge under our foundation causes compensatory actions in the ankle, hip, knee, and spine, and can knock our natural gait pattern off-kilter—and it does this in an instant!" Chronic health problems such as arthritis, nerve damage, and osteoporosis are all associated with spending years and decades in positive-heeled shoes.

An elevated heel also severely compromises the function of the Achilles tendon, which plays a central role in impact absorption and force production during walking and running. An elevated heel prevents the Achilles tendon from lengthening fully and coiling, which is how it provides springlike energy for forward propulsion in every stride. Over time, your Achilles—the largest and most powerful tendon in the body—becomes weakened, shortened, and more vulnerable to injury.

A strong Achilles tendon is essential to the health of your foot as well as to all manner of everyday movements and athletic performance. Evolutionary anthropologists and exercise physiologists go so far as to assert that the Achilles is the key to human running prowess and one of the most distinguishing anatomical characteristics of humans. Chimpanzees, gorillas, and others in our evolutionary family who lack a robust Achilles tendon and a prominent longitudinal arch are consequently ill-suited for both sprinting and long-distance running.

British computational primatologist Bill Sellers believes that the development of a strong Achilles tendon was the primary evolutionary adaptation that allowed humans to become hunters instead of herbivores! The ability of the Achilles tendon to provide elastic energy storage—the Achilles can store and return around 35 percent of its kinetic energy; the arches can store and return around 17 percent—is believed to be the reason why humans can run more than 80 percent faster than apes. When our human functionality is compromised by shoes, this results in a huge loss of performance—increasing our oxygen uptake requirement by an estimated 30–40 percent.

The development of a strong Achilles tendon was the primary evolutionary adaptation that allowed humans to become hunters instead of herbivores.

The functionality and resiliency of the Achilles is a huge freaking deal, yet we are knowingly causing its atrophy and dysfunction every day when we slip on shoes with elevated heels. Remember that Bill Bowerman's original reason for elevating the heel in a running shoe was to help his elite runners minimize the abuse they absorbed while pushing the limits of human endurance and musculoskeletal resiliency—basically, he was doing damage control for Kenny

Moore's Olympic dream. This is completely different from helping mere mortals achieve full range of motion and functionality in their Achilles tendons.

There's another reason to avoid shoes with a significant drop from heel to midfoot: they encourage poor posture. When you stand in an elevated-heel shoe, it forces your center of gravity to load over the balls of your feet instead of over your heels. This causes a chain reaction of adverse compensations, including a tucked pelvis, a hyperextended lumbar spine, a curved thoracic spine, forward-hunched shoulders, and a compressed cervical spine.

Humans are designed to stand with their body weight loaded over the heels—the calcaneus bone is extremely dense for just this reason. Optimal posture starts with, and is reliant upon, the weight of the legs, torso, and head loading over the heels. As soon as you slip on shoes with an elevated heel, you are forced into bad posture, and it's hard to correct it even if you try. The most important and beneficial attribute of a so-called "minimalist" shoe is a flat sole, meaning that there is no difference in elevation between the heel and toe—a zero drop.

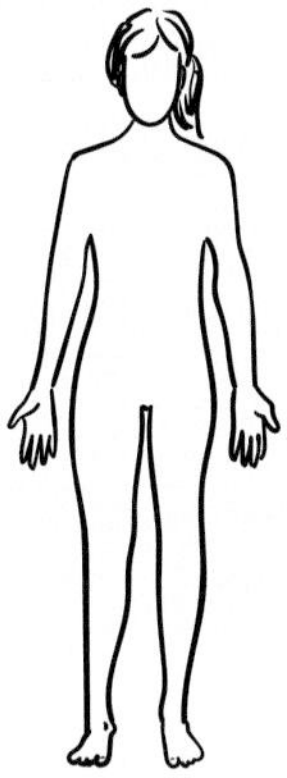

CHECK YOUR POSTURE

Stand with your bare feet facing forward and rock your body weight onto your heel bones. Flick your toes off the ground to confirm your position. Then roll your shoulders backwards in a circular motion so that they end in perfect vertical alignment with your spine and your ears. Stand with your palms facing forward and outward to help you maintain this upper-body alignment. Notice that your head, spinal column, pelvis, legs, and feet feel more balanced and comfortable when everything is loaded on your calcaneus.

Excessive Cushioning

An elevated, heavily cushioned sole promotes inefficient walking and running technique and actually worsens the impact trauma of each stride significantly—the exact opposite of the prevailing marketing claims. Even when you go for a leisurely jog, you generate an impact force of two to three times your body weight with each stride. The miraculous human body is highly adapted to handle such a load with grace and efficiency—especially the foot, which handles most of the load. But running in cushy elevated shoes prevents the foot from doing its job of absorbing impact, balancing moving body weight, and harnessing energy for an explosive takeoff.

Instead, cushy shoes allow a poorly conditioned recreational runner to execute a highly inefficient and jarring heel-first landing. This causes impact forces to be inappropriately distributed through the shins, knees, thighs, hips, pelvis, and lower back.

A Pinched Midfoot and Toes

All shoes inhibit the functionality of the midfoot and toes by encasing them in a single chamber that is typically far too narrow. Even wide-width shoes typically get narrower in the toe area to achieve a stylish look. That's right: one of the main design flaws of modern shoes exists purely for appearance's sake. The streamlined toe box seen in both women's and men's dress shoes dates back centuries to the time when peasants wore wide-toed work shoes and aristocrats sported stylish shoes with pointed toes. The narrow front area of today's athletic shoe is touted as providing stability for the foot by pinching the toes together: just look at soccer and football cleats, track-and-field spikes, and rock-climbing shoes. The truth is that a narrow toe area can have the opposite effect by inhibiting toe splay upon landing and the individual articulation of each digit through the stride pattern, which provides natural stability and force production.

When the metatarsals are pressed together and the toes encased, they are prevented from achieving their dynamic range of motion. They cannot expand sideways to absorb impact properly, and the big toe cannot independently and fully dorsiflex, which activates the glutes during running. Instead, toe-box restriction causes a loss of kinetic energy and a harmful dispersion of impact trauma into the lower extremities. Plantar fasciitis is also exacerbated by the loss of circulation throughout the plantar fascia region when the big toe is wedged in with the second toe. What's more, many foot maladies, including blisters, corns, bunions, osteomas, hammertoes, plantar warts, dermatitis, fungus, ingrown toenails, athlete's foot, and debilitating arthritis and tendinosis, are caused by forcing your feet to squeeze into tight compartments. Consequently, many minimalist shoes tout a "wide toe box" feature to alleviate crowding in the midfoot and toe areas. Wide toe boxes are better than tight toe boxes, but the most authentic barefoot-style shoe has individual slots for each toe. This allows each toe to articulate individually on several planes with no crowding or pinching.

Toe-box restriction causes a loss of kinetic energy and a harmful dispersion of impact trauma into the lower extremities.

A Rigid Sole and Excessive Arch Support

We've long been led to believe that the rigid soles and reinforced arches found in hiking boots, Birkenstock sandals, flip-flops with a rigid contour design, geriatric shoes, and nurse's shoes—are design features that increase comfort, relieve pain, and prevent injury. This is categorically untrue, validated by extensive research. A rigid or contoured sole and custom orthotics indeed relieve workload and minimize range of motion for your arch, metatarsals, and Achilles tendon. This might provide temporary relief for inflamed and traumatized joints or tissues, just as a plaster cast does. However, relying upon designer shoes and foot-support products is certain to cause further atrophy and pain over time.

Plantar fasciitis, an extremely common condition, is exacerbated and can even be caused by overstressing weak arches, Achilles tendons, and calf muscles during routine repetitive activity such as standing, walking, and running. The typical plantar fasciitis treatment protocol—rest and more arch support—is often unsuccessful over the long term because it results in further atrophy of the tendons and muscles involved and does not address the root cause. As soon as exercise is resumed after a plantar fasciitis–induced layoff, the painful condition typically returns—often worse than it was before—because of atrophy and the reduced blood flow and oxygen exchange during the layoff.

Shoes are almost always the leading cause of plantar fasciitis. Note that this includes making an abrupt switch to minimalist shoes without proper acclimation. It's true: a lifetime of wearing restrictive shoes weakens and overstresses your plantar fascia, but trying to correct it cold turkey can also overstress your plantar fascia. Minimalist shoes with a flat, flexible, minimally cushioned sole get your arches back in the game, but it's important to transition gradually to avoid straining atrophied arch muscles and connective tissue.

Toe Spring

Most running shoes have a distinct upward curvature of the sole, typically around fifteen degrees, starting around midfoot and heading toward the toes. This feature is known as toe spring, or rocker geometry. A toe spring is apparent when a shoe rests on the ground and the toe box is slightly elevated off the ground. This is advertised as minimizing impact trauma and facilitating a rocking motion while walking. Toe spring is also believed to improve performance for fast runners by preloading the toes into a dorsiflexed, energy-coiled position. For example, the carbon plates in energy-return "super shoes" (see page 76) have a pronounced toe spring, and research suggests that this is one of the key reasons why the shoes improve performance.

Toe spring is also a prominent feature of track-and-field spikes, which also have a rigid sole and a negative drop—in this case, the toes are higher than the heel because of the plastic plate that anchors the metal spikes on the forefoot area. These attributes deliver significant performance benefits in comparison to regular shoes, which weigh more and mute much of a runner's potential explosiveness. Alas, the feet and lower-body muscles and joints take a beating in spikes, so they are best saved for competition and occasional race-prep workouts.

It might be hard to accept the fact that your feet also take a beating in comfortable running shoes, but it's true. Preloading your toes into a coiled position in toe-spring shoes does provide a significant performance benefit, but it prevents the toes from working through their typical range of motion. Over time, this can cause atrophy to important muscles and connective tissues in the foot. What's more, a toe-spring design may actually transfer an excessive and inappropriate burden of impact absorption and propulsion to the highly vulnerable plantar fascia by forcing it into a stretched position. Toe spring is also believed to disperse impact force away from the foot, thus overburdening the knees and hips.

Kinetic Chains—Life on a Balance Beam Instead of on the Ground

Virtually everything we do as humans involves contact with the ground. The incredibly dense nerve endings on the bottoms of the feet send information to the brain with every step we take. When you put weight on your forward foot in a walking or running stride, the brain starts calculating the firmness, contour, available traction, and potential obstacles of whatever is underfoot. It senses how your step will affect your balance and forward propulsion, then gracefully executes the next stride. Thanks to the data dump from your foot, your nervous system understands how to splay the toes, dorsiflex the ankle and toes, flatten and tighten the arch, coil the Achilles, bend the knee, rotate the hip, pump the arms, and so forth. The neurofeedback from the foot initiates the complex and interconnected movement of what we call a kinetic chain.

This term describes the mechanism by which muscles, joints, and connective tissue interact to enable movements such as throwing, lifting, jumping, bending, and extending the body in various directions. There is an assortment of distinct kinetic chains involving groups of muscles and joints throughout the body, each named for the way it connects to the spine. The five major kinetic chains are intrinsic, deep longitudinal, lateral, posterior, and anterior.

For example, throwing a ball is not just a matter of cocking your arm back and letting it fly. The power for a throw originates in the lower body, because you must generate rotational kinetic energy through the uncoiling of the feet, legs, hips, and torso, synchronized with the forceful uncoiling of the shoulder, elbow, hand, and fingers. Rotational kinetic energy is the conversion of elastic energy, or energy stored by the temporary compression of muscles and joints, into energy output—for a running stride, jumping, throwing, and other physical efforts.

Similarly, the pull of a dead lift is not merely an effort from isolated muscle groups such as the lats and the hamstrings but also a synchronized application of force by a complex kinetic chain that starts with the bottoms of your feet and extends through the entire lower body and upper body—mainly the posterior chain, along the back side of your body. The involvement of so many parts of the body is why the dead lift is often lauded as one of the most effective exercises.

The kinetic chain for most athletic movements starts with the feet: throwing, deadlifting, running, jumping, swinging a golf club—you name it. Try throwing something while barefoot and pay attention to the way you gracefully engage the various bones, muscles, and connective tissue in your feet to achieve weight transfer and the harnessing of the energy needed to throw the object. Even balancing on one leg requires a complex kinetic-chain operation: the arch, metatarsals, and muscles of the lower leg, upper leg, hips, and back all work together to steady your body weight over one foot.

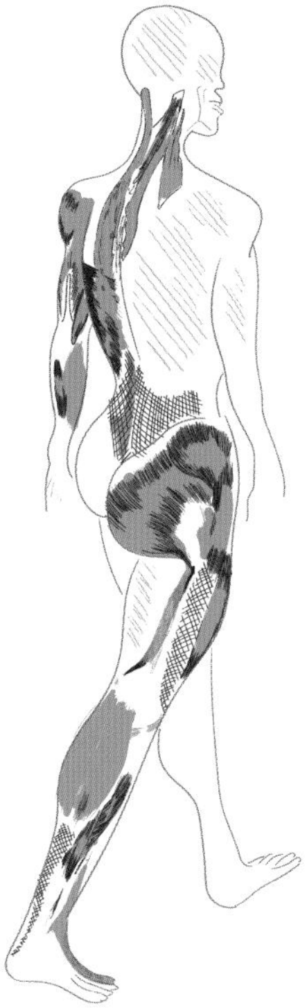

Virtually all complex kinetic-chain activity starts with the feet delivering precise neurofeedback to the brain.

Shoes with restrictive toe boxes, excess cushioning, rigid stability features, and elevated heels cause problems during walking, hiking, running, and other athletic endeavors by cutting you off from the neurofeedback the brain needs to organize kinetic-chain activity. Without it, the brain has to piece together the story in a haphazard manner. When it is forced to guess how to flex or extend the ankles, knees, and hips, the body becomes unstable and vulnerable.

Think about occasions when you lost your balance and fell. Typically, these miscalculations are the result of inhibited neurofeedback. For example, imagine that you're walking down a sidewalk in shoes, fail to notice a banana peel, and slip on it and fall to the ground. If you had been walking in bare feet, the sensation of landing on the unusual texture of the banana peel would be vastly more distinct and intense. Perhaps this feedback would have allowed you to take the necessary corrective action to prevent a fall.

Another example is the common skiing injury nicknamed tib/fib—a broken leg occurring just above the top of a ski or snowboard boot. The boots completely immobilize the ankle and foot by design, making the athlete vulnerable to severe injuries of this nature.

When you wear a shoe with excess cushioning and an elevated heel, you essentially disengage your ankles and feet from the kinetic chain, thereby forcing all complex movements to start from above the feet. This leaves your ankles incredibly vulnerable to turning and spraining and increases the risk of knee, hip, and lower back injuries. If you've ever turned an ankle when wearing running shoes, you can appreciate the dangers of being perched on a platform above the ground. In fact, encasing your feet in running shoes is kinda like running, playing soccer, even raking leaves in the yard while perched on a balance beam instead of on the ground.

Encasing your feet in running shoes is kinda like running, playing soccer, even raking leaves in the yard while perched on a balance beam instead of on the ground.

You may ask, "Why don't I notice the inherent danger and dysfunction caused by cushy shoes when I'm wearing them?" The answer is that the shoes disrupt your awareness of kinetic-chain activity. You are blissfully floating along on a cloud of muted proprioception. When the stable base provided by your feet is compromised, the slightest misstep—a basketball player landing on part of another player's shoe, a trail runner landing on an exposed rock or tree root—can cause the ankle to violently flip sideways.

By contrast, it's far more difficult to flip an ankle when you're barefoot because your foot is closer and more responsive to the ground and is thus able to react and disperse the unnatural impact efficiently. If you want to test this theory, go barefoot or don some five-toe minimalist shoes and take a leisurely walk on an extremely uneven surface, such as a rock bed. Or walk sideways across a steep incline or on a floor scattered with Lego pieces. Your foot and shoe will conform perfectly to every uneven landing and help you keep your balance and minimize impact trauma.

Granted, it's still possible to turn your ankle while barefoot or wearing minimalist shoes, but guess what—your ankle is vastly more mobile and resilient than your knee, so turning your ankle can occasionally be a way for your body to spare the knee from injury. The knee is a hinge joint, designed to move only in flexion and extension on a single plane, although it can handle just a bit of medial and lateral rotation, too. The ankle joint complex, on the other hand, has three bones and three joints and can move on the sagittal (dorsiflexion and plantar flexion), frontal (inversion and eversion), and transverse (abduction and adduction) planes, making it a so-called universal joint.

Your feet and ankles do an exceptional job of receiving sensory input from the ground and initiating the appropriate kinetic-chain activity during everything from standing upright to navigating a rocky trail descent. We want our ankles involved in the game at all times, even at the risk of turning them.

CHECK YOUR BALANCE

If you are feeling generally skeptical at this point that shoes are the enemy, try this little experiment. Stand in your favorite pair of casual or athletic shoes and try to balance on one leg—with your eyes closed. Most of us will find this to be incredibly hard. Then stand on one leg barefoot, close your eyes, and notice how efficiently and dynamically your arch, individual toes and metatarsals, and calcaneus absorb and disperse the subtle muscle contractions and weight shifts needed to keep you in balance. All manner of complex kinetic-chain activity must emanate from fully functional feet, otherwise you will inappropriately disperse impact loads, develop dysfunctional movement patterns, and suffer from chronic injuries.

The Dreaded Heel Strike and Overstriding

Perhaps the worst problem with elevated, cushioned shoes is that they enable a novice runner to strike the ground with a variety of imperfections and inefficiencies. Chief among them is the jarring, braking, heel-first landing called a heel strike. Elevated, cushioned shoes facilitate this technique error by destroying proprioception and providing sufficient cushioning in the heel to make it possible. It is virtually impossible to heel-strike while running barefoot because it's too painful.

Note that shoes *allow* a heel strike, but of course they don't *cause* heel strike. Novice and/or poorly trained joggers who don cushioned shoes have an inclination to heel-strike for an assortment of reasons, including

- a cadence (strides per minute) that is too slow for proper running;
- insufficient forward lean of the trunk (experts recommend hinging forward eight to ten degrees from the hip, keeping the spine straight, of course) and/or insufficient forward lean of the ankles (thanks to poor ankle flexibility);
- poor glute activation resulting from weak glutes and/or a lack of forward lean;
- poor hip extension in the push-off phase, resulting from weak and/or tight hip flexors, often prompted by sitting frequently in daily life; and
- a tendency for contralateral pelvic drop, a condition in which the airborne hip drops below the hip contacting the ground (thanks to weak musculature, causing pelvic instability under impact load). A 2018 study published in the *American Journal of Sports Medicine* revealed that each degree of hip drop increased injury risk by 80 percent.

It's important to realize, however, that because the biomechanics of walking differ from those of running, a heel-first landing is appropriate for the human walking gait. Your dense and cross-reinforced calcaneus can handle the impact load of a walking stride because impact is never more than your body weight. Still, an elevated shoe interferes with a proper heel strike so that even your walking form is compromised.

* * *

It's been said that nine-year-olds are the world's most natural runners because they haven't yet gotten screwed up by the weakness and dysfunction caused by sedentary lifestyle patterns. If you're well past your tweens, or if you otherwise lack the innate ability to take off down the street with excellent stride mechanics and vertical force production, you are likely to adopt an overstriding pattern when you hit the road wearing typical running shoes. While overstriding gives you a sensation of traveling forward and feels comfortable in cushioned shoes, it causes excessive and inappropriately dispersed impact forces and results in a significant braking effect with each stride. Furthermore, compromised proprioception causes runners to bounce up and down in cushioned shoes. This further increases the risk of impact trauma in comparison to running barefoot or in minimalist shoes.

Overstriding is revealed when the tibia forms an acute angle relative to the ground instead of the ideal near-ninety-degree angle at impact. This positions the foot in front of the pelvis instead of under it. When you overstride, in order to take the next step, your center of gravity must shift forward into the liftoff phase, only to lag behind again with the very next heel strike.

Beyond the braking effects, a heel strike causes your foot to stay in contact with the ground longer than necessary and compromises the potential changeover of elastic energy into rotational kinetic energy, which is what propels you forward. Instead, around 10 percent of the impact trauma is absorbed into the cushioned heel of the sole, while the other 90 percent dissipates inappropriately throughout your lower extremities. When you your foot strikes the ground during a running stride, two forces act upon the body—normal force, caused by the ground pushing up against your foot, and gravitational force, caused by gravity pulling your body weight down toward the ground. Overstriding increases both forces significantly. Using a complex mathematical calculation based on the forces acting upon a hypothetical 110-pound person, impact trauma can be measured at 3.7 times body weight in cushioned shoes versus 3.0 times body weight in minimalist shoes or in bare feet.

Essentially, cushioned shoes enable lazy running mechanics in people ill suited for running because of the reasons listed previously. They squander potential kinetic energy—unless you like applying force to squoosh your heel foam on every stride instead of applying force to run faster—facilitate imbalanced landings because of compromised proprioception, and allow for an inefficient fluctuation in your center of gravity. It's hard enough to run 26.2 miles, but it's even harder when a good chunk of your muscular and cardiovascular power is allocated to braking.

Daniel Lieberman, a professor of human evolutionary biology at Harvard University, author of *Exercised*, and a leading expert in barefoot running, published landmark research in a 2010 article titled "Foot Strike Patterns and Collision Forces in Habitually Barefoot Versus Shod Runners." This research revealed that heel-striking and overstriding inefficiency is exhibited by at least 80 percent and perhaps up to 95 percent of all recreational joggers and runners. Lieberman also found that impact load is actually *seven times* greater when a person heel-strikes in cushioned shoes than when he executes an efficient midfoot landing in bare feet. It further revealed that "[an inefficient heel strike is] essentially the same as hitting your heel with a hammer with two times your body weight." Remember, even the most robust heel cushioning will damp only around 10 percent of impact force.

Consider that a typical jogger will take an average of nine hundred strides per mile, so a 150-pound person running five miles is going to absorb some 1.3 million (two times the body weight at slow jogging) to two million (three times the body weight at steady running) pounds of force. When you inefficiently absorb millions of pounds of impact forces on every run, you are bound to incur microtraumas to the muscles, joints, and connective tissue. And with repetitive microtraumas, you develop inflammation, stiffness, and diminished mobility and blood flow. When activity continues on impaired joints and tissue, eventually the damage becomes severe enough to become a full-blown overuse injury. Why don't you notice this jarring impact on every stride? Because the cushioned shoe compromises your proprioception.

DON'T BE SUCH A HEEL ABOUT THE DETAILS

Equating heel strike with overstriding is potentially misleading. It's possible to run efficiently with what might appear to be a heel strike or a flat-footed strike, in which the entire foot lands at once. Among elite runners, who have short ground-contact time, there is a razor-thin difference between what might appear to be a midfoot strike, a flat-foot strike, and even a slightly heel-first strike. The reason heel-striking gets a bad rap in general is that almost everyone who overstrides is heel-striking. It's possible to overstride with a midfoot strike, but it's much more difficult.

Overall, the position of your foot and tibia upon landing are more important than what part of the foot you land on. Some coaches and performance experts suggest that you focus more on your tibia angle and foot position in relation to your pelvis than on what part of your foot strikes the ground first. However, it might be easier, especially for a novice, to develop kinesthetic awareness of a midfoot landing, which strongly promotes a vertical tibia landing, than to try to sense the tibia angle at foot strike in real time.

Another nuance to appreciate relates to the common recommendation to strike the ground directly underneath your center of gravity. This is an excellent general suggestion for everyone from endurance runners to Olympic sprinters. However, high-speed motion-capture cameras reveal that elite runners actually land slightly forward of their center of gravity but with their tibias still in vertical alignment with the ground.

Steve Magness explains the phenomenon on *The Science of Running*:

> *There has to be energy storage before there can be energy release . . . When you land slightly in front of the COG [center of gravity] . . . the body has time to absorb the impacts and move into a propulsion phase. If somehow you were able to land directly under your COG, you'd waste part of the time in which you could be applying propulsive forces to the ground because part of that time would be spent absorbing the passive forces.*

When Magness did high-speed motion-capture video analysis on his own stride, he noticed that his initial foot strike occurred around twenty-seven centimeters in front of his center of gravity and that it took .086 seconds for the foot to get directly underneath his COG.

Video analysis of many elite athletes consistently reveals this forward foot-strike pattern. Sprint coaches exhort you to think about "scraping the gum" or "pawing back" to encourage a powerful backward thrusting motion upon foot strike. This advice is intended to prevent lazily allowing the foot to land forward of the center of gravity and thus compromising power—or, worse, cause a braking effect. However, it's virtually impossible and undesirable to achieve a precise center-of-gravity landing. You'd have to be bent far forward or chop your stride inappropriately to touch down directly under it.

The Stress of Fractures

With the lack of proprioception in cushioned shoes, you don't get an immediate penalty resulting from poor technique and cannot sense the inefficient dispersion of impact trauma throughout the lower extremities. Instead, as you rack up the miles in comfortable shoes, you sustain "microtraumas" to the sensitive muscles, joints, and connective tissues in your lower body. Microtraumas result in inflammation, stiffness, and diminished mobility and blood flow to affected areas. When activity continues on weakened joints and connective tissue, you eventually develop a full-blown overuse injury.

The most egregious example of an overuse injury is a stress fracture—a tiny crack in a weight-bearing bone resulting from continually subjecting a traumatized and painful area to additional impact trauma. To put it another way, they're caused by a cumulative deficiency in the bone's capacity to repair itself from the microtraumas and repetitive impacts it endures daily. The tibia and the metatarsals are common sites for stress fractures in runners.

But your bones are not supposed to wear down and crack under pressure. In fact, Wolff's law, posited by the German anatomist and surgeon Julius Wolff in the late nineteenth century, asserts that when you apply appropriate loads to a healthy bone—by running, jumping, and lifting weights, for example—the bone will respond by becoming thicker and stronger over time.

Wolff's law also asserts that inactivity makes bones less dense and weaker. However, bones can become vulnerable when the surrounding muscles and connective tissue are compromised by microtrauma, inflammation, stiffness, and consequent poor functionality. It's critical for runners to grok this concept lest they labor under the misconception that a stress fracture is caused by bad luck—like catching a cold at a holiday party. On the contrary, stress fractures are invariably the result of a completely idiotic, obsessive, and dogged insistence on continuing to subject an obviously traumatized and increasingly severely and locally painful area of the body to more impact trauma. Granted, poor dietary habits, low vitamin D, and amenorrhea are also contributing factors to stress fractures, but the number one cause is overtraining.

The most egregious example of an overuse injury is a stress fracture—a tiny crack in a weight-bearing bone resulting from continually subjecting a traumatized and painful area to additional impact trauma.

The symptoms leading up to a stress fracture are quite distinct and worsen gradually, giving an athlete plenty of advance warning. Hence all those who sustain a stress fracture truly deserve to wear a dunce cap for the duration of their layoff—usually six to eight weeks. The journey to the common tibial stress fracture typically starts with shin splints along the medial (interior) bone line. Shin splints can manifest themselves as either a sharp localized pain or a dull ache. The condition begins with pain while running and typically progresses to persistent pain during the day that worsens after long periods of stillness or upon awakening in the morning.

You can continue to run on shin splints if you thoroughly warm up the traumatized tendons and/or wear cushioned shoes. Maybe you'll even mask any remaining sensations of pain with anti-inflammatory drugs so you can get your mileage in. Then, with continued abuse, the resiliency of your bone will weaken to the point where you experience a hot spot, also known as a stress reaction. This is a pinpoint location on the bone that becomes painful and extremely sensitive to the touch, especially at the completion of a training session.

If you immediately cease all impact-related activity, the bone will likely heal relatively quickly. Time to eat nutrient-dense animal protein, supplement with collagen peptides and vitamin C, do some corrective stretching and strengthening exercises, switch to no-impact activities such as cycling and rowing, and walk around barefoot or in minimalist shoes as much as possible. Walking will deliver an excellent strengthening effect and improve circulation to the injured areas without any impact trauma. If you insist on continuing to run with a hot spot, though, a fissure will likely develop and become a full-blown stress fracture.

I know: assigning a dunce cap is a little harsh, and hindsight after an overuse injury is always twenty-twenty. Many endurance runners have come to believe that feeling hobbled and banged up is a normal and expected part of the game and that feeling better after an extensive warm-up constitutes a green light to proceed with a workout. Although a gentle warm-up and cooldown are certainly essential and highly beneficial, it's time to dispel the myth that you can have distinct localized pain upon awakening or after sitting a while but carry on with training by warming up extensively and masking symptoms with nonsteroidal anti-inflammatories. The sports medicine physician Dr. Kathryn Gollotto, medical provider for the US Ski and Snowboard team, reminds us, "The tendons fool you when they become inflamed." Dr. Gollotto has surgically repaired enough overuse injuries for us to take her warning very seriously.

The best time to monitor the status of overuse issues is when you take your first steps in the morning. This is a sobering insight for longtime athletes like me who come to accept that limping and shuffling for a bit in the morning until you limber up with some gentle movement is normal. The National Institutes of Health reports that stress fractures comprise 15–20 percent of all running injuries. There is no reason that this should be the case: warning signs of a stress fracture arise over a long period of time, with increasing intensity and pain. These signs should compel athletes to take early corrective action.

The stress-fracture epidemic is another reason why walking should become a central element of most endurance runners' training schedule. It's extremely unlikely that one will sustain a stress fracture when engaging in an activity with a maximum impact load of one's own body weight. Remember, somewhere around half of all runners are injured every year, and around a fifth of those injuries are stress fractures. Spending more time walking, and doing low- or no-impact cross-training such as cycling, swimming, and cardio machines, will build musculoskeletal resiliency so you are less likely to get injured when you do run.

The Silly Full Circle of Running-Shoe Fads

In 2004, Nike made an impressive effort to enliven a stodgy running-shoe industry by introducing a novel model called the Nike Free. The design was inspired by video analysis of some of the world's top athletes running barefoot in practice. The Free had an extremely flexible sole made with a weblike formation of numerous tiny squares of loosely connected EVA foam. The checkerboard squares could move far more dynamically than a typical sole made of a single piece of EVA foam. As Nike explained with great fanfare, the Free enabled a dynamic range of motion akin to being barefoot. Models of the Free were introduced for running as well as cross-training. Even though the Free still had an elevated heel and encased the toes in a constricting box, Nike deserves credit for creating a stepping stone toward barefoot-inspired running and cross-training. Nike Frees have not transformed the shoe industry, because longtime runners tend to be passionately devoted to their favorite brands and models. It's also possible that a profit-minded public corporation such as Nike may have deliberately decided to deemphasize the Free because of its potential to cannibalize sales of its many larger and more lucrative lines of traditional running and cross-training shoes.

In 2006, another disrupter came to market in the form of Vibram Five Fingers, the original ultraminimalist shoe with individual toe slots. The first models were nothing more than Lycra sock material sewn to a thin rubber sole. The Vibram marketing pitch was spot-on: elevated, cushioned shoes cause dysfunction, while a barefoot lifestyle is the ultimate expression of health and functionality. Vibram enjoyed initial success out of the gate, as forward-thinking fitness enthusiasts started wearing them for walking, hiking, jogging, gym workouts, and everyday life. The popularity of the *Born to Run* book was a huge catalyst for Vibram Five Fingers, and sales grew to $160 million annually by 2012. If hoopsters wanted to "be like Mike," runners wanted to "be like the Tarahumara." Vibram Five

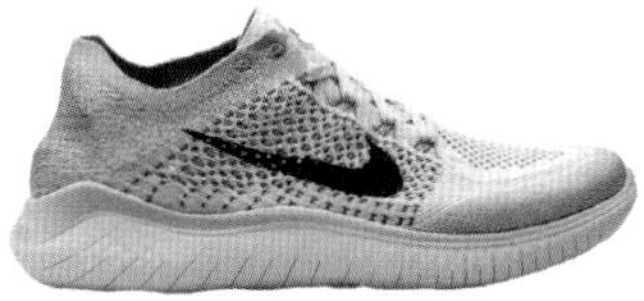

Nike Free's flexible sole gets the runner closer to barefoot.

Fingers sales at their peak were still a very small slice of the multibillion-dollar running-shoe market, but they were a true industry-transforming phenomenon.

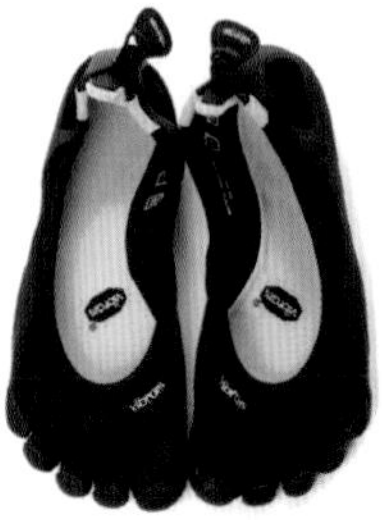

Vibram Five Fingers was the original barefoot-inspired shoe.

Unfortunately, then came the speed bumps. Like other fads, the barefoot-shoe fad lost its core message, scientific rationale, and best practices under an avalanche of marketing hype. Vibram and its customer base failed to respect the fact that virtually everyone who tried the shoes was incredibly ill-prepared for such an abrupt transition after years and decades of wearing elevated, restrictive footwear. If we were to rewind the clock to 2006, I'd exhort all runners to walk around in their Vibrams as much as possible, but please: don't run in them!

Predictably, the early wave of Vibram popularity took a huge hit in the form of a baseless but reputation-damaging class-action lawsuit filed in 2012. The plaintiffs contended that Vibram engaged in deceptive marketing and false advertising when claiming that the shoes could help strengthen feet and improve range of motion, posture, and balance. As the plaintiffs' argument went, there was no scientific evidence to validate that a barefoot-style shoe improves foot health and that it can actually have a negative impact because of increased stress to the lower extremities and exposure to debris. Vibram settled the lawsuit without paying any fines by setting aside around $4 million so that unsatisfied customers could receive partial refunds. The settlement agreement may have saved Vibram some bucks in litigation, but it was disastrous from a PR standpoint because it was seemingly an admission of guilt. Of course, subsequently, an increasing amount of research has confirmed that barefoot-like or minimalist shoes do in fact have the potential to generate all the aforementioned benefits when worn appropriately.

Sales of Vibram Five Fingers tanked in the ensuing years. They have since climbed back somewhat from the nadir, but only to the $20–$25 million range in 2021 and 2022. (The Five Fingers shoe line is a small division of the much larger Vibram corporation, whose main business is selling sole technology for hiking boots and other performance footwear.)

Despite Vibram's commercial troubles, it definitely succeeded in forcing runners to consider the merits of getting the human foot back to its natural functionality. Alas, industry insiders believe that the emergence of the so-called maximalist shoe movement that thrives today was buoyed by a rebound reaction to the Vibram crash-and-burn spectacle. As the oversimplified thinking goes, runners get injured in regular shoes, and they get injured in minimalist shoes, so what about . . . super-cushioned shoes? At last, a solution to consumer "pain points"! In 2010, an upstart brand called Hoka One One released a Mafate model that had two to three times the amount of cushioning of other running shoes. The brand and the maximalist concept quickly became a sensation, and Hoka became the fastest-growing running-shoe brand in the world over the following decade.

How were these crazy and extreme ideas able to make huge inroads against the superpowers of the running-shoe world, with their massive marketing budgets, decades of customer loyalty, and endorsement deals with the world's top professional runners? Considering the consistently high injury rates among runners, perhaps the industry has always been primed for disruption. What a ridiculous journey—driven by marketing hype, false promises, and uninformed, gullible consumers.

Over the past half century, we've been lured to, in succession,

- plunge into a high-risk, high-impact sport with ill-prepared feet and bodies;
- experience chronic musculoskeletal destruction through the use of elevated, cushioned shoes;
- abruptly switch to a barefoot-like shoe ("If a 104-pound Tarahumara can run all day with tire treads strapped to his feet, I can surely do a 50k trail run in Vibrams . . . after all, humans are born to run, right?");
- continue to experience an embarrassing rate of chronic overuse injuries; and
- pop for exciting new maximalist shoes that feel comfortable but, according to numerous highly respected research studies, do not reduce impact trauma or the risk of overuse injury one iota.

What About the New Energy-Return Super Shoes?

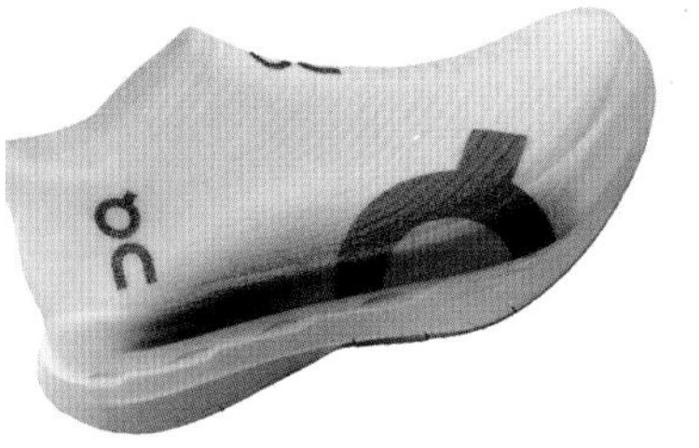

The Cloudboom Strike LS shoe from the Swiss company On derives the "LS" part of its name from "light spray," because the snug-fitting microfilament upper appears to be sprayed onto the foot.

You've probably heard about the sensational recent innovation in running-shoe design known as super shoes. These are maximally cushioned shoes made with extra-thick, ultra-lightweight, highly resilient foam midsoles and a stiff curved carbon-fiber plate embedded in the foam. Super shoes are purported to deliver an "energy return" effect in which the foam and carbon plate harness energy upon impact and then act as levers or springs upon takeoff. These shoes debuted in 2016 with the release of the Nike Vaporfly 4% model. Today, all major shoe companies offer super shoes.

In 2024, another innovation arrived in the form of a space-age "spray-on" super shoe from the Swiss company On. The shoe is made with a single semitranslucent synthetic monofilament almost a mile long that is extruded by a robot arm and customized to fit skintight around one's foot. This snug monofilament upper is then heat-fused to a foam-rubber and carbon-fiber sole.

Unlike other running shoes hyped by decades of marketing blather, super shoes really work. Exercise physiology studies reveal that elite runners can achieve as much as a 4 percent improvement in running economy with super shoes compared to the previous racing shoes worn by elite runners. Interestingly, running barefoot delivers the same 4 percent improvement in running economy, so super shoes essentially provide protection from the elements, traction, and comfort while getting one close to the ultimate efficiency delivered by bare feet.

Running economy is the metabolic, cardiorespiratory, biomechanical, and neuromuscular efficiency of a runner at any given pace. Running economy is similar to the highly touted performance and longevity marker VO2 max (see page 176) in that both are measured by oxygen consumption in milliliters per minute per kilogram of body weight. But running economy measures steady-state *sub-*

maximal oxygen consumption, while VO2 max measures *maximum* oxygen consumption. A runner with a low VO2 max and superior running economy might theoretically defeat a runner with a high VO2 max.

Improving running economy by 4 percent with energy-return shoes generates a whopping 2–3 percent improvement in race times. Super shoes have helped elite long-distance runners shatter world records, both on the road and on the track (the advanced foam and carbon plate technology is included in track spikes, too). Eliud Kipchoge's 1:59 marathon in 2019 was run in super shoes, as was Ruth Chepngetich's sensational 2:09 in Chicago in 2024, which shattered the female record. This 4 percent improvement in running economy essentially constitutes the difference between winning Olympic marathon gold and coming in fourteenth place. For example, Kipchoge won at the 2016 Rio games with 2:08, while the fourteenth-place time was 2:13. Since 2016, the top fifty male marathoners in the world have improved around 2 percent, while the top fifty females have improved around 2.6 percent.

Contrary to super-shoe hype, though, super shoes do not magically return extra energy beyond what's generated by your vertical force production—they are not springs. They do, however, squander less energy than regular shoes do. Shoes with typical EVA foam return 50–70 percent of the kinetic energy generated by your foot strike and push-off, and the rest is absorbed (squandered) into the sole. The new energy-return EVA and carbon-plate shoes return more than 85 percent of the energy. However, this increase only offers marginal performance improvement. So how do super shoes (and super spikes on the track) confer such a remarkable advantage? Surprisingly, scientists don't know for sure and caution against the reductionist thinking that seeks to isolate a single feature as the main performance enhancer.

Disparate opinions are emerging from continued extensive research on super shoes. The "teeter-totter" theory, advanced by respected Canadian-Swiss biomechanics researcher Benno Nigg, proposes that the curved, rigid sole improves the joint mechanics of the ankle and toes: vertical force production into the ground is transferred upward on the heel, generating propulsion with less effort—i.e., more economy.

Researchers at the University of Colorado propose that the toe spring offers a substantial performance advantage. Preloading the toes into a dorsiflexed, energy-coiled position relieves the toes and the small muscles of the foot from having to balance moving body weight and proceed through their typical range of motion during the stride pattern. It's like a bench-press spotter lifting the bar six inches off your chest and then asking you to hoist it from a position of better leverage—i.e., with straighter arms. There is also speculation that the incredibly high forty-millimeter sole thickness effectively increases the length of your lower limbs, which theoretically could increase stride length. Even an increase of less than one inch can save a couple of minutes over the course of a marathon. Finally, the comprehensive energy return features and are believed to minimize overall musculoskeletal trauma associated with running. You are less "beat up" running in super shoes. Theoretically, athletes can do harder workouts, recover faster, and thus perform better in competition.

But before you get excited and go drop $500 for a pair of super shoes, realize that you have to run pretty fast before experiencing any advantage. Seriously: $500 is the retail price of the Adidas Adizero Adios Pro Evo 1 ultralight five-ounce racing shoes, which are designed to be worn for just one marathon race before disintegrating—no joke. Can you say, "Formula 1 tires"?

In addition, experts also propose that there exists a speed threshold at which the carbon plate can provide an advantage and below which the plate can hinder running economy. Elite runners can improve running economy by 4 percent because they generate sufficient ground reaction force to trigger the mechanical advantages offered by the sole and benefit from the improved energy return. Average runners, on the other hand, benefit much less than that, and slow runners will not benefit at all and might even experience a decline in running economy. Research conducted by scientists at St. Edward's University, in Austin, Texas, reveals that running an 8:03-per-mile pace in super shoes delivers a 1.6 percent improvement in running economy while running a 9:40-per-mile pace improves running economy by 0.9 percent. If you run slower than ten minutes per mile, the shoes won't help—sorry. There is also significant disparity in the responsiveness to the shoes among individual runners and individual shoe models: some enjoy an improvement of 4 percent; others have *lost* 1 percent of their running economy.

There are pros and cons to super shoes from a big-picture perspective, so runners should use them judiciously. The same attributes that provide a performance advantage can also lead to atrophy in important muscles and connective tissues in the foot. A 2023 study conducted by researchers in Germany and the United States revealed an increased incidence of navicular stress fractures in athletes wearing carbon-plate shoes, believed to be caused by novel impact forces (the feet were accustomed to regular shoes) as well as the runners' increased hours of training at faster speeds.

Consequently, experts recommend wearing super shoes only for races or challenging workouts with high impact load. Even elite runners use regular shoes for most routine training sessions, especially long runs and recovery runs. Here I'm sneaking in a recommendation to go barefoot or wear minimalist shoes in everyday life to improve foot functionality, strength, and range of motion. Then, when you lace up any kind of athletic shoe, you will be better adapted to withstand the beating that your feet will most certainly take when wearing modern shoes. I'll describe in detail how to improve foot functionality and transition to a barefoot-inspired lifestyle in chapter 8.

CHAPTER 4
The Catastrophe of Chronic Cardio

THE SHOCK-VALUE INSIGHTS I've offered up to this point—shoes cause injury; running keeps you fat; most runners are better off walking—pale in comparison to the insights we can glean from the extreme exercise hypothesis. This hypothesis states that the longer and/or more competitive one's endurance journey is, the more one runs the risk of hormonal, immune, musculoskeletal, and metabolic problems as well as serious heart problems.

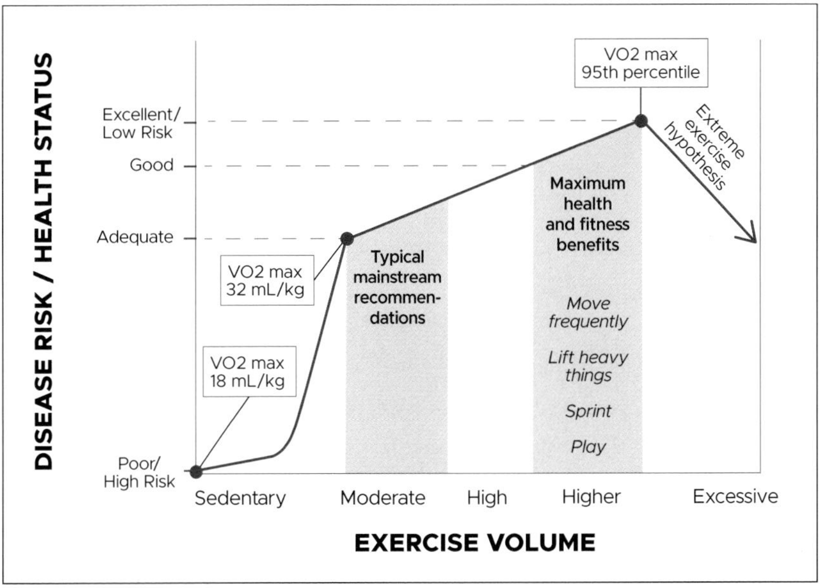

Going from inactive to moderately active delivers massive health benefits. But engaging in too much cardio increases the risk of of burnout and disease.

The hypothesis is laid out in the graph on page 81, showing the relationship of energy expenditure to health outcomes. Going from inactive to active brings a quick and noticeable increase in health, vitality, and disease prevention. Soon a sweet spot is reached—the optimal amount of energy one should expend for overall health and protection from cardiovascular disease. Beyond that, people who take exercise to the extreme and put in years and decades of long mileage at paces above the fat max heart rate actually increase their risk of accelerated aging and disease.

The sweet spot where one optimizes cardiovascular health and minimizes disease risk is shockingly low in comparison to what's advocated in the struggle-and-suffer marketing hype the fitness industry shoves down our throats. Dr. James O'Keefe, a cardiologist in Kansas City, Missouri (watch his viral 2012 TEDx talk "Run for Your Life! At a Comfortable Pace, and Not Too Far"), and coauthor of four books, including *The Forever Young Diet & Lifestyle*, suggests that running two to five days per week at around a ten-minute-per-mile pace, for a total of ten to fifteen miles a week (that's a total running time of around one to two and a half hours a week), will help you become bulletproof against cardiovascular disease. The highly regarded Copenhagen City Heart Study backs this up, suggesting that just one to two and a half hours a week of cardio will generate a 44 percent reduction in mortality risk compared with being inactive. Dr. Benjamin Levine, director of the Institute for Exercise and Environmental Medicine at the University of Texas Southwestern Medical Center, reports that the benefits of exercise for lowering blood pressure, regulating blood sugar, and lowering overall disease risk continue to accrue with an exercise regimen of five to eight hours per week.

Realize that Dr. O'Keefe's reference to a ten-minute-per-mile pace is intended as a general guideline. His main point is that a little cardio goes a long way. It's essential to individualize your approach so that the almost all your steady-state cardiovascular exercise is below your fat max heart rate. Although running ten-minute miles will help keep well-trained runners honest, the majority of people will likely have to go significantly slower to feel comfortable and remain at or below fat max heart rate for the duration of the workout.

Remember, if a forty-year-old can run one mile in ten minutes at a fat max heart rate of 140 (using the popular 180-minus-age calculation), staying under 140 for a five-mile outing will require a much slower pace than ten minutes per mile—probably eleven and a half or twelve minutes per mile. Hence, for most runners, going for an "easy five-miler" means walking or alternating jogging with walking, not jogging at a steady pace. The aerobic benefits and disease protection are still there for the taking, without the huge risk of overuse injuries, burnout, and cardiovascular damage caused by running.

I'd call one to two and a half hours of weekly cardio the bare minimum to try to ensure that you won't die early from lifestyle-related disease. If you're doing five to eight hours weekly, you're living an active, energetic, fit lifestyle. If you start to accumulate more than eight hours a week of cardio, Dr. Levine asserts that "you're not training for health, you're training for performance." This doesn't mean that additional exercise is unhealthful, just that the returns are marginal compared to the immediate benefits of going from inactive to active and potentially diminish when you overdo it. If you insist on a big commitment to endurance exercise, it's critical to do it correctly so you can avoid the risks associated with chronic cardio. This will help you continue to accrue health benefits as you become more active.

What's enough? And what's too much? Well, developing broad-based supreme fitness is the single best longevity strategy known to mankind, and a primal-inspired approach of blending extensive low-level movement, regular resistance exercise, and occasional all-out sprints has been scientifically validated as the most effective protocol. I'll cover this further in chapter 9.

It's also clear that there are many people with a huge devotion to and passion for serious endurance training who enjoy a variety of incidental benefits, such as happiness, fulfillment, focus, discipline, and camaraderie with their fellow enthusiasts. These folks may be unwilling to allocate more time and energy to pumping iron and sprinting and less time to a steady slog on the roads.

If that's you, I get ya. I've been that guy whose life revolves around his endurance training and racing. Remember, I ditched my goal of going to medical school and moved across the country so I could put in big miles in pursuit of my Olympic dream. I can also appreciate the incredible joy and value of spending time in nature, exercising your body, and pursuing daunting endurance goals that teleport you out of your comfort zone and into the arena of peak performance and personal-growth breakthroughs. After all, there are few sports where you can actually toe the same starting line as Eliud Kipchoge, Sifan Hassan, Courtney Dauwalter, and Kristian Blummenfelt (the Olympic gold medalist and ironman triathlon world champion from Norway).

The maxim that more activity is better can be true provided that the exercise is sensible, enjoyable, and not overly stressful. Researchers using the massive database of the Cooper Institute Longitudinal Study conducted another landmark study in 2019 involving sixty-six so-called extraordinary exercisers. This group had been active for decades and reported working out for thirty-five hours a week. Considered the most extreme exercisers ever studied, they showed no increased risk of heart disease or any other long-term problems associated with their activity levels.

The maxim that more activity is better can be true provided that the exercise is sensible, enjoyable, and not overly stressful.

Researchers surmised that extreme exercisers were engaging in lots of health-boosting, comfortably paced (below fat max) movement—"effortful but not exhaustive," according to study coauthor Dr. Laura DeFina. After all, it's simply not possible to hammer out thirty-five hours of chronic cardio per week unless are a Tour de France cyclist or elite ironman triathlete. The *British Journal of Sports Medicine* published a review of forty-eight papers on exercise and health conveying a similar message: "Mortality risk was lower at physical activity levels well above the recommended target range. Further, there was no threshold beyond which lifespan was compromised." Of course, to reap maximum benefits from an active lifestyle, you must avoid chronic cardio as well as overly grueling events that can overwhelm your system and cause illness and burnout. In the vast majority of cases, this means slowing down your pace, most likely to a walk, to maximize fat burning and minimize stress to the cardiovascular, endocrine, immune, and digestive systems.

A Heartfelt Case Against Chronic Cardio

The heart is an amazing organ that works nonstop your entire life and answers every demand to go above and beyond baseline function during physical exercise. The heart definitely appreciates a good workout and will adapt by becoming larger, stronger, more efficient, and more resilient—if you allow for proper recovery. The responsive heart also helps your muscles and organs go beyond baseline on demand and develop a critical longevity marker called organ reserve. Maintaining excellent functional capacity in your organs is the essence of aging gracefully, and it all starts with the heart—then you gotta use those lungs and muscles to keep fit!

Remember: any muscle challenged to perform a vigorous workout, including the heart and its arteries, will stretch, inflame, engorge with blood, and experience oxidative stress and microtrauma from the effort. For example, when a fit endurance athlete maintains an all-out racing effort for one hour, the heart rate can triple from resting rate. An hourlong race or practice race, a.k.a. a time trial, also causes stroke volume (the amount of blood pumped per heartbeat) to increase to thirty to forty liters per minute from three to five liters per minute at rest.

With a sensible, aerobic-focused cardio program, good nutrition, adequate recovery time, and a stress-balanced lifestyle, an endurance athlete will develop a bigger, stronger heart, just as a bodybuilder will develop huge guns from doing tons of curls in the gym. A well-trained athlete's heart can be twice or even three times as large as a sedentary person's—desirably so, in most cases—with a lower resting heart rate, higher stroke volume, and improved vagal tone—a measure of the heart's capacity to handle stress and promote rest and recovery. Vagal tone is also represented by a heart-rate variability, or HRV, score. HRV measures the variation in beat-to-beat intervals of the heart, with a greater variation indicating a robust cardiovascular system and improved stress-rest balance.

However, just as too much exercise stress can cause a tear in the biceps or a stress fracture in the tibia, an overtrained heart can sustain serious and irreversible damage. I'm not talking about what happens to a mere weekend jogger: I'm talking about what happens to a runner who obsessively logs fifty miles week in and week out for years and decades; who goes out the day after a marathon for an "easy jog," thinking it supports recovery; or who enters three marathons a year instead of perhaps three marathons in a lifetime (gulp: I raced more than twenty marathons, and ran another ten marathons in training, all before the age of thirty-five). This is what happens to a triathlete who squeezes workouts into every spare moment: running in the dark at 6:00 a.m., swimming during a lunch break, rushing back to the office with wet hair to chomp down a burrito, and heading out on weekends for hundred-mile bike rides. This is what happens to a racing cyclist who jumps into aggressive pack rides a few times a week, pedals solo for hours to maintain high weekly mileage, and competes in Masters cycling races for decades.

Most of us can walk our way to health, avoiding the huge risk of overuse injuries, burnout, and cardiovascular damage caused by running.

Don't even get me started on the potential adverse long-term health effects among those who participate in extreme events that don't allow for sleep or extend for several days, such as the two-hundred-mile trail races that have risen in popularity ("When running a hundred miles just ain't enough"). Other such events include multiday expedition races involving multimodal transportation (hiking, running, orienteering, mountain biking, rock climbing, rappelling, kayaking), such as the Eco-Challenge, the Primal Quest, the Raid Gauloises, and the many smaller races patterned after these events. There are also FKT (fastest known time) solo efforts across lengthy routes such as the Pacific Crest Trail, the Appalachian Trail, and the Colorado Trail; bicycle stage races modeled after the Tour de France; and relay races such as the 198-mile Hood to Coast run, in Oregon.

Scientific research reveals that serious heart conditions are occurring with shocking regularity among longtime competitive marathoners, ultramarathoners, triathletes, racing cyclists, long-distance cyclists, and cross-country ski racers. Medical experts are now referring to the heart troubles associated with extreme exercise as runner's cardiomyopathy, or Pheidippides cardiomyopathy. To be clear, the Pheidippides phenomenon is not applicable to walkers, hikers, backpackers, trekkers, and touring cyclists who spend hours or even days exercising at comfortable heart rates—for example, those involved in large-participation, multiday bike rides such as the festival-style RAGBRAI, a fifty-year-old 460-mile ride across Iowa (twenty thousand riders complete the full course; four thousand more riders complete shorter distances), or those pedaling down the Pacific Coast in the summer carrying supplies on panniers for nightly tent camping.

Leisurely paced cardiovascular exercise is universally regarded as healthful and longevity-promoting. It's also been proved that short bouts of high-intensity effort, such as sprinting, strength training, team sports, explosive sports, and stop-and-start ball sports, do not carry the risk of scarring, inflammation, and arrhythmia that a long-term pattern of medium-to-difficult steady-state workouts does. No, you really have to suffer at a brisk pace for years and decades, pushing through obvious symptoms of fatigue, injury, illness, and burnout, to blow out your heart.

Engaging in chronic cardio for years and decades can prompt an assortment of pathological structural and electrical changes to a healthy heart, including a stiffening of the atria, right ventricle, and major arteries; a scarring and thickening (a.k.a. fibrosis) of the heart muscle itself; an accumulation of calcified and noncalcified plaque in the arteries; high blood pressure; and a singeing and searing of the walls of the arteries from repeatedly overstressing the cardiovascular system with insufficient recovery time. That's right: this is the same high blood pressure and hardening of the arteries that you think you're running away from with your devotion to endurance training. Alas, if you keep running long enough and keep pushing the pace, you will potentially complete a loop that lands you on a couch next to your lazy, junk food–eating next-door neighbor.

A study of longtime marathoners—those who finished a minimum of twenty-five marathons over the previous twenty-five years—showed an average calcified plaque volume, also known as a coronary artery calcium (CAC) score or Agatston score, of 274 versus an average volume of 169 in a sedentary control group. For reference, a CAC score over 300 is considered indicative of a very high risk for heart disease; 100 suggests an elevated risk; below 50 is considered safe; and zero is a great score—clean pipes from clean living and sensible fitness pursuits.

The right ventricle is particularly vulnerable to damage from chronic cardio, because it typically pumps against the low-resistance lungs and is far less muscular than the left ventricle. When the delicate right ventricle is repeatedly stretched and scarred from overuse, it is no longer able to contract efficiently—like a worn rubber band. While a scarred hamstring is a bummer for your fitness goals, scarred heart tissue can cause disruption to the electrical impulses that flow through it and cause arrhythmias. Endurance athletes are particularly susceptible to atrial fibrillation as well as premature ventricular contractions, atrial flutter, ventricular fibrillation, ventricular tachycardia, atrial tachycardia, and hypertrophic cardiomyopathy. In the worst cases, athletes will experience sudden cardiac death during exercise, even when their blood work and routine screenings such as EKGs show no evidence of atherosclerosis or other risk factors. Many athletic types have gone in for routine screenings to discover significant blockages of the major arteries, despite their impressive fitness credentials.

Dr. O'Keefe cites research showing that longtime hard-training endurance athletes have a 500–800 percent increased risk of atrial fibrillation. This increased risk was verified in a 2019 study of more than 208,000 Swedish cross-country skiers who had been participating for more than a decade in the popular fifty-six-mile Vasaloppet event, held in Dalarna, Sweden. The study found that those racers who had the most finishes and the fastest times also had the highest risk of arrhythmias. Interestingly, this was only for males; female athletes have a much lower risk of arrhythmias in general. Dr. O'Keefe himself has experienced heart problems associated with his devotion to endurance exercise, commenting, "I've been an exercise addict my whole life. There's a subconscious logic that says if some is good, more is better . . . But that's absolutely wrong when it comes to exercise."

In 2023, Australian cardiology researcher André La Gerche, an elite amateur marathoner with a 2:29 personal best, began conducting landmark research on high-performing athletes from Australia and Belgium. He nicknamed his study Athletic Framingham, after the highly regarded Framingham Heart Study, the longest and largest epidemiological study in medical history, which has been tracking residents of Framingham, Massachusetts, since 1948. Professor La Gerche's study puts hundreds of high-level endurance athletes through intensive heart examinations and repeats them at two, five, ten, and twenty-five-year intervals. He's doing a bit of timeline shortcutting by studying some elderly ex-athletes to provide a model of the way athletic hearts age in general. He reports that 12 percent of elite athletes in their thirties and forties have scar tissue in their hearts but that the significance of this is still unknown. He also takes strong exception to extremists on both sides of the debate—the endurance zealots who refuse to acknowledge the clear risks of chronic cardio as well as the alarmists who cite the tragedies in order to condemn endurance exercise in general. "Most cases of atrial fibrillation fit into the nuisance category rather than the scary category. But it's there. We can't ignore that," says Professor La Gerche.

In 2006, I published a treatise titled "A Case Against Cardio" on my friend Art De Vany's blog. The article garnered so much attention that it served as the inspiration to start my own blog, *Mark's Daily Apple*. Since I first made my case against cardio, I've been keeping a private registry of superfit folks who have irreparably damaged their hearts or come to a tragic early demise. Something that resonated strongly from my article included my nonscientific speculation that these occasional strange cases of heart misfortunes among hard-core endurance athletes resulted from more than just genetics or random bad luck. The registry has become a morbid fascination of mine, especially after I landed on it myself in my early sixties.

I developed PVCs—premature ventricular contractions, something I attribute to years of abusing my heart and body as an extreme endurance athlete. Well, I do tend to go overboard with my competitive intensity—trying to reign supreme on my local fitness club's scoreboards for the VersaClimber and rope pull machines, on fat-tire beach bike rides that include stretches of going full tilt in soft sand (just to stay upright!), and on the Ultimate Frisbee pitch against the young bucks. I've basically revved my heart up to its maximum three to four times a week for my entire adult life. After my diagnosis, I took medication to suppress my maximum heart rate for five years, but today I am cleared to exercise without restriction. I'm fortunate to report that my PVCs are firmly in the nuisance category—I'm occasionally awakened from sleep by a pounding "catch-up" heartbeat, but that's about it.

My reaction—taking ownership of my role in causing this condition—contrasts sharply with those of many endurance-athlete cardiac patients when they first land in the hospital or get their first diagnosis of disease or, God forbid, when their families have to be debriefed after a sudden fatality. Often, the party line is that the athletes' misfortunes are attributable to genetics. This raises my hackles, especially when I hear the preposterous but common conjecture that a patient's high fitness level—a "strong heart"—spared him or her a worse fate. I think this brazenly disregards the huge risk factor that overexercising presents in relation to these conditions—whatever one's genetic predispositions are.

As I wrote in my 2009 book, *The Primal Blueprint*, your genes are not your destiny. Genetic predispositions—for obesity, alcoholism, flat feet, or atrial fibrillation—are certainly real. However, in order for the genes that cause dysfunction and disease to be expressed, your lifestyle behaviors have to provide them with signals to do so. If you don't consume alcohol, for example, you won't become an alcoholic. If you don't scar your right ventricle and burn the walls of your arteries by doing decades of chronic cardio, you are unlikely to develop atrial fibrillation and can surely build a better heart by forming sensible exercise habits.

Today, the science behind runner's cardiomyopathy is attracting increased attention among cardiologists as well as among hard-core exercise enthusiasts with years and decades of experience. As Dr. O'Keefe explains,

> The fitness patterns for conferring longevity and robust lifelong cardiovascular health are distinctly different from the patterns that develop peak performance and marathon or superhuman endurance. Extreme endurance training and racing can take a toll on your long-term cardiovascular health. For the daily workout, it may be best to have more fun and endure less suffering in order to attain ideal heart health.

According to a study led by Dr. O'Keefe and published by National Institutes of Health, high-risk endurance athletes are training way beyond the sweet spot of a few hours a week, as proposed by O'Keefe's research and the Copenhagen City Heart Study—more like one and a half to five hours a *day*—and at heart rates slightly to significantly above comfortable fat max pace. These are the guys flying by you on the trail with a terse "On your left!" warning. All told, they are expending five to ten times more energy than the typical level recommended for disease prevention.

Your overall weekly exercise energy expenditure can be quantified by multiplying exercise time by your activities' MET—metabolic equivalent of task. The MET scale ranks activities by how strenuous they are. Resting in bed has a value of 1 MET; brisk walking has a value of 5 METs; running a ten-minute mile has a value of 10 METs; running a seven-and-a-half-minute mile has a value of 13.5 METs; sprinting has a value of 30 METs. Extreme endurance athletes such as marathon racers and ironman triathletes typically accumulate 200–300 METs in a week. As Dr. O'Keefe's NIH study asserts, "Humans are not genetically adapted for protracted, sustained, and extreme aerobic exercise efforts." Any endurance athlete who has experienced heart irregularities would be well advised to read the many informative and often harrowing books and articles on the subject, such as Dr. John Mandrola's *The Haywire Heart*, the NIH study led by Dr. O'Keefe, and the many personal accounts published online.

How Chronic Cardio Can Damage Mitochondria

Mitochondria are energy-producing organelles found inside most of your cells. They convert oxygen and food calories into adenosine triphosphate, or ATP, which powers the cells' metabolic activities (see page 151). Many health and medical experts contend that mitochondrial health is equivalent to overall health, because mitochondria produce the majority of the body's energy and help regulate cell growth and cell death. Healthy mitochondrial function translates into an active, energetic, healthy human—and healthy animals and plants. Poor mitochondrial function drives systemic inflammation, oxidative stress, diabetes, heart disease, cancer and other diseases, accelerated aging, and, ultimately, death. Essentially, if your mitochondria don't function well, you cannot create enough energy to power your heart, lungs, or organs.

Appropriate doses of regular exercise help increase the quality and function of the mitochondria throughout your body. Exercise also stimulates the production of new mitochondria—a process called mitochondrial biogenesis. Short bouts of high-intensity exercise are especially effective for mitochondrial biogenesis, because briefly depleting your cells of energy signals the body to make more mitochondria. This helps you process more oxygen and generate more energy during future workouts as part of the adaptive response to training.

One of the by-products of producing cellular energy is the production of reactive oxygen species, a.k.a. free radicals. Just as your car spews exhaust when you turn it on and your chimney spews smoke when you light a fire, your body spews free radicals when you expend energy. The problem arises when mitochondria are overwhelmed by chronic stress, smoking, environmental pollution, processed foods, excessive exercise energy demands, and/or aging. When worn-out mitochondria produce an excess of free radicals and a shortage of energy, chronic inflammation and disease are the result. And when you exceed your stress capacity with exercise and plunge into chronic patterns, you promote a condition known as exercise-induced mitochondrial dysfunction.

Serbian researcher Dr. Sergej Ostojic, a biomedical scientist with expertise in mitochondrial dysfunction and exercise physiology, published an analysis proposing that

> exercise-induced mitochondrial dysfunction (EIMD) might be a key proxy for negative outcomes of exhaustive exercise, being a pathophysiological substrate of heart abnormalities, chronic fatigue syndrome (CFS) or muscle degeneration. It's all about dose response with mitochondria. Too much exercise stress is harmful, but a sensible exercise program featuring extensive low-level cardio; regular brief, intense resistance workouts; and occasional all-out sprints is an excellent catalyst for mitochondrial biogenesis and mitochondrial health in general, and thus a tremendous boost for general health and longevity.

Dr. Peter Attia, too, describes what happens in the cells when they are overstressed by exercise demands:

> When mitochondria are heated up too frequently for too long, proteins become denatured . . . and mitochondrial DNA leaks out of cells. This phenomenon is highly problematic because mitochondrial DNA is perceived as a foreign agent by your body. They are different from cellular DNA and strikingly similar to bacteria cells. When mitochondrial DNA leaks into the bloodstream, your immune system is confused into launching an attack against a perceived invader. This triggers an inflammatory autoimmune response . . . a sustained pattern of which accelerates aging and disease risk.

If you have symptoms such as unusual muscle weakness or fatigue during workouts, persistent achy muscles after workouts, intense soreness and stiffness in the forty-eight hours after workouts, mood disturbances, or chronic fatigue, don't pass them off as the normal consequences of athletic effort. There's a difference between being physically fatigued and experiencing dysregulated immune, cardiovascular, and hormonal function. Learn to know the difference. If you are training earnestly, you can expect occasional transient muscle soreness, but it shouldn't be severe or chronic. You will likely need to sleep more and rest more during challenging training cycles, but you should not experience disturbances in your everyday energy levels or cognitive focus. Fortunately, research reveals that mitochondrial dysfunction can correct itself quickly when stressors are minimized, such as by resting when you experience overtraining symptoms.

Acute Damage from Extreme Endurance Exercise

Running a marathon is no picnic, but it won't kill ya. The true health risks come from chronic activity as opposed to occasional magnificent endurance feats that you are well prepared for and bring a huge sense of accomplishment and satisfaction. I'm all in favor of the latter. Pushing beyond the comfort, convenience, and luxury that many of us experience in modern life to pursue daunting physical challenges makes for a rich, meaningful life. We build camaraderie and self-confidence and get a refreshing break from the mundane aspects of our daily routine when we go all-in for the bucket-list items. In fact, when aspiring marathoners ask me for guidance, I don't try to dissuade them—that's a waste of energy. Instead, I suggest that they run two marathons in a lifetime. The goal of the first one is to finish, and the goal of the second is to improve your previous time. Then retire—or at least pursue your performance goals by running much shorter races that are less inherently health-destructive.

Alas, we must be cognizant of just how acutely destructive extreme endurance events are so we can carefully manage the risk and reduce the frequency of our participation to the bare minimum. Do only what's necessary to float your boat—that is, if you insist on floating your boat with a wholly artificial modern construct that is fundamentally misaligned with human health. Don't forget: the 26.2-mile marathon distance was standardized based on fabrications by a nineteenth-century poet, and the Ironman triathlon distances—a 2.4-mile swim, a 112-mile bike ride, and a 26.2-mile run—were conjured under the influence of "bravado and beer" (to quote a *New York Times* article on the subject). Some military men based in Hawaii were arguing at an awards banquet over which of three existing individual events of the aforementioned distances was the toughest organized endurance competition in Hawaii: the Waikiki RoughWater Swim, the Around Oahu Race on bicycles, or the Honolulu Marathon. To settle matters, a small group of intrepid souls endeavored to try all three in one day in 1978, intent on finishing and being crowned an "iron man."

It's a great story, and perhaps a great bucket-list achievement for those so inclined. What's troubling today are the hundreds of millions of corporate marketing dollars and tons of social media influencers irresponsibly glamorizing extreme endurance events as the ultimate athletic accomplishment—hallmarks of a healthy, fit, adventurous, focused, and disciplined lifestyle. I'll argue that truly excelling in a local community 5k race is just as laudable an athletic achievement as plodding along all day and into the night on the lava fields or shuffling along for the forty-two kilometers of a marathon.

If you were to go directly from crossing a marathon finish line to the nearest emergency room and have blood drawn, you would have the same lab results as someone suffering a myocardial infarction—a heart attack.

When we push our limits and complete a marathon or an ironman, numerous critical health, immune, inflammatory, and cardiac biomarkers get temporarily blown off the charts, even in the best-prepared athletes. The free radicals produced from your extreme effort temporarily overwhelm the capacity of your system to buffer oxidative stress. For a short time in the aftermath, damage and destruction win out over the extremely powerful and effective homeostatic mechanisms that keep us alive and healthy under normal circumstances. If you were to go directly from crossing a marathon finish line to the nearest emergency room and have blood drawn, you would have the same lab results as someone suffering a myocardial infarction—a heart attack.

Stress hormones such as cortisol, norepinephrine, and adrenaline are spiked and remain elevated for a week or more because of the severity of what the human nervous system perceives to be a life-or-death experience. In men, this sustained elevation of stress hormones will cause testosterone to plummet (cortisol antagonizes sex hormones), lowering mood, energy, libido, and cognitive function and delaying recovery. Inflammatory markers will be sky-high. These include

- high-sensitivity C-reactive protein, the preeminent marker of the general inflammatory state of the body;
- creatine kinase, an enzyme stored in muscle tissue that leaks into the bloodstream after overexertion;
- creatine kinase–myocardial band, which leaks into the bloodstream after damage to the heart muscle;
- cardiac troponin I, a regulatory protein whose levels increase—and can stay increased for months—when the heart is overstressed and lacking oxygen;
- B-type natriuretic peptide, a neurohormone secreted in the ventricles in response to volume expansion and pressure overload and a reliable indicator of heart failure; and
- myoglobin, a protein found in the heart that elevates when muscle is damaged.

Exhausted endurance performers experience assorted other problems, too. A study published in the *American Journal of Kidney Diseases* revealed that a stunning 82 percent of marathon finishers experience acute kidney injury. This is a temporary condition resulting from fluid and sodium losses during the effort in which the kidneys have difficulty filtering waste from the bloodstream.

The kidneys can also be harmed by a condition called rhabdomyolysis. Rhabdo, as it's called in the extreme fitness community, occurs when muscle tissue damaged by overexertion, overheating, or excess impact trauma releases its proteins and electrolytes into the bloodstream instead of containing them inside cells, where they belong. One of the proteins released is myoglobin, a large molecule that can clog up the delicate tubules in the kidneys and cause renal failure. High levels of potassium in the blood from rhabdo can also trigger arrhythmias or cardiac arrest. The early stages of rhabdo are revealed by persistent intense muscle aches or swelling and dark red or muddy brown urine. Rhabdo typically kicks in twenty-four to seventy-two hours after an extreme effort and is identified by elevated creatine kinase levels in the bloodstream. It requires immediate medical attention and can cause permanent damage or even be fatal if left unchecked.

IS RUNNING THE TOUGHEST SPORT?

We can have some fun debating who the fittest all-around athletes are, what the most competitive sport is, which athletes have the best cardiovascular conditioning, what the world's toughest athletic event is, and so forth, but I contend that endurance running is the single most physiologically and psychologically stressful athletic activity known to mankind.

This is for an assortment of reasons:

- it generates an impact of two to three times your body weight with every stride;
- when you're wearing cushioned shoes, running destroys proprioception, so you can't discern the amount of impact trauma you are dispersing throughout your body;
- it's mostly continuous, with no breaks or variation of technique or even effort level, which prevents potential physical and mental refreshment;
- it places huge demands on the feet and the largest muscle groups in the body by requiring repetitive movements that modern humans are generally ill-adapted for
- it places huge demands on the heart in a repetitive and prolonged manner that can lead to inflammation, scarring, and arrhythmias; and
- it places huge demands on the psyche and the emotions, requiring us to ignore our human instinct to stop and urging us instead to carry on suffering to the finish line.

Swimmers, cross-country skiers, triathletes, and Tour de France riders are all amazing cardiovascular machines, and they suffer as much as or more than any runner in pursuit of peak performance—and they often suffer for longer periods of time. Actually, Nordic skiing generates the greatest cardiovascular demand of any sport, because it uses the largest number of muscles in the upper and lower body. However, the aforementioned sports generate little to no weight-bearing or impact trauma.

CrossFit Games contenders, boxers, MMA fighters, Olympic decathletes and heptathletes, soccer players, and basketball players are supremely conditioned both aerobically and anaerobically in addition to being capable of performing incredibly complex physical maneuvers. They get a ton of votes for best all-around athletes. Athletes in major team contact sports such as football, rugby, and hockey exhibit mental and physical toughness and complex skills. Endurance runners, on the other hand, won't get any votes for all-around athleticism, nor do they use much in the way of gross or fine motor skills. Running ranks as the most simple, accessible, and easy to learn of all sporting activities, but the overall stress quotient is a huge deal.

Recreational runners can easily overtrain because the entry barrier to the sport is so low. This is thanks to cushioned shoes, simplicity of technique, the struggle-and-suffer ethos of endurance running culture, and the marketing hype that promotes extreme endurance events as a worthwhile goal. It's time to consider aligning your fitness goals and workouts with health, vitality, and longevity. At least MMA fighters and NFL players acknowledge the disconnect between their fitness pursuits and their general health. What's more, you can't even participate in these sports on a recreational level.

The Athlete's Paradox: Suppressed Immune Function

When you conduct sensible workouts within your capacity, you generate a manageable level of free radicals as a consequence of burning calories, kind of like a bit of smoke coming off your campfire. This is because the presence of free radicals, or oxidative stress, prompts the body to boost production of internally manufactured antioxidants such as glutathione, superoxide dismutase, and catalase. With an appropriate dose of exercise and other hormetic stressors (in which you administer a small, beneficial amount of something that can be harmful in large doses)—including hot sauna, cold plunging, and even consuming the natural plant toxins in your kale smoothie—you fine-tune the body's antioxidant and anti-inflammatory defense mechanisms. Research has shown that the benefits of an antioxidant defense response from a vigorous workout can last for up to three days.

Unfortunately, the immune system takes a beating from chronic exercise patterns as well as individual extreme efforts beyond your capacity. When your free radical production exceeds your body's capacity to neutralize it, you accelerate the cellular aging process. Extensive research reveals that both the innate and adaptive immune systems are suppressed for three to seventy-two hours after an extreme athletic effort. This happens when overworked muscles release of large amounts of both pro-inflammatory and anti-inflammatory cytokine proteins into the bloodstream, which temporarily compromises normal immune function. During the COVID-19 pandemic, you may have heard about the "cytokine storm" that causes immunocompromised people to fare poorly when they contract the virus. This storm is an inappropriate overreaction by the immune system to a threat, whether it be COVID-19 or a marathon.

While regular, sensible exercise helps improve immunity, extreme efforts do the opposite. This constitutes what's known as the athlete's paradox—too much of a good thing. For example, interleukin-6, released from muscle tissue in response to exercise, is lauded for its role in optimizing the immune response. It can exert either a pro-inflammatory or anti-inflammatory influence depending on what's needed in a given situation. But when massive amounts of interleukin-6 and other cytokines are released after a marathon, they temporarily weaken the body's defenses against microbes and pathogens.

Essentially, your immune system is vulnerable because it's super busy trying to deal with emergencies, including the elevation of body temperature (runners can burn a 102-degree fever during a race), postexercise hypothermia (your extremities cool rapidly when you stop running, lowering your core temperature), muscle damage, dehydration, electrolyte depletion, and assorted other issues. A marathon is such an ordeal that it takes a week or longer for your immune, digestive, and reproductive systems to return to normal. Furthermore, the huge and sustained elevation of cortisol in the bloodstream also kills immune function in the spirit of liquidating your assets for peak performance (see page 38).

In everyday life, you ideally want to be in inflammatory balance—homeostasis. You certainly don't want the low-grade chronic inflammation prompted by inactivity and other adverse lifestyle practices, nor do you want to overwhelm your defenses with a cytokine storm. Ideally, from a starting point of homeostasis, you might trigger desirable acute inflammation to deal with things like a bee sting, a sprained ankle, or a workout within your capabilities. Afterward, you quickly recalibrate to homeostasis. For example, your muscles will release an appropriate amount of interleukin-6 after a sensible workout, which delivers anti-inflammatory and regenerative effects, including influencing the release of other anti-inflammatory cytokines such as interleukin-10 and inhibiting the release of the pro-inflammatory cytokine TNF-alpha.

Dr. David Nieman, director of the human performance laboratory at Appalachian State University and accomplished (2:37) marathoner, is a leading researcher of the effects of hard running on immunity. After a frustrating case of the flu derailed his preparations for an important race, he was inspired to conduct a study of two thousand runners at the 1987 Los Angeles Marathon. Dr. Nieman's study revealed that 13 percent of his subjects fell ill in the week following the marathon, compared to just 2 percent of the non-marathoning population. Imagine: 260 of his two thousand study subjects were moaning and sniffling under the covers instead of applying a fresh 26.2 decal to their car bumpers and basking in accolades at the office. At this rate of postmarathon immune disturbances, we're talking about 6,682 boxes of Benadryl flying off the shelves after 51,402 people finished the 2023 New York City Marathon. Postmarathon acute illness is so commonplace that aspiring first-timers are often told to expect to catch a cold in the days after their accomplishment.

Several strategies to try to mitigate the inflammatory and immune damage caused by running a marathon have been tested. Interestingly, by far the most effective is the practice of ingesting sufficient carbohydrates during the effort, typically in the form of quick-energy sports drinks and energy gels at a recommended rate of up to three hundred calories an hour. Getting some onboard calories during sustained efforts can help minimize the stress-hormone spike, but digestion can be problematic during exercise, as I'll discuss shortly. Your body gets the message that it has sufficient fuel and can tone down inflammatory emergency operations such as gluconeogenesis.

Running and Leaky Gut

A sensible exercise program helps promote the formation of healthy gut bacteria and increases microbial diversity. A healthy gut promotes a healthy body—improving digestion, nutrient assimilation, inflammation, and immune function as well as preventing obesity-related pathologies and boosting many other aspects of general health. Exercise increases production of the short-chain fatty acid butyrate, which is part of the mucus that protects and strengthens the gut lining. Exercise also helps improve gastric motility and gastric emptying by increasing blood flow and strengthening muscles in the gastrointestinal tract. Walking after meals helps food move through the digestive tract more efficiently and reduces bloating, particularly for people with irritable bowel syndrome. A 2017 Italian study about the effect of exercise on gut health offered this insight: "In fact, stable and enriched microflora diversity is indispensable to the homeostasis and normal gut physiology contributing also to suitable signaling along the brain-gut axis and to the healthy status of the individual."

That's the good news. It's also the case that your digestive system takes a beating from extreme exercise: recall the high frequency of gastric distress among ironman triathletes. The problem is greatly exacerbated when an athlete tries to process sugary drinks, bars, and gels on a minimally functional digestive system. Australian researcher Ricardo Costa, PhD, explains that significant gut disturbances occur surprisingly easily after just two hours of low-intensity effort at 60 percent of VO2 max—well below fat max. Things can be even worse for marathon runners because of the fast pace—the pounding and jarring the digestive tract is subjected to during a marathon is more severe than it is for someone shuffling through the final leg of an Ironman—to say nothing of ultramarathon runners, who, because of the race's extreme duration and their need for lots of onboard calories amid constant impact trauma, perhaps suffer worst of all.

During vigorous exercise, the increase in the body's core temperature prompts inflammation and permeability of the intestinal lining, which is necessary and expected in order to dissipate heat. Furthermore, blood supply is diverted from the digestive tract to meet the high demands of the heart and the muscles, causing further dysfunction and gut permeability. These effects are greatly magnified when exercising in warm or hot weather, which Dr. Costa asserts is anything over eighty-six degrees Fahrenheit. Inhibited gut function during hard, sustained exercise is the reason why runners commonly experience flatulence, bloating, stomach cramps, and diarrhea—not just in the aftermath of a marathon but also in daily life.

Chronic gut inflammation and permeability can also be caused by consuming gluten and other plant toxins that can irritate the gut lining in sensitive people. This condition is known as leaky gut syndrome, and it's being blamed for a variety of downstream autoimmune and inflammatory conditions. Normally, the tiny, delicate microvilli lining the small intestine form tight junctions that allow only desired nutrients (carbohydrates, protein, fatty acids, vitamins, and minerals) to enter the bloodstream and keep out unwanted bacteria and pathogens. In someone who has leaky gut syndrome, the tight junctions become inflamed and permeable, and undesirable agents enter the bloodstream that are not supposed to, including undigested food, bacteria, mucus, and dead white blood cells.

As a consequence of undesirable shit (literally) getting into your bloodstream, the immune system becomes confused and attacks itself—not just in the digestive tract but also throughout the body. This can cause gut problems such as irritable bowel syndrome, ulcerative colitis, gastritis, and celiac disease as well as systemic issues such as rheumatoid arthritis, dermatitis, acne, rosacea, psoriasis, Hashimoto's disease, Graves disease, type 1 diabetes, lupus, and multiple sclerosis. Leaky gut also contributes to the systemic inflammation that many health experts now believe is the root cause of the majority of cancers and other diseases. Dr. Robert Lustig cites research stating that 93 percent of Americans suffer from chronic inflammation caused by leaky gut syndrome.

Get in Shape—the Right Way—or Else!

Marathon racing is destructive enough for those who are extremely fit and well prepared. But today—unlike the early days of the running boom, when greyhounds shod in Onitsuka Tiger Marathons comprised the vast majority of participants—the people who toe the line today are neither fit nor well prepared. A huge chunk of the field starts races in a state of chronic inflammation and mild immune suppression caused by overtraining and perhaps other counterproductive lifestyle practices, including poor diet, insufficient sleep, and too much stress. Yep: that extra twenty-mile run you put in two weeks before the big race—the one your ego needed to feel "ready"—likely pushed your body over the edge and into deficits. Many other competitors start the race insufficiently prepared, perhaps because they ramped up from an unfit baseline too quickly—like charity runners who take a six-month crash course. These athletes' inflammatory and immune systems will become overwhelmed by the effort.

Doing almost all your steady-state cardio at or below fat max heart rate, also known as the aerobic zone, while less endorphin-inducing and ego-satisfying than pushing the pace, allows cardiovascular endurance to progress steadily over time without interruption by the fatigue, depletion, overuse injuries, and minor illnesses that most runners contract during preparation periods. If marathon aspirants ditch chronic cardio and instead do a ton of walking, along with perhaps an occasional 10k or a 13.1-mile running race, and if they sprinkle in some high-intensity strength and sprint workouts, they will be better prepared and less destroyed afterward.

You can see the difference between poorly prepared participants and well-prepared participants if you peruse the postmarathon press conferences with elite runners on YouTube. They will be all cleaned up and dressed stylishly in their sponsor-logo sweat suits, enthusiastically recounting the race just hours after finishing in two hours and change. The next day, they'll head out for an easy five-mile jog to loosen up the legs. Even while running at breakneck speed for twenty-six miles, they'll fare better physiologically than almost all the recreational participants shuffling to the finish line.

Indeed, a study of sixty amateur finishers of the 2004 and 2005 Boston Marathon, led by Harvard cardiologist Dr. Tomas Neilan and Florida cardiologist Dr. Malissa Wood, revealed that acute heart damage was lowest or absent in those who trained forty-five miles a week or more. Those who ran thirty-five miles or less—a distance that's widely regarded as insufficient preparation for a marathon—showed diastolic dysfunction, increased pulmonary pressures, right ventricular dysfunction, and high levels of troponin, B-type natriuretic peptide, and myoglobin. As Dr. Wood remarked, "If even the healthiest hearts after a marathon leak a heart enzyme or demonstrate reduced pumping function, those with sick hearts will have trouble." If you're gonna go long, you have to long in training, and at a comfortable pace. This will enable you to build a phenomenal aerobic and musculoskeletal system and mitigate the inevitable damage from extreme endurance challenges.

The Folly of Fixx

Jim Fixx, the aforementioned author credited with catalyzing the running boom, collapsed and died during a run in 1984 in Vermont at the age of fifty-two. Fixx's misfortune caused him to transition posthumously from running-boom pioneer to the butt of jokes told by heavyset stand-up comics and gloating sedentary types at cocktail gatherings everywhere, citing Fixx's fate as their rationale for avoiding exercise. This carried on for decades, seemingly validated anytime there was a news report warning of the dangers of extreme exercise. Fixx's autopsy revealed that one of his coronary arteries was 95 percent blocked, another was 85 percent blocked, and another was 70 percent blocked. It was speculated that Fixx likely suffered a few minor heart attacks in the weeks preceding his fatal run and ignored the obvious accordant symptoms.

The backstory behind Fixx's rise to fame is compelling. At age thirty-five, he was smoking two packs of cigarettes a day, weighed 220 pounds, and was haunted by the specter of his father, who suffered a heart attack at thirty-five and died of heart disease at forty-three. One day, inspired by the desire to rehab a tennis injury, Fixx took off running down the road. He lost sixty-one pounds in short order and was soon logging eighty-mile weeks, writing bestselling books and training logs, and traveling the world promoting the running boom.

Beyond Fixx's dramatic and tragic roadside demise, his legacy was further shaped by his brazen and aggressive promotion of the irresponsible running dogma of the day, including the Bassler hypothesis, advanced by California pathologist Tom Bassler, MD. Bassler, president of the now defunct American Medical Jogging Association in the late 1960s, proposed that if you could break four hours in a marathon and didn't smoke, you would have "100 percent immunity from coronary heart disease." Not quite, as it turns out, but Dr. Bassler was working with the available medical intelligence of the day, so he was not a crackpot by any means. Fixx, whose best marathon time was 3:15, gleefully endorsed the cheeky adage that "if the furnace is hot enough, anything will burn"—meaning you can eat indiscriminately provided that you burn the calories on the road. This became a mantra in running circles and remains so to this day. I contend that one of the most prominent factors motivating runners to slog through their weekly miles is to earn "vouchers" so they can consume extra calories—especially reward foods. Yep, digging a hole to install a ladder . . .

Besides being glib about fueling his mileage with fast food and sugar, Fixx went out of his way to shout down sensible dissenting opinions. Fixx famously phoned Dr. Nathan Pritikin to criticize a chapter in Pritikin's 1985 book, *Diet for Runners*. The late Dr. Pritikin, who emerged in the 1970s as the father of reversing heart disease through diet with his ultra-low-fat Pritikin diet and Pritikin Longevity Centers, recounted the conversation. "Jim thought the chapter [titled "Run and Die on the American Diet"] was hysterical in tone and would frighten a lot of runners. I told him that was my intention. I hoped it would frighten them into changing their diets. I explained that it is better to be hysterical before someone dies than after."

Six months after their conversation, Fixx was found dead just fifty yards from the lodge where he was staying, so it's apparent that he had completed his run and was in the process of cooling down. According to Dr. Kenneth Cooper, this is the period of time most conducive to arrhythmias because the heart is going through ventricular defibrillation in attempt to return to its resting rate.

The "anything will burn" adage actually originated in a 1978 cult-favorite novel titled *Once a Runner*, by John L. Parker Jr. Parker described the protagonist, Quenton Cassidy, as a collegiate runner training feverishly to break the four-minute mile: "He was not a health nut, was not out to mold himself a stylishly slim body. He did not live on nuts and berries; if the furnace was hot enough, anything would burn, even Big Macs." If you're keeping score at home, you'll know that this is at least the fourth example of running lore that emerged from fiction, joining the idea that a four-hour marathon earns you immunity status, the notion that running shoes prevent injury, and the legend of Pheidippides's "Rejoice, we conquer" run from Marathon to Athens.

Fixx was certainly not killed by chronic cardio alone but by a combination of serious risk factors, including his history of smoking and obesity, a penchant for shoveling junk food into his furnace, extremely unlucky genetics, a brazen refusal to acknowledge his preexisting risk factors, and—as science proved in the decades following his death—his eighty miles a week on the roads. The aforementioned Dr. Kenneth Cooper of *Aerobics* fame wrote extensively about the Fixx case in 1986. In 1984, months before his death, Fixx actually stayed at the Cooper Institute in Dallas to write a piece for *Sports Illustrated* about Dr. Cooper's breakthrough work. Dr. Cooper tried to persuade Fixx to undergo the battery of tests offered at the institute, which Fixx adamantly refused to do. Dr. Cooper expressed remorse for not "forcing the issue" and speculated that Fixx may have already known he was ill. Many heart attack victims experience the telltale warning signs in the days and weeks preceding their events. Six weeks before he died, Fixx reportedly mentioned to a friend that he was having chest pains.

Dr. Cooper was compelled to posit that there is a "Jim Fixx syndrome" characterized by a "myth of invulnerability" that many runners bought into. Despite Fixx's fatal obstinance and the ridicule heaped on him posthumously, we must acknowledge that his personal transformation and ability to share it with the masses was a fantastic catalyst for increasing awareness of the benefits of an active lifestyle. Fixx inspired many people to quit smoking and start moving and was a huge boost for the running boom and the concurrent fitness boom, which gave rise to aerobics, Nautilus machines, health club chains, and other cultural trends of the Me Decade. Ideally, he and others could have taken a page from the late great fitness icon Jack LaLanne. One of LaLanne's famous sound bites was "Exercise is king, and nutrition is queen. Put them together and you've got a kingdom."

We must also acknowledge that mainstream nutrition and medical opinion in the 1970s was laughably primitive. Remember, the US surgeon general only told us to quit smoking in 1964. Dr. Cooper's advocacy of the cardiovascular stress test as a means to assess heart disease risk was met with aggressive opposition from other cardiologists, who feared it was unnecessary and too dangerous. This conjures the memory of Oxford medical student Roger Bannister, who in 1954 became the first person to break the four-minute mile. Bannister persevered amid naysayers in his orbit, including many of the world's leading medical scientists. With the world record stalled at 4:01 for nine years before Bannister's feat, experts actually speculated that elite milers had reached the physiological limitations of the human body and that one's heart might explode in an effort to run a mile in less than four minutes.

Don't Have a Heart Attack Worrying About Heart Attacks

In the interest of being fair and balanced here, I must acknowledge that serious heart damage is mostly happening among a small number of hard-charging, long-duration endurance athletes who are unlucky and/or genetically predisposed to cardiac problems. In 2021, Alex Hutchinson, PhD, former elite Canadian 1,500-meter runner, author of *Endure*, and leading endurance sports science journalist, wrote an article for his popular Sweat Science series in *Outside* magazine called "There's New Evidence on Heart Health in Endurance Athletes." The overall message is one of caution against the alarmist commentary on the subject. Hutchinson cites research to support his contention that "the fitter you are, the longer you're expected to live, and there's no evidence whatsoever that the pattern reverses once you get really, really fit."

While research supporting the Pheidippides syndrome continues to accumulate, Hutchinson reminds us that "there's still lots to learn about exactly what's happening with calcium in the arteries, arrhythmias, and heart scarring." One example is the aforementioned elevated coronary artery calcium scores found in serious endurance athletes. Their calcium deposits seem to be mostly the kind that are stable and less likely to rupture than the noncalcified plaque that's implicated in heart attacks. According to Dr. Brian Olshansky, an Iowa heart rhythm specialist and devoted runner, a serious runner's fivefold increased risk of atrial fibrillation takes him or her from a 0.3 percent risk to just 1.5 percent.

Furthermore, most cases of atrial fibrillation are highly treatable, either by curtailing overly stressful exercise or by undergoing an ablation. An ablation is a minor surgical procedure in which the scarred tissue responsible for faulty electrical signaling is destroyed, either by burning it with a radio-frequency catheter or by freezing it with a balloon filled with refrigerant. Hutchinson's article also explains that when fit specimens develop atrial fibrillation or calcification, they fare much better than unfit folks with similar conditions. That's comforting, but who wants to be the fittest guy in the cardiologist's waiting room?

Regarding the young team-sport athletes who occasionally collapse on the court or the field: these incidents are almost all caused by genetic conditions, not by the adverse effects of athletic training regimens—even though the cardiac events typically occur during strenuous exercise. While these misfortunes often draw headlines, they are extremely rare, and overall risks are minimal, even for athletes diagnosed with heart abnormalities.

Consider a study presented to the American College of Cardiology in 2023 that analyzed seventy-six athletes playing at the NCAA Division I level or the professional level who were diagnosed with a genetic heart condition. Over the course of seven years, only three athletes suffered cardiac episodes related to their diagnosis, and these were mild cases of fainting. Even with a formal diagnosis of serious abnormalities—athletes are usually diagnosed following examinations performed after minor complaints such as heart palpitations—95 percent of athletes had no problem, and no one died. However, three-quarters of them were disqualified from sports and told to avoid heavy exertion before eventually being cleared.

To minimize your risk of contracting today's number one killer (16 percent of global deaths result from heart disease), my suggestion is to get as fit as you possibly can, *but do it the right way*. Swap out chronic cardio in favor of broad-based fitness. This means (1) doing almost all your steady-state cardio at or below fat max, (2) being consistent with resistance workouts—In his book *Outlive*, Dr. Peter Attia recommends that half your exercise hours be devoted to strength training—

and (3) building competency with explosive, all-out sprinting. Even if endurance racing is your competitive focus, I promise that you will be pleasantly surprised to discover that building strength and speed will improve your marathon time.

In the hundreds of races and triathlons I competed in, at no time could I ever admit that I was having fun.

My evolution from a skinny, sickly, chronically injured, and constantly fatigued endurance freak in my youth to an all-around athlete has been one of the great joys of my life. I relish every element of my fitness lifestyle and every minute of my workouts and competitive efforts—yep, even when my muscles burn riding the fat-tire bike in soft sand and when my Ultimate Frisbee team is getting torched by the opposition. By contrast, I can assure you that in the hundreds of races and triathlons I competed in, at no time could I ever admit that I was having fun. My entire endurance experience was one of pain management. I still have fond memories of my racing days, an incredibly intense period that honed my focus, discipline, and resilience in the face of all manner of adversity. However, all these benefits still accrue now that I pursue broad-based fitness and athletic goals with a sensible approach.

* * *

I appreciate the reasonable attitude of Alex Hutchinson as well as Professor La Gerche's admonition to neither smugly dismiss the risks of chronic cardio nor blow them out of proportion. But beyond your cardiology risk profile, it's important to point out that chronic cardio is no fun on many other levels. It's essentially an immersion in a moderately to highly addictive lifestyle, one in which a person's happiness and self-esteem often depend upon getting a scheduled workout in, getting a regular hit of endorphins, or getting a desired race result. Endurance freaks are continually teetering on the edge of breakdown and often have diminished energy, motivation, and joie de vivre because they have allocated too much energy to workouts.

How can you tell if you've allocated too much energy to workouts? If you have a five-year-old budding soccer star who asks if you want to go outside and kick the ball around and you answer, "Maybe later" because you need to rest for or from your workout, you might have a problem. I predict you will be filled with deep remorse and regret a year or a decade in the future—however long it takes to awaken to the fact that there will never again be another U6 soccer season for your little grandbaby. As the popular New Age author Dan Millman says in his 1980 classic, *Way of the Peaceful Warrior*, "There are no ordinary moments in life." If you want more food for thought, look up the lyrics to the Harry Chapin song "Cat's in the Cradle" if it's not on your current playlist.

Don't worry: from here on out I'm going to cover how to do things the right way—leading a healthful, active, fit lifestyle and steering clear of potential trouble. If you, dear reader, have been going way beyond the modest recommendations offered by Dr. O'Keefe, Dr. Levine, the Copenhagen City Heart Study, and my Primal Blueprint plan, and/or if you have been routinely exceeding your fat max heart rate during your steady-state cardio workouts, it's time to pay attention and strongly consider slowing down.

Interestingly, many hard-core endurance freaks diagnosed with arrhythmias have put their conditions into remission by simply backing off, and that includes me. After my diagnosis of PVCs, I resolved to dial back my maximum efforts by 5 percent. One thing I've noticed is that I'm probably fitter overall now than I was before, because I never cross that line into cellular destruction, oxidative damage, and delayed recovery caused by pushing too hard and combining that pushing with jet travel and work stress.

If you're inclined to dismiss the concerns about extreme endurance exercise as not applicable to your comparatively modest training routine and performance goals, I must warn you that the fight-or-flight response in the body is identical regardless of the stimulus. A hard-charging professional working fifty-hour weeks who dabbles in triathlon training for ten hours a week and has family responsibilities on top of that has an overall life-stress score similar to that of a professional triathlete who trains thirty hours a week and spends the rest of his or her time eating, sleeping, and relaxing.

Following are some symptoms of heart irregularities that warrant medical attention. This is not intended to be construed as medical or personal advice, but I think it's helpful nonetheless. Contact your doctor if you experience

- an unexpectedly rapid or irregular heartbeat—often you can feel abnormal pulsations in your chest, such as a quick flutter of fast beats before the heart returns to a steady rhythm (a good heart-rate-variability app, such as BradBeat HRV, can reveal irregularities that warrant a medical consultation);
- tightness, pressure, or heaviness in the chest;
- lightheadedness, faintness, dizziness, or blacking out;
- shortness of breath;
- uncharacteristically low energy or a string of poor performances in workouts and races;
- uncharacteristic irritability;
- swelling in the abdomen, legs, or feet; and
- discomfort with exertion that goes away with rest.

If and when you seek medical attention, it's extremely important to find a professional who is familiar with the athletic heart. In Dr. Mandrola's book *The Haywire Heart*, he cites real-life examples of cardiologists and electrophysiologists who have misinterpreted test results in athletes because of a lack of experience or familiarity with the unique attributes and risk factors associated with hard-core endurance training. I have had countless adverse experiences with the mainstream medical community, many of whom saw me as an ordinary patient instead of a high-performing athlete with an extreme devotion to health and peak performance. So if you feel at all discounted or dismissed when you mention your training regimen or concerns as an athlete, get a second or third opinion.

CHAPTER 5
The Ordeal of the Obligate Runner

Now it's time to deliver the straight scoop and not pull any punches for the sake of being polite or politically correct. It's time to have "that talk" about your endurance pursuits.

I contend that the endurance community is filled with many well-intentioned people who are suffering inappropriately and ingloriously. This suffering might be driven by the flawed childhood programming that many experts believe is the root cause of the majority of our psychological problems in adult life. There are many people for whom running has become a form of self-torture, either because of poorly regulated type A drives or low self-esteem or both. There are others for whom running serves as a distraction, a way to avoid confronting dysfunctional relationships and/or career circumstances. What better way to run from your problems and/or avoid acknowledging and healing from the "little-t" traumas of life?

I'm singling out endurance sports because the potential drawbacks associated with a sport of suffering is not applicable to surfers, golfers, or adult league basketball players. I'm here to encourage you to use your fitness pursuits as a vehicle for empowerment, happiness, satisfaction, and freedom from self-limiting beliefs and behavior patterns. It's time to do it right!

In 1955, Roger Bannister offered this profound thought in his autobiography, *The Four Minute Mile*: "Sport [i.e., running] . . . illustrates a universal truth that most of us find effort and struggle deeply satisfying, harnessing almost primeval instincts to fight, to survive." He was referring to his valiant struggle to be the first to break the unthinkable four-minute-mile barrier. He most certainly was not referring to showing up a at half-marathon with a 101-degree fever because you already paid your entry fee or immersing yourself in a hectic, high-stress lifestyle in which you bite off more than you can chew and train beyond your physical capacities. In Bannister's book—written when he retired from racing in order to continue his medical studies, despite the fact that he was only twenty-five years old and at the top of the running world—he explained that pursuing ambitious goals that require discipline, sacrifice, and the overcoming of fears and insecurities will result in fulfillment and personal growth—regardless of the result.

If you're a highly motivated, goal-oriented, type A guy or gal, I want to ask you right now: How's your struggle going? Are you layering in so much stress that everything you do entails unnecessary and inappropriate struggle? Don't worry: you can be honest with me here. If your answer is yes, or "Maybe a little," it's okay—we'll work on a solution together. In fact, unnecessary, inappropriate suffering seems to be the norm in the endurance community and has been for decades. Back in the early 1980s, with the running boom at its height, the late psychiatrist Alayne Yates and her colleagues at the University of Arizona Health Sciences Center coined the term "obligate runner" to mean "those for whom running is a compulsive drive that preempts fulfillment in other life areas or who run to the point of inflicting physical damage on their bodies." Yates and her team described obligate runners as those who run at least forty miles a week, typically become "unequivocally committed" between the ages of thirty and fifty, are generally unfulfilled in their careers or personal lives, are "troubled by diminished physical attractiveness," and use running as "an aid toward the denial of aging, physical dissolution, and death."

Overuse injuries are devastating to obligate runners, because so much of their identities are wrapped up in being a runner. They center their days around running—not just by carving out time on the calendar but also by devoting a huge percentage of their physical and emotional energy to their workouts. In 1983, Dr. Kenneth Callen, then a psychiatrist at Oregon Health Sciences University, surveyed nearly five hundred runners and determined that "twenty-five percent state that they have experienced emotional problems associated with running. In almost every instance, the problem is one of depression, anger, or frustration associated with not being able to run due to an injury." Among injured runners, Dr. Yates observed, "Not surprisingly, they continued to run in spite of illness, which was often denied, or contraindications, such as arrhythmias, atherosclerotic heart disease, or stress fractures. Such unreasonable dedication has resulted in permanent disability or even death."

Obligate runners are "those for whom running is a compulsive drive that preempts fulfillment in other life areas or who run to the point of inflicting physical damage on their bodies."

A 1983 study led by Dr. Yates and published in the *New England Journal of Medicine* was titled "Running—An Analogue of Anorexia?" Researchers theorized that both runners' and anorexics' dangerous yet "partially successful" behavior (i.e., exhibiting the celebrated attributes of focus and discipline but resulting in poor health) is motivated by the desire to form an identity. Both types of people typically come from affluent socioeconomic backgrounds and are hard-driving, compulsively athletic, and obsessed with food and body composition. Distinct personality attributes of both include "inhibition of [the expression of] anger, extraordinarily high self-expectations, tolerance of physical discomfort, denial of potentially serious debility, and a tendency toward depression . . . Their singular commitment to running [began] at a time of heightened anxiety, depression, and identity diffusion." The researchers observed that "obligatory runners and anorexic women must continue to prove themselves by running or dieting, as if they were not able to form an enduring or absolute sense of who they are," and that their obsessions provide them with "a clear identity that differentiates them from other less dedicated people."

I know the obligate runner archetype well and have been one myself. I would have never compared myself to an anorexic, but I did develop a disordered relationship with food in my obsession with slamming down enough calories to perform and recover. Those were the days when carbo-loading reigned supreme. Buoyed by popular books like *Eat to Win* and *The Pritikin Program for Diet and Exercise*, runners, and the health-conscious population in general, came to view dietary fat as the enemy, as if eating fat would make us fat. Consequently, I would go to ridiculous lengths to consume between six hundred and a thousand grams of carbohydrates every day—that's between 2,400 and four thousand calories just in carbs—and eat more than five thousand total calories daily. I've joked previously about endurance athletes downing a Ben & Jerry's pint when they get depleted or dysregulated, but my jam was to clean out an entire half gallon of rocky road to reward myself after a great workout or race result. Other times, I recall attempts to reach "racing weight" that entailed skipping meals and restricting portion sizes while I concurrently ran long and ran hard. Eating disorder? Who, me?!

For me, my day had far less value if I didn't run. If I performed poorly—not just in big races but also in routine training sessions—I'd stew in negative thoughts until I redeemed myself with a good performance. This might be rewarded with mass quantities of fried chicken embryos (had to drop a *Saturday Night Live* Coneheads reference in here), pizza, beer, and rocky road, about which I might feel guilty the following day and put in a few extra miles . . . you get the picture. I remember sitting down with my training diary on Sunday evenings to total my mileage and being compelled a few times to head out for a quick one- or two-mile jog through the neighborhood in order to reach that hallowed hundred-mile benchmark—my twenty-two-mile run that same morning notwithstanding. I exuded what Dr. Yates's research team described as "grim asceticism." By contrast, my current favored endeavors—stand-up paddling, giving it my all on the Ultimate Frisbee pitch, fat-tire beach cycling, long hikes in the mountains, even hoisting heavy weights in the gym—are all about fun, a deep reverence for the process, and the unbridled expression of my adventurous and competitive spirit.

Harmonious Passion Versus Unhealthful Obsession

A 2015 Italian study of nearly seven hundred marathoners published in the *Scandinavian Journal of Medicine & Science in Sports* revealed that runners who develop unhealthful obsessions about their training perform worse than those who are "harmoniously passionate" about it. The Italian sports psychologist and study lead, Fabio Lucidi, explains that obsessed runners, as opposed to harmoniously passionate runners, suffer from more injuries, more worry, more negative self-perception, and more general unhappiness, all of which hamper performance. Meanwhile, well-adjusted runners handle race-day stress better and have a more positive attitude about training. Dr. Lucidi contends that the nature of one's motivation is the driving factor: intrinsic motivation is more (intrinsically!) healthful than becoming obsessed with external recognition and tangible results. Granted, it's perfectly fine to set specific performance goals and celebrate success, but it's surely a problem when you become despondent about falling short of expectations.

Dr. Lucidi suggests asking yourself some important questions to help determine if you're drifting away from harmonious passion toward unhealthful obsession. First, do you feel compelled to run? Or do you do so willingly? These questions are similar to the ones used to determine whether a person is addicted to food, gambling, or alcohol. Lucidi observes about obsessive runners, "They often ruminate excessively and fail to disengage from risky or unsuitable tasks." Continuing to run all the way into a stress fracture surely qualifies as risky and unsuitable.

Next, Dr. Lucidi wants to know whether running is your top priority in life. Even if you're gunning for the Olympics, it really doesn't have to be and shouldn't be. Elite runners are certainly all-in with their devotion to training and peak performance, but every single one of them values the athletic lifestyle, camaraderie, and the capacity to inspire others in addition to their passion for competing, winning prizes, and setting records. The elites are always striving for balance in their personal lives because they desperately need those weekend camping trips and postseason stays at tropical resorts in order to handle the intense pressure and massive training loads that come with the career.

If you envision elite athletes as living and breathing practice times and competitive results, you are sorely mistaken. This is a fallacy that's been propagated by Rocky Balboa and other Hollywood "athletes" and perhaps by recreational competitors seeking justification for tuning out real life. Elite endurance athletes are definitely blue-collar: they punch the clock and put in an incredibly hard day's work, but they know how to disengage, watch Netflix, go to the pub with their mates, bake cookies, visit relatives in nursing homes, and linger in bed on Sunday mornings for extra rest and crossword puzzles. It's not uncommon to see elite endurance athletes cultivating hobbies such as art, music, and photography or immersing themselves in family life.

On occasion, an athlete with a demanding full-time career will be able to perform at the elite level. American marathoner Bob Kempainen ran in two Olympics and won the 1994 Boston Marathon in an American record time of 2:08 while going through medical school. At times he juggled eighty-hour hospital workweeks with one-hundred-plus-mile training weeks. Scottish middle-distance runner Laura Muir, the silver medalist in the 2020 Olympics and bronze medalist in the 2022 world championships, studied in and graduated from veterinary school in tandem with the rise of her international career. As Muir says, "Sport is so unpredictable . . . if your career's cut short, it's good to have something to fall back on, and to continue in something you love to do." Running can certainly be a harmonious passion, a social centerpiece, a source of great joy, and a way to integrate discipline, focus, and structure into your daily life, but it probably shouldn't be your top priority. "To have a harmonious passion for running means to build a personal identity that allows one to maintain one's [other] priorities and agenda while still considering running a central part of . . . life," explains Dr. Lucidi.

Also, Dr. Lucidi wants you to ask yourself if running has become your "core identity." If so, big trouble awaits when your attach your self-esteem and happiness to your results. Beware of attaching your self-esteem to the outcome and instead appreciate the *process* of pursuing meaningful goals and leading a fit lifestyle. Personal growth results from both success and failure.

Don't worry: it's okay to put a 26.2 sticker on your car, linger in endurance chat rooms online, publish your postworkout data to Instagram, and make running the centerpiece of your social life. However, it's also important to cultivate other hobbies. Resolve to nurture personal relationships outside of running and add other fitness activities to your schedule, including walking, hiking, cycling, water sports, winter sports, and high-intensity resistance and sprint workouts.

In addition, check on the general state of your energy and mood. If you're too physically and emotionally exhausted to do much more than log your weekly mileage, or if you're uninterested in engaging with work or family life, you've entered the ranks of the obligate runner. These are the dads who politely decline to play with their children during their precious afternoon "recovery" time, are too tired for a night on the town with their significant others, and are wallflowers at any social gathering not dominated by fellow runners and running conversation. "Obsession . . . does not produce psychological gains and may even facilitate some deleterious effects, such as burnout and overtraining," warns Dr. Lucidi.

Professor Sisson's Competitive Intensity 2.0

Pushing my body to the limit and being highly competitive for my entire life has brought me tremendous satisfaction, contentment, confidence, focus, and discipline. These traits were originally forged largely through endurance sports, and they have served me well as a husband, parent, friend, businessman, and role model. Granted, my longevity prospects would be better if I had run only half my lifetime mileage, lifted only to 90 percent capacity in the gym, competed with a 10 percent reduction in effort and intensity, and perhaps applied that extra time and energy to yoga, meditation, tai chi, and other stuff I recommend but have never tried. However, from a psychological perspective, I'd be less confident, less focused, less happy, less everything—a shell of my true self.

That said, my extreme endurance pursuits have given me lots of fodder for reflection in the decades since, centered on the prevailing theme of "What was I thinking?" I must admit that my penchant to suffer and endure on the racecourse has caused some fallout in real life. Physically, my athletic exploits have given me those pesky premature ventricular contractions, a huge permanent knot of scar tissue in one of my hamstrings, an increasingly bum hip that may have to be swapped for titanium someday, a stiff and scarred Achilles tendon, poor mobility in one shoulder, and assorted other battle scars. I've also endured toxic relationship dynamics and unfavorable business situations with a stiff upper lip that's been honed by my ability to endure the pain of hitting the wall in a marathon and still carry on for six more miles. Rather than having the courage and foresight to step off the course or correct course when it was essential to my well-being, I simply endured, to my extreme detriment.

In my entrepreneurial life, my default position has been to work really hard, sometimes to the extent of banging my head against the wall instead of being smarter and more strategic. My social media followers are aware of the great success of my Primal Kitchen enterprise, which was acquired by the Kraft Heinz Company for a sum that made me wealthy beyond my dreams. What people may not be aware of is the fate of the primal-themed fast-casual restaurant chain I started around the same time as my foray into healthful condiments.

Sometimes it's a great idea to soften up, give up, and redirect your energy and attention to something fresh and new.

I suffered from the get-go, making bad decisions, ignoring the writing on the wall, and digging myself into an ever-deeper financial and emotional hole, thanks to my endurance-athlete disposition. Marathoners know the level of pride involved with carrying on no matter what instead of dropping out: "Never give up"; "Stay hard,"; "Just do it,"; "There is no finish line." Well, sometimes it's a great idea to soften up, give up, and redirect your energy and attention to something fresh and new—lest you develop a stress fracture or a relationship fracture! My Sisson 2.0 take on the endurance-running hypothesis of evolutionary biology looks beyond the Achilles tendons, nuchal ligament, and other items on the list of genetic endurance attributes. It was obviously much more advantageous for our ancestors to leverage their genetic gifts for brainpower than their genetic gifts for endurance. If they hadn't, we might still be chasing antelopes on the savanna instead of building AI robots and plotting Mars missions.

Since I'm not the most mystical or metaphysical guy, I don't automatically embrace the idea that "it's all part of the journey that got me where I am today." No way. Of course, that statement is partly true for each of us, but I think it's bullshit to go and camp out there. I'm oriented toward disciplined critical thinking, honest self-assessment, and problem solving. I have tons of regret and frustration about my journey as a marathon runner and ironman triathlete. Even today, I reminisce about how much better I might have performed armed with my current knowledge about training, diet, recovery, mindset—and super shoes! I feel guilty that I allowed my competitive intensity to get the better of me during my career: it caused me to leave some great performances on the training ground and end my career too early. Bestselling author Brené Brown believes that "guilt is adaptive and helpful—it's holding something we've done or failed to do up against our values and feeling psychological discomfort."

I'm pouring my heart out to you here (by my standards, anyway) because I don't want you to make the same mistakes I made. I want you to experience your athletic endeavors as a means of personal growth rather than as another outlet for obsessive-compulsive behavior and unregulated ego demands. For example, an essential goal of parenting is to learn from the previous generation's mistakes, break free of dysfunctional family dynamics, and try to leverage your life experience to do the best you can. When my son, Kyle, was born, I couldn't wait to introduce him to the world of athletics, which has been the centerpiece of my life. You know—shower him with support, encouragement, and my vast knowledge of training to help him succeed. Deep down, my ego hoped that Kyle might come of age and aspire to be a chip off the ol' block. I remember envisioning being there for him every step of the way, ready with a stopwatch and sage advice about workout planning, marathon pacing, and honing the endurance mentality.

Well, Kyle turned out to be an athlete, all right, but in a completely different realm from mine. Beginning a young age, he was a natural at every sport he tried. He became an elite high school volleyball player, and can hang (in the air and on the ground) with professional-caliber Ultimate Frisbee players. Lately he has become a par golfer in just a few years of intense focus. Upon reflection, I'm grateful that he was able to naturally and intuitively shape his own athletic experience rather than robotically follow in his father's footsteps. Watch Kyle bomb a drive off the first tee or snowboard down a challenging run and you'll realize that it would have been tragic to waste that innate athletic ability on an obsessive devotion to weekly mileage. Similarly, every athlete I've ever coached has benefited from my wisdom born of suffering and failure. My playbook contains a healthy percentage of sayings that essentially boil down to "Do as I say, not as I do."

The Camaraderie of Streakers

Among the most serious longtime runners, there exists an eccentric subculture of "streak runners" who are dedicated to running at least one mile every single day, for better or for worse, in sickness and in health, till death do they part. Their badge of honor is the duration of their streaks, which they keep track of on the website run by the Streak Runners International organization (RunEveryDay.com). There you find tiered ranking categories with cute names such as Legends (forty- to forty-five-year-long streaks), Grand Masters (thirty-five to forty years), and so forth. Two hundred fifty runners are listed as having daily streaks lasting longer than twenty years, and more than 7,500 people are listed with active or retired streaks of a year or more. The organization is quite sophisticated, with a sixteen-person advisory board and extremely detailed record keeping as well as verification processes ("Show me your training log from 1978") and software to keep the streak counts automatically updated. The movement is compelling enough to warrant a 2022 article in the *New York Times* titled "The Rise of Daily Run Streakers. No, Not Those Streakers."

Six men have reached the milestone of running every single day for fifty years. Lois Bastien, eighty-seven years old in December of 2023, has the longest active female streak with forty-four years, a record she set in 2024. At the top of the rankings, with a fifty-four-year streak and counting (starting in 1969), is Jon Sutherland, seventy-three years old in May of 2019, a longtime Los Angeles–area runner whom I watched win local 10ks in the '70s and '80s. Forget the modest standard of having to shuffle at least one mile to officially keep your daily streak alive: Sutherland has run an average of ten miles every day for a half century—more than two hundred thousand miles! He has persevered through ten broken bones, including a broken back and pelvis, and a nasty bout with shingles that made his streak torturous for months.

The late Ron Hill of Great Britain—who shattered the world marathon record in 1970, then broke world records at ten miles, fifteen miles, and twenty-five kilometers, won the 1970 Boston Marathon, and ran 112 marathons under 2:50—set the previous streak standard of fifty-two years, from 1964 to 2017. His streak ended on January 30, 2017, when he reported that "after 400 meters my heart started to hurt and by the time I got to the one-mile point I thought I was going to die." Hill promptly had a stent implanted in a coronary artery. He survived four more years with an Alzheimer's diagnosis before passing away, in 2021.

There is a streaker in my South Beach neighborhood in Miami named Raven, a.k.a. Robert Kraft, who has run eight miles on the same out-and-back route on the packed sand starting at 5:30 p.m. every day for forty-eight years! Raven has accumulated some 144,000 miles on the sand and eight more during Hurricane Irma, in 2017, when he was forced to run 240 laps around his apartment to knock out his eight miles. The Raven is often joined by well-wishers on his daily jaunts and has become a beloved fixture of our beach community. When the beaches were closed to the public during the 2020 pandemic, he received special permission from city agencies to access the beach, and he ran 573 solitary miles over the course of seventy days.

I'm not here to denigrate the streak movement, because these runners have a tremendous sense of personal pride and deep camaraderie with fellow streakers (I'll try to write similar sentences until I make you laugh). A *Runners World* article about Jon Sutherland includes a video of an organized group run on the occasion of his streak's fiftieth anniversary. He was joined by many close friends and runners whom he coached, and he emphasized relationship building as the best part of his running journey. In a 2021 *Outside* magazine profile titled "The Minds and Habits of Master Streakers," several of the highest-ranked streakers made good arguments that theirs is a "healthy obsession." Sutherland explained, "I have a tremendous urge to run, to be moving. I think when I'm running. It's my church that I go to every day. When I get done I feel good about myself." In an ESPN.com article about him, he said, "That's kind of the inside joke among all the streakers—we tell each other how crazy we are, but we aren't. We're just people who have something we really enjoy and we do it."

Steve DeBoer, who at the time the article was published had the third-longest streak in the world, at fifty-two years, said, "Follow your passion (something positive, not necessarily running) and see how far it will take you, but don't let it take over your life." Sue Favor, third in the world among women with a thirty-nine-year streak at the time, said, "For me it's a bodily and emotion regulator. Running got me through depression, and a lot of other stuff." Steve Gathje said that the end of his streak of nearly forty-six years came after he battled extreme hip pain for a month before finally giving up: "Running used to make my life better, and now it was making it worse." About his streak, he explained, "It reduced stress, it was my own time. If I wasn't addicted to exercise, I'd be addicted to something harmful." Granted, having your daughter jog alongside you pushing your IV pole so you can get your run in right after an appendectomy (as Texan streaker Bill Anderson did) or shuffling along on a stress fracture for weeks of one-mile jaunts to maintain a streak (a common practice among streakers) is a more than a little goofy, but it seems the streakers at least have a clear understanding of both the benefits and the drawbacks of their extreme commitment to daily running. How could they not?

The stories of these streakers offer a good opportunity to reflect on the pros and cons of taking one's running passion to an extreme. I am certainly aware of the enormous payoff that awaits those of us who are brave enough to escape from the shackles of safe, comfortable, predictable modern life, explore the limits of physical and mental endurance, and feel that deep sense of elation, fulfillment, and satisfaction that comes from crossing the finish line. Clearly, once you unleash your adventurous spirit, there is a natural tendency to raise the bar and raise the stakes with each new experience. Imagine a new runner embarking on a life change and going out daily for a whole month, and then a year, and then three years—you can see the allure of becoming a streaker.

Few memories are more poignant to me than my first running success. As I worked through the quintessential teenage struggle to form an identity and find my place in the social hierarchy, knowing that I would never throw a winning touchdown pass or make a winning basket, I found breaking my first tape to be life-changing and life-affirming. Clearly, I was destined to come back for more and more—to the extent that I committed the brazen act a decade later of trading a medical-school track for a running track.

But the deeper and more extreme your passions, the more difficult the balancing act of life becomes. Psychotherapist Sepideh Saremi, of Redondo Beach, California, is the founder of the Run Walk Talk therapy technique. She conducts sessions with clients while walking or jogging down the beach. She describes herself as a type A personality and specializes in similarly high-achieving patients who are typically reluctant to seek help.

For those of us who are wired similarly, Saremi offers a few suggestions for successfully navigating passions that can drift into obsessions.

> I encourage anyone with a behavior that is taking over their life to take a breath and think about how that activity is a reflection of their values. Is running helping or hurting your relationship to your body? Is it causing you to feel closer to or more distant from important people in your life? Is it a source of pleasure or anxiety? People who become addicted to running typically feel extremely anxious, depressed, or distressed if they can't run due to illness, schedule, or other factors.

Obligatory Obligate Runner Stories

Jim Fixx (see page 104) is the poster boy for the obligate runner, thanks to the sordid details of his obsession—particularly his obstinate refusal, even when he was on Dr. Kenneth Cooper's doorstep, to be tested for the cardiovascular problems that must have been obvious to him at the time. If Fixx is the OG obligate runner, David Goggins is carrying the torch these days. Goggins is a former Navy SEAL, Army Ranger, and member of the Air Force Tactical Air Control Party. He is the only man to complete the rigorous training for all three and the only man to complete the notorious Navy SEAL BUD/S training course twice. He is an ultramarathoner, an ultradistance triathlete, the author of self-help books like *Can't Hurt Me* and *Never Finished*, and arguably most famous extreme endurance athlete on the planet. He was runner-up at the Ultraman World Championships, a three-day ultra-distance triathlon on the island of Hawaii that requires six miles of swimming, 190 miles of cycling, and fifty-two miles of running. He came in third at the infamous 135-mile Badwater Ultramarathon, for which runners in summertime Death Valley brave the globe's hottest temperatures to climb from below sea level to the finish line at the Mount Whitney trailhead, at 8,500 feet. He set a record running 204 miles in forty-eight hours. He's completed more than seventy ultramarathon runs, including fourteen hundred-milers and a five-hundred-mile ultramarathon bike race.

Goggins is widely admired for overcoming serious trauma, abuse, and racial discrimination in childhood and excelling in his wide-ranging military career. He ballooned to nearly three hundred pounds and got back to ripped on two separate occasions. He also uses his extreme athletic exploits to promote confidence, discipline, and empowerment and raise funds for the families of fallen soldiers. He commands six-figure speaking fees: his pearls of wisdom include "You are in danger of living a life so comfortable and soft that you will die without ever realizing your true potential" and "It's a lot more than mind over matter. It takes relentless self-discipline to schedule suffering into your day every day."

In his books and numerous podcast appearances, Goggins admits that he peeled the skin off the inside of his hands and contracted rhabdomyolysis while setting a world record of four thousand pull-ups in seventeen hours. He says that he entered his first hundred-mile race near his home in San Diego on extremely minimal training, having never completed a marathon and weighing 240 pounds at the time. He made it to mile 70 before collapsing in exhaustion. With his then fiancée attending to him in a lawn chair at the race site, he lost control of his bowels and bladder. But since you can't hurt him and he's never finished, he somehow willed himself to go thirty more miles to the finish line—logging an impressive time of just under nineteen hours to boot. The story continues with his being too weak to ascend a flight of stairs to his apartment. His fiancée had to drag him up the stairs and into the shower, where he again started "peeing Coca-Cola." Knowing that this was a sign of rhabdo and potentially fatal kidney failure, his nurse-fiancée begged him to go to the hospital. To this he replied, "Just let me enjoy this pain I'm in." Two weeks later, Goggins ran the Las Vegas Marathon in 3:08. A month after that, he ran another hundred-miler, landing in a wheelchair after the finish.

Over the course of two appearances on Joe Rogan's podcast in 2018, Goggins regaled the host with descriptions of these and other superhuman exploits and his "stay hard" philosophy. Potentially lost in the shuffle were Goggins's breezy mentions of the numerous stress fractures he continued to run on during military training and the regimen of replacement hormones he takes to cover for his torched adrenal, thyroid, and endocrine systems. "A lot of my injuries I just pushed through . . . I just duct tape it up . . . One way or another it's gonna heal, but it's not gonna heal right; it's gonna heal all jacked up and crooked. I'm a crooked, jacked-up dude, but I can still get it done."

I don't mean to throw shade on this incredibly energetic and likable bloke who's also the reigning king of inspirational, expertly placed f-bombs. But it's important to acknowledge that you don't need to abuse yourself to access a portal to personal growth. Goggins makes an effort to qualify his message accordingly: "I'm not saying be me and run 204 miles at one time. But start to learn how the mind is powerful." You might also want to filter out some of his nonscientific nuggets, such as his assertion that he only needs three to four hours of sleep a night because it's "high-quality sleep." Or his widely touted and occasionally memed 40 percent rule: "When your mind and body are starting to tire and you feel like giving up, you're only at 40 percent of what you are truly capable of achieving." Here I'll reference the 40 percent mark of my failed restaurant venture as an excellent time to give up!

Take what you need from his message to get your ass off the couch and get going. Take what you need from his aphorisms to keep going when you feel like giving up but are actually poised for a breakthrough performance. However, I'm going to counter here with a 70 percent rule: When you're 70 percent done with an extreme challenge and at your limit, stop before you compel your partner to clean up your mess.

Kathy Ormsby's story is a little more sobering than "stay hard" Goggins's. Ormsby was competing in the 1986 NCAA championship women's 10,000 meters at Indiana University as the reigning NCAA record holder in the event. With a couple of miles left in the race, she was in fourth place, running on the track down the back straightaway approaching the curve. Instead of turning with the pack, though, she continued straight. Without breaking stride, she ducked under a railing, ascended some stairs, and left the stadium. Few in the sparse crowd noticed besides her parents and coach. She then crossed a softball field, climbed a seven-foot fence, continued down a main thoroughfare, and jumped headfirst off a bridge over the White River. She fell thirty-five feet onto a marshy riverbank, an unsuccessful suicide attempt that left her a paraplegic.

Ormsby was a straight-A student, a model teammate and citizen. One teammate described her as a "perfectionist." "The whole team loved her," said her best friend and teammate, Patty Metzler. Ormsby has struggled to pinpoint what prompted her seemingly spontaneous act. A decade later, a newspaper interview related that Ormsby was "convinced that what happened resulted from the unhappy confluence of physical, mental, emotional, and spiritual factors with stress, pressure, heat, fatigue, delicate chemical balances altered by extremes of exertion, and a misguided sense of personal responsibility." Indeed, Ormsby experienced panic attacks in her three previous races so severe that they caused her lose consciousness. As she said about the incident, "It was like something snapped . . . It's like I was out of control . . . Why, I don't know . . . I'll always wonder a little, but now I'm at peace with it. I don't want to analyze it anymore." Shortly after the accident, the deeply religious Ormsby speculated that it was part of God's plan. Her father shared a similar sentiment but offered, "I believe, though, that it had something to do with the pressure that is put on young people to succeed."

Metzler reflects, "Competing at that level is so intense and difficult. You push yourself to great extremes and you want to maintain that, and when you don't, you become your own worst enemy. The body and the mind have to work together to make a good athlete, and when there's a break anywhere, you can have problems . . . [Ormsby] talked about being scared because she had run so well at Penn Relays and then everybody expected her to win nationals. She was under a lot of pressure." In a *Los Angeles Times* feature story about the incident, Ormsby's teammate Connie Jo Robinson described the sentiments that she fielded from Ormsby's comrades from other schools: "No one asked why. No one. They just said, 'We're praying for her,' and gave us cards. They didn't need to know why. They know why. We're all in the same boat. We feel the same pressure."

Sadly, Ormsby's incident was not unprecedented. In 1982, Mary Wazeter, a national-caliber distance runner at Georgetown University who had been hospitalized for anorexia and had attempted suicide several times, jumped off a railroad bridge near her home of Wilkes-Barre, Pennsylvania, and became a paraplegic. Now known as Mary Mannhardt, an author (*Dark Marathon* and *Client to Clinician*), speaker, and licensed professional counselor, she specializes in women's issues, including depression, eating disorders, codependency, stress management, obsessive-compulsive disorder, and bipolar disorder.

Detoxing from the Runner's High

When you brazenly chase the runner's high on the regular, you are bound to pay a severe price in the form of what we might call the runner's crash. This is the exhaustion of your fight-or-flight mechanisms: you start to produce lower-than-baseline levels of important hormones such as cortisol, dopamine, and catecholamine. You also produce less adrenaline and noradrenaline, which you need to support everyday alertness, energy, and metabolic and cognitive function.

Consequently, you develop dysregulated immune function, appetite, mood, energy levels, sleep cycles, and stress management. You exist in a state of endorphin deficiency—characterized by persistent aches and pains, sleep difficulties, mood swings, and depression—and can develop chronic system-wide inflammation. This is the condition that drives the stubborn visceral fat I discussed in chapter 2, the chronic overuse injuries I discussed in chapter 3, and the acute and long-term cardiovascular, immune, digestive, and endocrine problems I discussed in chapter 4.

Liquidating your assets in pursuit of the runner's high leaves you with insufficient resources for effective cell reproduction, repair, and growth. Your heart gets bigger and stronger, but it also can develop the scarring and compromised electrical signaling that causes arrhythmias. The microtraumas in your lower extremities develop into Achilles tendinitis, plantar fasciitis, shin splints, or chondromalacia, a.k.a. runner's knee. Routine exposure to viruses and pathogens can overwhelm your exhausted immune system and leave you vulnerable to colds and the flu.

Liquidating your assets in pursuit of the runner's high leaves you with insufficient resources for effective cell reproduction, repair, and growth.

None of that sounds like fun, but we must all acknowledge how difficult it is to resist the powerful pull of instant gratification in favor of a sensible long-term approach to fitness, health, and life in general. The problem is worse than ever today, since the inexorable technological progress of modern life makes it easy to indulge in all manner of instant gratifications, anytime, to destructive excess. In Dr. Robert Lustig's 2017 book, *The Hacking of the American Mind*, he makes a compelling case that profit-seeking corporate entities are strongly to blame for turning us all into dopamine addicts. Perhaps the most prominent and novel example in recent years is the addictive allure of mobile technology and social media, which are hijacking our collective attention spans. In other books, including *Fat Chance* and *Metabolical*, Dr. Lustig asserts that sugary sweets and treats and processed foods do this, too. He also contends that our minds are hacked by cigarettes and vaping, caffeine, marijuana and other recreational drugs, antidepressants and prescription painkillers, gambling, video games, pornography, sex, shopping, and, yes, chronic exercise.

Dr. Lustig explains that when we routinely and excessively flood the dopamine pathways with quick-hit, easily accessible pleasures, we block the receptors for serotonin and oxytocin. These neurotransmitters are associated with happiness, contentment, fulfillment, a sense of purpose, bonding with others, and other high-minded stuff. We experience a rich and meaningful life when we persevere through long-term challenges that have deep meaning to us, achieve the highest expression of our talents, and contribute to society. We don't have to be constantly rewarded, praised, recognized, or entertained in order to light up our serotonin pathways.

Serotonin can be generated by toiling over a book manuscript, taking a leisurely walk on the beach and marveling at pelican dives or sand crab digs, or shopping at the farmers market and preparing a home-cooked meal—in stark contrast to the dopamine hit one gets from greasy takeout delivered by DoorDash. As Dr. Lustig says, "There is nothing that will improve your health, your well-being, your achievement, your sense of accomplishment, your sense of community, and the health and happiness of your family as much as cooking yourself and enjoying a meal with others." Serotonin gives us a feeling that we have accomplished enough, possess enough, and can relax and appreciate the everyday, non-glitzy activities of life. These include caring for an infant, punching the clock every day at the factory as a valued member of the operation, or enjoying a walk or jog without timing it, judging it, or pushing yourself into a zone of discomfort.

Nurturing a harmonious balance in brain neurochemicals enables us to work hard, appreciate and celebrate our successes, have lots of fun while keeping our priorities straight, and prioritize interpersonal relationships and core life responsibilities over consumerism, instant gratification, and getting stuck on the so-called hedonic treadmill, on which one nourishes an incessant desire to achieve and consume. Instead of experiencing contentment, our hacked minds suffer from addiction, anxiety, depression, and chronic disease, thanks to the health-destructive long-term consequences of these instant-gratification vices. Dr. Lustig puts it even more bluntly: "The more pleasure we seek, the less happy we get. Wall Street, Madison Avenue, Las Vegas, Silicon Valley, and Washington DC have conflated pleasure with happiness so that we don't know the difference. In the process society has become fat, sick, stupid, and broke."

Understand that dopamine is not inherently bad: it's the chronic flooding of dopamine receptors at the expense of the serotonin and oxytocin pathways that's the problem. Also, dopamine is technically not the reward or instant-gratification neurotransmitter that it's often said to be. Dopamine is more accurately categorized as a motivation neurotransmitter, because it forms an imprint in the brain that compels us to repeatedly engage in behaviors that result in success, survival, and, yes, pleasure. Serotonin leaves us content and not wanting more; dopamine drives us to seek more. Hence mental, physical, and emotional well-being depend upon a healthy balance between the four major brain neurotransmitters:

- GABA (gamma-aminobutyric acid), an inhibitory neurotransmitter, which has a calming effect;
- acetylcholine, an excitatory neurotransmitter, associated with arousal, focus, learning, and memory;
- serotonin, an inhibitory neurotransmitter, which regulates emotions, mood, appetite, pain, sexuality, and sleep; and
- dopamine, which is both excitatory and inhibitory depending on the neurons it's targeting.

Obviously, sex delivers a huge dopamine hit, which ensures that we propagate the species. When our ancestors discovered a beehive or took down a beast on a persistence hunt, they experienced surges of dopamine that wired in these rewarding behaviors so they would be repeated. Unfortunately, unlike our ancestors, who strove mightily to light up their dopamine pathways, dopamine flooding happens too easily and frequently today. Dr. John Gray, author of the *Men Are from Mars, Women Are from Venus* franchise and often regarded as the number one bestselling relationship author of all time, argues that the ominous combination of video games and pornography is particularly devastating to young men. These two vices satisfy men's most prominent testosterone-fueled biological drives: acquiring a mate and conquering the competitive environment. Consequently, with reliable dopamine flooding available at the click of a button, one can do whatever one wants in Grandma's basement without any motivation to tackle the real-world challenges of relationships and careers.

Thanks to incredibly clever, often sinister, profit-seeking corporate forces, we have become addicts, according to the clinical definition. We erode our potential for happiness and contentment by flooding our dopamine pathways and blocking our serotonin and oxytocin pathways. Consequently, we develop a dependence on our vices of choice—not for the pleasurable high we enjoyed at first but just to feel normal. One example is the obligate runner heading out for a run every day despite a worsening case of shin splints. Another is the video-game and porn addict wasting his nights away in the basement at the expense of his career and relationship potential. Yet another is the person who absentmindedly scrolls through social media when she's bored and depressed, making her even more bored and depressed.

Serotonin leaves us content and not wanting more; dopamine drives us to seek more.

The healthful way to optimize brain neurotransmitters and enjoy both an exciting and fulfilling life is to persevere through difficulty to reach the highest expression of your talents—pursuing your calling and making a contribution to society. Persevering through difficulty and even setbacks makes all the difference, because working for success delivers a *sustained* elevation of dopamine, followed by a graceful return to baseline. By contrast, instant-gratification dopamine hacks prompt a spike, followed by a crash and withdrawal symptoms. Furthermore, healthful dopamine-boosting behaviors do not flood the dopamine receptors: they allow for a sustained release of other mood-balancing chemicals such as serotonin, oxytocin, and vasopressin without a corresponding crash.

When Roger Bannister caught his breath at the finish line and heard the public address announcer declare his winning time of "three minutes . . ." (the rest was famously drowned out by the crowd), you can bet he was flooded with dopamine, serotonin, and oxytocin that remained there long into a celebratory evening. If you have the patience, restraint, and long-term commitment required to develop an aerobic base, you will get fitter, faster, and more resistant to injury and burnout. You'll still enjoy plenty of instant-gratification highs from peak performance as well as long-term contentment from doing things right and achieving the highest expression of your talents.

Cultivating an Enjoyable Approach to Fitness

If any of the ominous commentary in this chapter hits home, consider implementing some strategies to transition from unhealthful obsession into harmonious passion. The legendary middle-distance runner Sebastian Coe—who set twelve world records, won unprecedented back-to-back Olympic gold medals in the 1,500 meters (1980 and 1984), went on to serve in the British Parliament and chair the 2012 London Olympic organizing committee, and is currently serving his third term as the popular president of World Athletics, the global track-and-field governing body—captured the essence of being super competitive while maintaining a healthy perspective: "Competing is exciting and winning is exhilarating, but the true prize will always be the self-knowledge and understanding that you have gained along the way." Pair this with Roger Bannister's message that "the essence of sports is that while you're doing it, nothing else matters, but after you stop, there is a place, generally not very important, where you would put it," and you have an ideal athletic disposition.

I also favor advice from Ashley Merryman, coauthor with Po Bronson of *Top Dog: The Science of Winning and Losing*. She contends that that our competitive focus should be on making an effort toward improvement. Merryman makes a sharp distinction between this ideal and merely expending effort, explaining that the latter simply isn't good enough. It snares many devoted endurance athletes who doggedly accumulate the maximum possible weekly mileage on the disastrously flawed assumption that mere miles translates into competitive success. Banging your head against the wall with an ill-advised, ineffective strategy is not going to support health, nor will it bring satisfaction or happiness. If you're gonna lace 'em up and spend a tremendous amount of time and energy on your harmonious passion, following are some tips for doing it the right way.

Get Over Yourself

Regardless of how accomplished you are, people don't care about your performance as much as you think they do. Even athletes who win Olympic gold medals and set world records are eventually relegated to retirement, replaced by new stars, and forced to reckon with a less exciting life. It's hard to put on blinders and ignore the powerful pull of social comparison and external accolades, but it's essential to your happiness and well-being, athletic and otherwise.

Morgan Housel, author of *The Psychology of Money*, notes that our consumer purchases are strongly influenced by a deep-seated desire to signal wealth, but the observers we signal to don't care in the manner that we perceive them to. Instead, Housel suggests that "people often bypass admiring you, not because they don't think wealth is admirable, but because they use your wealth as a benchmark for their own desire to be liked and admired . . . People look at the Ferrari, and don't pay attention to who's driving the Ferrari . . . Spending money to show people how much money you have is the fastest way to have less money."

Mark Manson, author of the 2016 runaway bestseller *The Subtle Art of Not Giving a F*ck*, proposes that "self-worth is an illusion, and actually a form of persistent low level narcissism." Instead, he suggests that true freedom and well-being can be had by "seeing your life as a series of decisions and actions, and trying to maintain an identity defined by as little as possible." This advice is particularly meaningful for a fitness enthusiast. Every day, you can wake up and decide to recommit to a fitness lifestyle, to your planned workout, and to your specific performance goals—yes, it's okay to set goals and celebrate success. But resolve to stop short of wrapping your identity and your self-worth around being a runner, especially a runner of a certain pedigree. Instead, resolve to focus your efforts on improvement. This will bring personal growth, satisfaction, and meaning to your life. In Japanese sporting culture, there exists an ideal called *doryoku*, translated as "honor in the effort." This suggests that sports is not about just winning or getting to the finish line by any means necessary. It's about pursuing your goals in an honorable manner every step of the way.

Sports is not about just winning or getting to the finish line by any means necessary. It's about pursuing your goals in an honorable manner every step of the way.

Put Endorphins in Perspective

Endorphins—literally, endogenous morphine—are a group of peptides that act on the opiate receptors in your brain. They are classified as both neurotransmitters and hormones because they deliver pain-killing effects to the brain and body that are eighteen to thirty-three times more potent than pharmaceutical morphine. Endorphins are part of our evolution-honed survival mechanisms and are released into the bloodstream in response to extreme exercise. The harder and longer your push yourself, the bigger the endorphin rush.

Although florid articles on fitness websites may refer to endorphins as "reward chemicals," their main evolutionarily honed purpose is actually to ensure that your death is as peaceful as possible—or to keep you going when you're starving and exhausted but still need to chase prey in hopes of surviving. When you're about to succumb to a predator, endorphins flood your bloodstream to mercifully allow you go out on a blissful note instead of a terrifying note. Endorphins are what the zebra secretes as it lies down and accepts its fate after fighting the good fight against the lion. It's certainly acceptable to enjoy an occasional endorphin high from your extreme exercise efforts, but it's important to acknowledge the drawbacks of pursuing them to addictive excess.

I can trace the end of my elite running career to a single week in 1980, when I ran a hard twenty-miler each day for five consecutive days. Running just slower than a six-minute pace, I was deep in the groove and felt euphoric, not exhausted, at the end of each run. Physiologically, my bloodstream was becoming bathed in ever-increasing levels of endorphins as the week progressed. In an evolutionary sense, I was running myself to death—not literally and not because I was running from a predator but because my racing career was dying of unregulated competitive intensity. Wouldn't you know it, the wheels quickly came off after the hundred-mile binge when I aggravated a chronically inflamed hip injury. I never trained at the same level again, Realizing I was broken as a runner, I turned to triathlon as a means of extending my endorphin addiction another few years. When the smoke cleared, the hip took twenty-five years to fully heal from mild chronic pain and inflammation. A couple of decades later, it's now reaching its expiration date. When I share this story with other hard-core long-term endurance athletes, they shake their heads in understanding, not surprise.

Balance Your Inner Goggins with Your Inner Bannister

Dr. Art De Vany, a mentor of mine in the ancestral health movement, author of *The New Evolution Diet*, and an extremely fit specimen well into his eighties, said, "Modern life leaves our minds restless and underutilized because we are confined, inactive, and comfortable." Point taken. I urge you to get out there and challenge your body to get fitter, stronger, faster, and more active overall. Each time you complete a challenge outside your comfort zone, you have by definition expanded that comfort zone. In doing so, you become more resistant to all manner of stress, anxiety, tension, uncertainty, and conflict. However, don't get caught up in the endurance community's glorification of inappropriate and inglorious suffering. This disgraces the beautiful message from Roger Bannister and misappropriates the most astute takeaways from David Goggins: push yourself beyond the confines of your self-limiting beliefs for a personal growth experience—without, ideally, needing any duct tape.

Your fitness pursuits can indeed be the ultimate vehicle for personal growth. However, with an ill-advised, indiscriminate, addictive, self-flagellating approach, they can instead give voice and purchase to the dark side of your personality. The key is to align your behavior with your values and beliefs. In a 2015 *New York Times* article called "The Moral Bucket List," journalist David Brooks wrote that people "on the road to inner light" have lives that "often follow a pattern of defeat, recognition, redemption. They have moments of pain and suffering. But they turn those moments into occasions of radical self-understanding."

Develop an Effective Fitness Strategy

Whether you have no particular competitive goals or are at the other end of the spectrum and have a list of markers you want to hit, it's important to implement a thoughtful, custom-designed strategy in order to avoid overtraining and burnout. Have you developed a comprehensive fitness plan through consultation with experts and/or trial and error? Does your training fit conveniently into your daily life so that you are not shortchanging your other key responsibilities? Ashley Merryman urges us to "focus on process and progress, not results and rewards," and to regularly look at our performance and ask ourselves, "Is this working or not working?"

As the original obligate runner–anorexia analogue research from Dr. Yates at the University of Arizona suggests, it's likely that many in the fitness community tend to look around at their inactive, unfit, and overfat fellow citizens with a smug sense of superiority. As if burning tons of calories and collecting lots of medals is enough—"Look how much fitter I am than today's average person!" This perspective might be preventing you from honest self-examination and inhibiting your personal growth. Regardless of your finishing times, and regardless of whether you're the fastest person in your neighborhood, aspire to do things right: be prepared, be sensible, and come up with a well-formulated plan that's still flexible and allows you to make changes on the fly when necessary.

Focus on process and progress,
not results and rewards.

For example, if you're going out for an adventurous, all-day hike in the mountains, spend some time studying a map. Choose appropriate attire and prepare for unforeseen challenges by packing emergency gear and establishing communication backup plans. Stories of outdoor adventures gone bad play well on social media and at social gatherings, but I'd like you to put them in the same dunce-cap category as stress fractures. If your endeavor is a simple five-mile morning jog, spend a few minutes doing warm-up mobility and flexibility drills.

Warm up and cool down methodically and monitor your heart rate so you achieve the intended benefits of the workout. If you feel those annoying shin splints flare up early into the run, slow to a walk, turn around, and head home. *Doryoku*!

Set Realistic, Sensible Goals

First, let's talk about how far and how often you think you need to run to experience personal growth and self-satisfaction. Do you really have to train for and complete a 26.2-mile event to feel whole? Can you acknowledge the profound influence that marketing hype has on your psyche? Can you understand that you've been socialized by your fellow runners, running-industry marketing dollars, Hollywood movies, and the commercial glitz of the Olympics to worship the marathon as the ultimate accomplishment in long-distance running? Remember Morgan Housel's observation that "people often bypass admiring you" and Mark Manson's suggestion to "try to maintain an identity defined by as little as possible."

Craig Virgin is one the greatest American long-distance runners ever, a two-time winner of the World Athletics Cross-Country Championships in 1980 and 1981. He's the only American ever to win this prestigious event, which purists contend is harder to win than an Olympic gold in any single track and field event because all the world's top distance runners toe the line over the twelve-kilometer course. Virgin, a 2:10 marathoner (and Boston runner-up in 1981), has some choice comments about the marathon distance being the preeminent goal in the running community:

> If you want to slog through a marathon to say you did it once, fine. But there are two forms of satisfaction in running. Number one is going a distance you've never gone before. The next logical goal should be "How much faster can I get?" . . . Just running the distance, hammering your legs four or five or six hours—if that's your first marathon, that's okay, but if it's your third or fourth that's just stupid.

Virgin is especially critical of charity running programs: "They're just getting people fit enough to do the Bataan Death March."

Truly Recover Mind and Body

Recovery doesn't just mean running fewer miles at a lower heart rate. It's essential to give your mind a break from nonstop rumination about the current state of your fitness, the quality of your recent workouts, and your future competitive prospects. When you take a break to focus on recovery, make it a complete mind-body disengagement. Make a deliberate effort to not think or talk about your fitness endeavors. Don't weigh yourself on that cruise vacation. Leave your GPS watch and heart-rate monitor at home when you head out for a casual hike with relatives. Take a break from running-related social media. Make a deliberate effort to work on your hobbies, spend time with friends, and enjoy experiences that get you away from sitting around and musing about running. Do what people who have high-drama jobs, including first responders, do: make your home a sanctuary, away from the intense (albeit positive and exciting) energy you experience as soon as you meet the running group at the trailhead.

Indulge in Self-Care

Get regular sports massages, try out some temperature therapy such as sauna or cold plunging, and try some advanced healing techniques such as photobiomodulation (red-light therapy) and leg-compression boots. Seek out self-care and graciously accept some pampering to balance all that hard work.

Nourish Yourself

Resolve to eat nutrient-dense, easy-to-digest foods and quit the silly game of burning calories on the road in order to "get away with" chowing down on junk food. Yes, you can handle the extra calories better than an inactive person can, but is getting away with stuff an honorable way to approach your health and fitness goals—let alone life in general? Remember, if you have even a bit of visceral fat, you are not getting away with anything. Instead, understand that your requirement for nutritious food vastly exceeds that of a sedentary person because you demand so much more from your body. Of course, you deserve a treat now and then, but be highly selective when you indulge. Make a sincere commitment to fueling your body with the best nutrition you can find.

Serve Others

A surefire way to emerge from the clutches of an unhealthful obsession is to serve others. If you're injured and feeling sorry for yourself because you're going to miss your planned race, how about contacting the organizer and offering to volunteer at a water station on race day? There you can experience camaraderie with your fellow runners from a fresh new perspective.

Seek Support

Too often even close-knit training groups can cook up negative competitive energy instead of exhibiting true togetherness and offering moral support to one another. This is especially the case now that social-media comparison culture is in full bloom. Build a support team of trusted confidantes—both in your running world and outside of it—and be open and receptive to their feedback and guidance.

If you believe you meet the criteria for an eating disorder or an addiction to running, please seek professional help. Quick litmus test: Do you feel guilty, anxious, or emotionally unstable when you don't run? Does running bring less joy than it did before? Has it become more of a "must do" than a mood booster?

Unfortunately, treating running addiction is not among the highest of society's priorities. In fact, there is extensive research and support for using running to treat drug addiction. Dr. Wendy Lynch, psychiatry professor at the University of Virginia School of Medicine and an expert on the neurobiological basis of addiction, said, "In the early stages of addiction, where dopamine is primarily motivating the drug use, exercise also activates dopamine release . . . [Running] could serve as an alternative to the drug reward and thereby prevent future drug use… We've shown that even modest amounts of exercise can reverse relapse vulnerability."

Trading a major addiction for a less destructive addiction is quite common and certainly represents progress. Alas, if your struggles pertain specifically to an unhealthful obsession with running, you might feel alone, unsupported, and misunderstood. After all, the drama and destruction generated by other addictions is much higher on the societal triage chart. What's more, with most of society struggling to be sufficiently active, those with the inclination to overexercise will not elicit much empathy. No matter: seek out the support you need, which is easier than ever with the internet as a resource.

Diversify Your Goals

Consider pursuing alternative forms of exercise that can help you cross over from unhealthful obsession to harmonious passion. This may not specifically address the root cause of your running addiction, but it can be a step in the right direction, just as when an addict pivots away from substance abuse and gets his dopamine hits from running. Many runners have made successful transitions into triathlon, where they can better balance the musculoskeletal load, become engrossed in the challenge of learning new technical skills and workout protocols, experience new training environments (especially with cycling), enjoy a more diverse training schedule, get decked out in new equipment and apparel, and generally extricate themselves from a situation in which running in a straight line is their sole athletic outlet. You can also experience a sense of freedom and relief by integrating walking into your training program. In part 2 of this book, you'll learn in detail how to embrace walking as an outstanding way to boost aerobic conditioning—and thus racing performance at all distances—without the risk of injury, burnout, and addiction that come from an unhealthful obsession with running.

PART II

EMBRACING THE *BORN TO WALK* LIFESTYLE

CHAPTER 6
Slowing Down and Building an Aerobic Base

Whew! That was a bit of a rough journey through the marketing hype, broken promises, and unintended consequences of the running boom. Thanks for hanging in there.

But before I regale you with tales of the amazing and wide-ranging benefits of a walking-inspired lifestyle and slowing down your cardio to an appropriate fat-burning pace, I want to acknowledge that slowing down is a tough commitment to make. After all, we don't get much encouragement, social media likes, or awards for doing so. Instead, we've been culturally conditioned to struggle, suffer, keep pushing, never give up, and so forth. These traits signal that you are tough, confident, resilient, fearless, and adventurous. They're wonderful traits, to be sure, especially if you're living an inactive, soft, predictable, and comfortable life that withers away both body and spirit. However, if you want to pursue daunting physical challenges, it's important to learn to do so the right way. Otherwise, you are completely missing the point. When one is addicted to suffering, fitness pursuits are no longer about health, balance, happiness, and peak performance. Instead, they become yet another outlet for obsessive-compulsive urges and other obligate runner personality traits.

If you love to pursue competitive running goals and have made training and racing a big part of your social life, I promise you can still go for it—I just want you to have a clear understanding of endurance physiology, be smart with your training—which might mean walking for part or most of your total mileage—and focus on foot functionality and correct running technique. You can keep wearing your favorite cushioned running shoes, but you should make a concerted effort to carefully transition to a barefoot-inspired lifestyle outside of workouts.

Since you've learned about the impact trauma and compromised form caused by heel-striking in cushioned shoes, I want you to start running with a well-crafted midfoot strike. A graceful midfoot strike with a slight forward lean of the torso might be a challenge if your sedentary routines and shuffling stride have deconditioned your hip flexors, glutes, and abdominals. But I'm going to assume that you exercise in order to improve your health and fitness *over time*. By the same token, I will assume that you are not training to inflict torture on your mind and body, suffer repeated overuse injuries, and carry excess visceral fat.

Slowing down is going to require bravely navigating past rigid beliefs and behavior patterns that you've developed through exposure to flawed science, marketing hype, and peer pressure.

Slowing down is going to require bravely navigating past rigid beliefs and behavior patterns that you've developed through exposure to flawed science, marketing hype, and peer pressure. I encourage you to open your mind to a new perspective, one that will allow you to steadily build your fitness without the risks and setbacks caused by overdoing it. Don't worry: I'm not asking you to suppress your competitive nature and join the nearest bird-watchers club. I'm saying that by slowing down and building an aerobic conditioning base, you can protect your health and achieve your fitness goals with less pain, struggle, and sacrifice than you thought possible.

Having an aerobic conditioning base means that you are efficient at burning fat during comfortably paced exercise. Because even the leanest among us can manufacture energy from their abundant fat stores, you can perform an assortment of athletic maneuvers for a sustained period of time without becoming exhausted. This includes steady-state cardio, of course, as well as CrossFit classes, soccer and basketball games, tennis matches, strength-training workouts, and any sort of sustained effort of more than a couple of minutes. Without an aerobic conditioning base, you become gassed sooner rather than later.

When a player desperately raises her hand to be subbed out of an adult league basketball game, and when an unfit traveler is hustling through an airport terminal and has to slow to a walk or stop to catch his breath, those people have exhausted their aerobic capacities. They are in oxygen debt—i.e., out of breath—and can no longer burn fat efficiently. Hence they are forced to transition to an anaerobic metabolism and rely on glucose, a quick-burning but scarce energy source.

Remember, the term "aerobic" means "with oxygen," and the term "anaerobic" means "without oxygen." The burning of fatty acids requires oxygen, while glucose can be burned without oxygen. Doing a circuit of weight machines at the gym and playing a tennis match are still cardio workouts because they place high demand on the cardiovascular system during both the aerobic endurance and anaerobic explosive efforts that happen during such activities. The aerobic system helps fatigued muscles and energy systems recover from bursts of anaerobic activity that happen during intense points in a tennis match or when your muscles are under load during a set of chest presses or lat pull-downs. Even when you're walking around the court collecting errant tennis balls, resting between sets at the gym, or catching your breath after a whistle on the court or field, you are still getting an aerobic workout because your heart rate is still probably double its resting rate.

When you get out of breath during sustained exercise, this is an indication that you have exceeded fat max heart rate and are now burning glucose. It sucks to miss a flight because you can't make it to the gate in time, but if you can't so much as climb a flight of stairs or walk to the mailbox without getting winded, your future survival prospects are dismal. This is why the Cooper Institute, Dr. Attia, and other fitness-minded experts place such an emphasis on aerobic activity and increasing VO2 max value (see page 176) for general health, vitality, disease prevention, and longevity.

The Fat-Burning Foundation

Here's the thing I desperately want you to completely understand, fully appreciate, and never forget: you can't reach your endurance potential without an outstanding aerobic conditioning base, and you build an aerobic conditioning base by exercising at a comfortable pace, one at which you primarily burn fatty acids for fuel. That's right: you have to slow down to get faster at all racing speeds, whether you're racing 800 meters or running a marathon or ultramarathon.

You can't reach your endurance potential without an outstanding aerobic conditioning base, and you build an aerobic conditioning base by exercising at a comfortable pace, one at which you primarily burn fatty acids for fuel.

"But Mark," you say. "That means I'll be burning fewer calories during my endurance walking than during my grinding endurance runs." Yep. It's time to reject once and for all the idea that you need to count calories in order to lose fat and become fit. It has been proved again and again by both research and practical experience that reducing calorie intake in order to lose fat is a flawed, ineffective strategy and that hormone optimization is the key to fat reduction. You have to slow down to get fitter, leaner, and faster because your aerobic base is the launching point from which you perform all high-intensity efforts and because aerobic exercise makes you a better fat burner at rest.

Interestingly, your base is what predicts your ultimate competitive potential. Did you know that the pedestal structure built to support the Statue of Liberty is taller, at 154 feet, than Miss Liberty herself, who is only 151 feet tall? Such a pedestal was necessary to support the 220-ton statue and to make it visible and prominent in the New York City skyline. I know the idea that slowing down to go faster conflicts with billions of dollars of marketing hype and Hollywood storylines declaring that you must struggle and suffer to go for the gold, but it's an unassailable fact of exercise physiology that a robust aerobic system is a prerequisite for a robust anaerobic system. Your aerobic-energy-producing enzymes and muscle fibers are intertwined with your fast-twitch muscle fibers (see page 152) and glycolytic enzymes, and the former supply the latter with the nutrients, blood, and oxygen they need to contract forcefully for short periods of time. Afterward, the aerobic-energy-producing enzymes replenish the energy and facilitate the removal of waste products from the muscles.

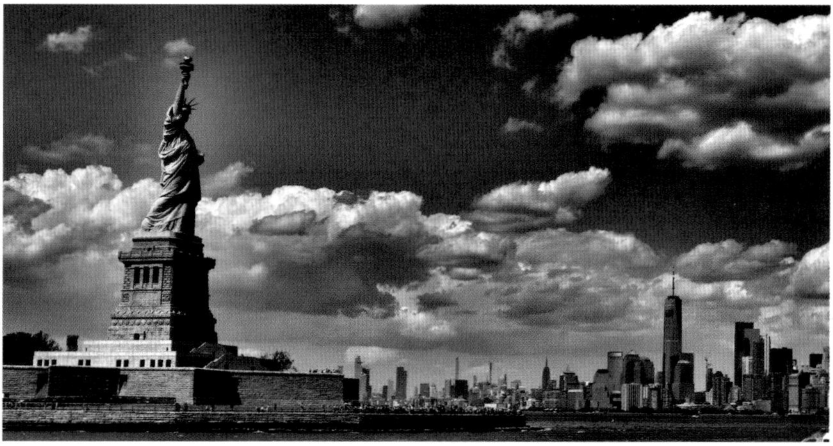

Building a base is important for everyone, even Miss Liberty.

It's also important to understand what really constitutes speed, i.e., anaerobic efforts, and what constitutes endurance, i.e., aerobic efforts, because the endurance lexicon is highly misleading. The term "speedwork" is routinely used inappropriately to describe any effort that's shorter and faster than a typical training session or one's preferred race distance. In fact, all sustained bouts of exercise lasting longer than just a few minutes are accurately characterized as aerobic endurance efforts and are predominantly aerobic to a surprising degree.

Research published by Dr. Paul Gastin when he was a senior lecturer at the Deakin University School of Exercise and Nutrition Sciences, in Australia, reveals that a ten-second sprint is 94 percent anaerobic; a one-minute and fifteen-second maximum effort is 50 percent aerobic and 50 percent anaerobic; and a maximum effort of six minutes is 79 percent aerobic and 21 percent anaerobic. An all-out effort lasting one hour—yes, even a Tour de France time trial with racers flying along at better than thirty miles an hour—is 98 percent aerobic! True endurance events lasting for several hours, such as marathons, ultramarathons, and long-distance triathlons and cycling events, are entirely aerobic—except for a possible sprint to the finish line for the cameras. These insights should be sufficient to spur corrections in the endurance world, where "sprint" triathlons last for an hour, marathoners enter 5k races to work on their "speed," and an "anaerobic session" often entails conducting numerous work intervals lasting two, three, or five minutes. Granted, you're going hard, but even a 5k is an endurance endeavor accomplished mainly by the aerobic system.

During very low-intensity exercise, such as leisurely walking, most of your energy (around 85 percent, in most cases) comes from free fatty acids circulating in the bloodstream. The remaining 15 percent comes from aerobic carbohydrate metabolism. Yes, carbs can be burned by both the aerobic and the anaerobic systems. As intensity drifts upward to near fat max heart rate, the body starts to mobilize fatty acids from triglycerides stored in muscle and adipose tissue. At around fat max, the contribution from fatty acids stored in muscle and tissue and fatty acids in the bloodstream is about even, and fat is burned at the highest possible rate per minute (i.e., fat max). At that point, fatty acids contribute around half of your caloric energy, and aerobic carbohydrate metabolism contributes the other half.

There can be significant variation in these ratios based on one's fitness level and aerobic competency. Hence descriptors such as "fat-burning workout" and "fat-burning zone" merely describe a relatively higher rate of fat oxidation compared to higher-intensity workouts, not a workout that is burning only fat. When you speed up beyond fat max, your rate of adenosine triphosphate, or ATP, utilization is too fast for the efficient and plentiful fat-burning system to keep up with demand, and you are forced to rely increasingly on aerobic carbohydrate metabolism and, with further increases in speed and effort, increasingly on anaerobic carbohydrate metabolism.

The relative contribution of the various energy systems is based on how much energy you need and for how long. This concept is the essence of elite sporting performance. When we watch the athletes racing around the track at the Olympic Games, they are desperately maxing out the capabilities of each energy system in succession, then tapping into a more sustainable energy system and maxing that out, all the while trying not to slow down. I'll explain this important concept in further detail in chapter 9.

AEROBIC SLOW-TWITCH MUSCLE FIBERS VERSUS ANAEROBIC FAST-TWITCH MUSCLE FIBERS

The aerobic system relies on slow-twitch muscle fibers, known as type 1, or red, fibers. They are rich in myoglobin for maximum blood and oxygen delivery, giving them a dark color. Aerobic metabolism requires a constant supply of oxygen in order for mitochondria to synthesize adenosine triphosphate (ATP)—the source of cellular energy in the body—slowly and steadily during comfortably paced endurance exercise. Aerobic respiration produces thirty-eight ATP molecules, using fatty acids as the fuel source.

By contrast, the anaerobic system synthesizes ATP very quickly during shorter-duration efforts requiring more immediate energy—such as a 100-meter all-out sprint—but it fatigues very quickly, too. Anaerobic respiration relies upon fast-twitch muscle fibers, known as type 2, or white, fibers and produces only two ATP molecules.

Type 2 fast-twitch fibers are pale in color because they have less myoglobin, less blood and oxygen, and lower mitochondrial density than type 1 fibers. These white fibers are the white meat of your body. Type 1 slow-twitch fibers are red in color because they are rich in myoglobin. These fibers are the dark meat of your body. If the two types were represented in campfires, aerobic respiration would be a bunch of big logs painstakingly nurtured to glow with warmth for hours. The anaerobic system would be twigs and wadded-up newspaper generating an instant but short-lived flare-up.

Type 2 fibers are classified as either type 2a, oxidative fast-twitch, or type 2b, glycolytic fast-twitch. Type 2a fibers can fire with or without oxygen and are recruited when exercise intensity switches from low to moderate and high. Type 2b, also known as type 2x, fibers are reserved for maximum power efforts. They don't use oxygen, and they fatigue extremely quickly. While one's ratio of slow-twitch to fast-twitch muscle fibers is largely genetic, type 2a fibers can become more endurance-adapted or more power-adapted based on training stimulus.

Running a marathon is predominantly a type 1, slow-twitch endeavor, but the grueling nature of the event eventually causes all types of fibers to be called into action. Type 2 fibers are more easily fatigued and glycogen-depleted and are more susceptible to damage from eccentric contractions caused by ground impact, especially downhill running. The symptoms of hitting the proverbial wall during a marathon, such as sharp muscle pain and heaviness—which often occur around mile 20—are driven by the exhaustion and depletion of type 2 fibers. These fibers had to be ushered into service in the first place because type 1 fibers were getting tired, especially if aerobic competency is inferior.

This is why you can see many if not most three-, four-, and five-hour marathon finishers shuffling through the finish chute and looking for cots to collapse into—and why you can see Ruth Chepngetich finishing the Chicago Marathon in world-record time, then immediately running back onto the course to high-five well-wishers lined along the route. Elite runners with an outstanding aerobic base can run fast and still be burning fat and using the slow-twitch fibers ideal for marathon running. If they need to sprint to the finish (as did Sifan Hassan en route to gold at the 2024 Paris Olympics marathon), their type 2 fibers are fresh enough to answer the demand.

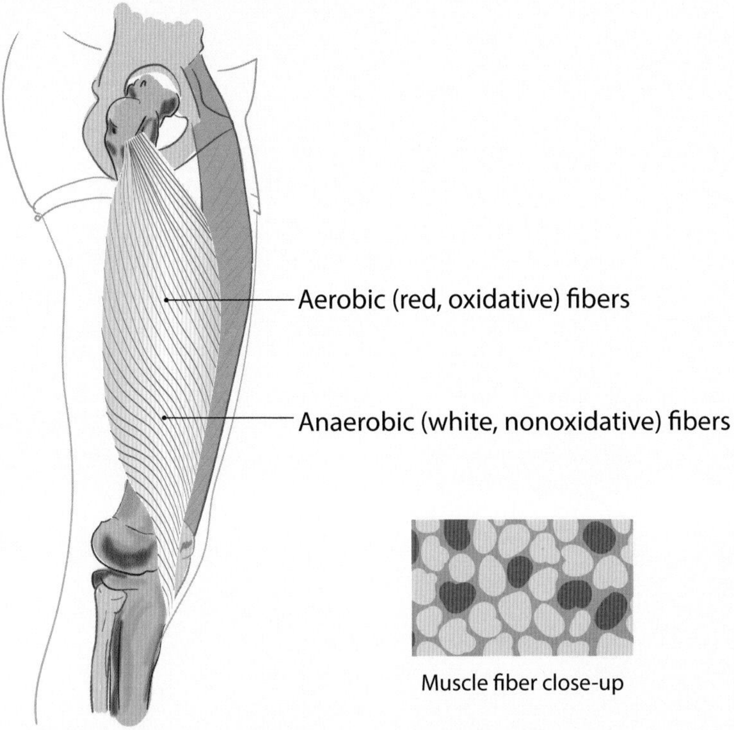

The quads are typically two-thirds fast-twitch (this varies by individual), but the oxidative fibers are intertwined.

Anaerobic System

Produces ATP quickly; fatigues quickly;
fast twitch; explosive performance . . . **big flames!**

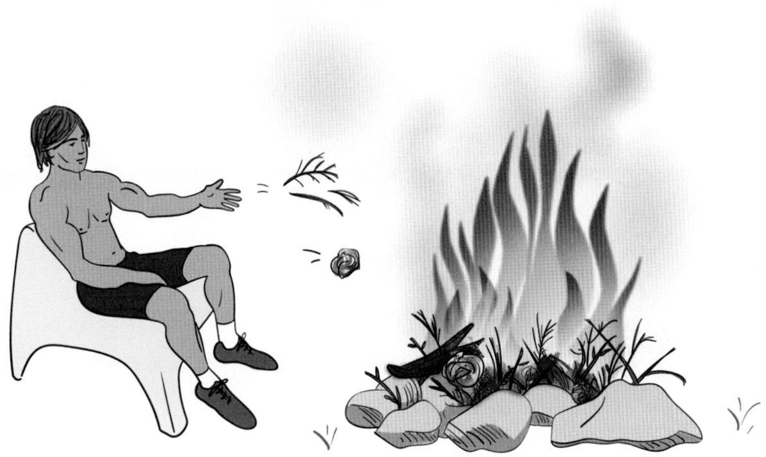

Aerobic System

Produces ATP slowly and plentifully;
slow twitch; endurance performance . . . **steady glow!**

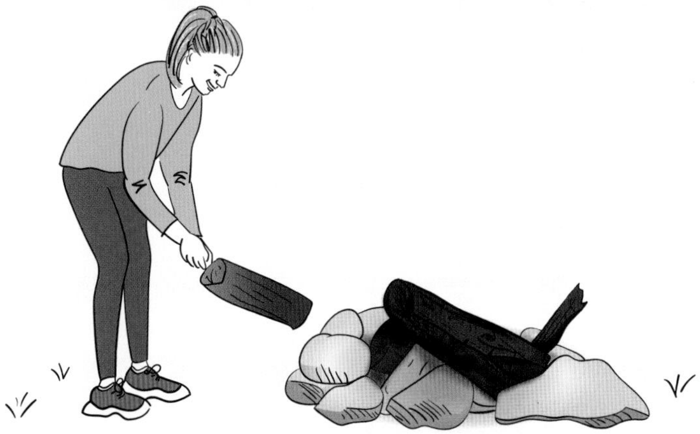

Determining Your Fat Max Heart Rate Accurately

Fat max heart rate is the upper limit for a properly conducted aerobic workout that is minimally stressful and emphasizes fat burning with a minimum of glucose burning. Training right at fat max is great, but excellent aerobic benefits are still obtained even when you exercise well below fat max. This is a highly disregarded aspect of endurance training that deserves to come into focus as you plan your training sessions and aspire to balance stress and rest.

When you exceed fat max heart rate, you of course burn more *total* calories than you would at or below fat max, but you burn fewer *fat* calories than you do at fat max. The body quickly and dramatically switches its emphasis to glucose burning (see the chart on page 155) to fuel harder efforts. A faster workout certainly stimulates your body to adapt to the new exertion level and improve your fitness, and it gives you a nice sweat and an endorphin buzz, but if this becomes the norm, you can trend toward being a sugar-burning machine instead of a fat-burning machine.

Fat max heart rate can be precisely identified during a performance test in an exercise physiology lab by the appearance of a nonlinear spike in ventilation on a graph of your oxygen consumption during exercise. The spike is called ventilatory threshold, or VT. Exceeding fat max is also associated with spikes in glucose metabolism, lactate accumulation, and the mobilization of type 2a muscle fibers. You will still be very comfortable, but your breathing will quicken to the point where you cannot comfortably converse. This threshold might be sensed as transitioning from an easy to a moderate degree of difficulty. In well-trained athletes, VT often occurs at around 77 percent of fat max heart rate, but it can occur at a lower percentage in unfit individuals.

After conducting field tests on hundreds of athletes over several years in the 1970s and 1980s, Dr. Philip Maffetone discovered that exceeding fat max—which he calls the maximum aerobic function, or MAF, heart rate—is characterized by a visible alteration in one's running gait. He contends that this is caused by increased stimulation of the hypothalamic-pituitary-adrenal, or HPA, axis and increased musculoskeletal load: more stress prompts a decrease in the grace and fluidity of the gait pattern. This can manifest itself as anything from poor posture (failure to preserve a straight and elongated spine through the stride pattern) to a hitch in the stride to a bit of tensing in the shoulder girdle or a straining of the facial muscles. In a cyclist who exceeds fat max while pedaling up a hill, you might see the shoulders go from stable to rocking laterally back and forth a bit.

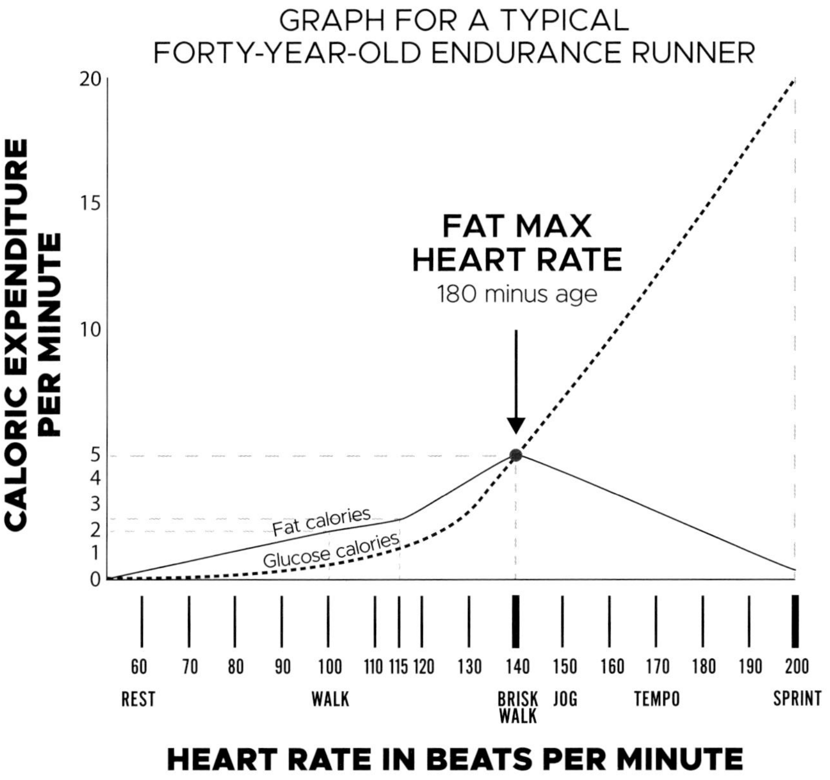

Since the ventilatory threshold cannot be pinpointed without laboratory testing, and since most athletes don't know their true maximum heart rate and therefore can't determine what 77 percent of it is, Dr. Maffetone's highly regarded 180-minus-age formula is the recommended way to calculate your fat max heart rate: subtract your age from 180, and that is your estimated fat max heart rate in beats per minute. For example, a fifty-year-old exerciser has an estimated fat max of 130 beats per minute (180 minus 50).

Following are an assortment of potential adjustments to your fat max number that attempt to account for the status of your general health and aerobic fitness. I adapted and expanded these guidelines from Dr. Maffetone's original adjustment factors.

- Subtract 20 if you eat a nutrient-deficient standard American diet heavy in processed foods. Your fat burning will be highly compromised right out of the gate.
- Subtract 10 if you are suffering from chronic overtraining, recovering from illness or surgery, or are taking prescription medications on an ongoing basis. Yep: all prescription drugs have side effects that warrant a lower fat max heart rate.
- Subtract 5 if you have suffered a recent injury or regression in training; if you get more than two colds or bouts of flu annually; if you suffer from allergies or asthma; if your training patterns are inconsistent or if you have recently returned to training; or if you are categorized as overfat by waist-to-height ratio. Be honest here: most devoted endurance athletes will have to begrudgingly subtract these 5 points.
- You need no adjustment if you have been training consistently—i.e., four times a week—for two years and are free from the aforementioned problems.
- Add 5 if you have had success in training and competition for two years or more.
- Add 10 if you are a fit, successful athlete over the age of sixty-five. Fit specimens age more gracefully and thus reduce maximum heart rate more gradually, which overrides the chronological-age variable in the formula.
- Fit, successful athletes over the age of forty-five can subtract two to three beats for every five years of aging over forty-five. For example, a fit sixty-year-old with a baseline fat max of 120 (180 minus 60) might try training at 129 beats per minute. That would be the fat max calculation for a forty-five-year-old—135—minus six beats, or two beats for every five-year-block between forty-five and sixty.

Dr. Maffetone also advises using common sense to potentially lower your fat max number—even temporarily—if you fall into a rut in training or get a minor illness or overuse injury.

Dr. Maffetone's highly regarded 180-minus-age formula is the recommended way to calculate your fat max heart rate.

It follows that you must use an accurate heart rate monitor to be able to monitor fat max pace during workouts. This is extremely important not just for serious competitive athletes, but also novices who have minimal aerobic conditioning and high risk of overexertion and burnout. If you find yourself without the ability to monitor your heart rate during exercise, there are a couple of on-the-go ways to estimate fat max during exercise. The talk test asks you to carry on a conversation or recite the alphabet while exercising without getting winded. Nasal breathing is another popular way to estimate when you reach fat max. The idea is that inhaling and exhaling entirely through the nose, keeping your mouth closed, should be sufficient to support fat max exercise, whereas exceeding fat max will likely prompt you to open your mouth to obtain enough oxygen. Remember: exceeding fat max is marked by a nonlinear spike in ventilation from the exercise physiology lab.

THE BENEFITS OF NASAL DIAPHRAGMATIC BREATHING

Nasal diaphragmatic breathing entails taking deep breaths with a full activation of the powerful diaphragm muscle, which engages the oxygen-rich lower lobes of the lungs for maximum respiratory efficiency. As practitioners of yoga and meditation know, breath control also has a huge influence on autonomic nervous system function. Nasal diaphragmatic breathing stimulates the parasympathetic nervous system, exerting a calming, relaxing influence and effectively making your workouts less stressful. By contrast, most exercisers tend to take shallow, panting breaths with an open mouth. This results in a less efficient exchange of oxygen by the upper lungs and stimulates the sympathetic nervous system, or fight-or-flight response, potentially making your workouts more stressful and more difficult to recover from.

Nasal breathing also helps warm and humidify the air and filter out pollutants such as allergens, bacteria, viruses, and industrial toxins. Warming the air with your nose is particularly important in freezing temperatures to prevent damage to the lungs and bronchial tubes. Air filtration is important for urban exercisers, too, who typically inhale large, unfiltered doses of particulate matter through the mouth.

In addition, nasal breathing stimulates the production of nitric oxide, a highly beneficial substance produced in the paranasal sinuses and nasal cavity. Nitric oxide is a potent vasodilator—it expands blood vessels and improves blood and oxygen exchange throughout your cardiovascular system.

There is yet another performance advantage to be gained through nasal diaphragmatic breathing and attempting to keep the mouth closed during moderate exercise. As explained in Patrick McKeown's book *The Oxygen Advantage*, inhaling the minimum amount of oxygen necessary will increase levels of carbon dioxide in the bloodstream. Tolerating higher carbon dioxide levels prompts your red blood cells (hemoglobin) to release oxygen to the working muscles and tissues throughout the body. This is a fundamental principle of biochemistry known at the Bohr effect. McKeown argues that most athletes are habitual overbreathers, reflexively sucking in more air than necessary and in the process developing poor carbon dioxide tolerance and causing red blood cells to hold on to oxygen instead of delivering it to the body parts that need it.

The idea that we breathe more than necessary can be validated by testing your blood oxygen level using an inexpensive pulse oximeter that attaches to your fingertips. A healthy person will typically have 96–99 percent oxygen saturation at sea level (it will a bit lower at high altitude). If your blood is always nearly fully saturated with oxygen, taking huge inhales is like overfilling a glass of water—unnecessary. Instead, McKeown suggests that you breathe through your nose only, as minimally as possible—but deeply, using the diaphragm—at all times, especially while sleeping. You can even honor this edict this as you work out. Breathe through your nose only during warm-up, cooldown, and recovery intervals. When it's time to perform, by all means open your mouth and inhale as much air as you need, but try to return quickly to nasal breathing. It seems paradoxical to try to inhale the minimum amount of oxygen necessary during exercise, but the Bohr effect cannot be disputed. Less sucking of air means more oxygen delivered to working muscles!

First calculate your estimated fat max heart rate using the 180-minus-age formula and the adjustment factors. Better yet, undergo a metabolic test to identify your true fat max. Then get a proper Bluetooth-enabled wireless heart-rate monitor that transmits to a companion device or smartwatch. Set an alarm at your fat max or, preferably, five beats below your fat max, and honor it at all times during steady-state aerobic training sessions. I know: this can be highly frustrating for you competitive types, because you are going to have to walk up hills, let your training partners carry on without you, and slow down in the latter stages of your workout in order to prioritize your heart rate over your inclination to doggedly adhere to a certain pace per mile for the entire workout.

Exceeding fat max by even a few beats, or even just a few times during brief energy spurts over the course of a long workout, can negate the intended benefits of the entire session.

It's essential to be highly disciplined and accurate with your fat max training. Exceeding fat max by even a few beats, or even just a few times during brief energy spurts over the course of a long workout, can negate the intended benefits of the entire session. Once you trigger that nonlinear spike in ventilation, stress hormone production, and glucose metabolism, it's difficult to recalibrate back to fat metabolism. Dr. Maffetone warns that undisciplined training can lead to fitness regression, injury, and burnout over time. Dr. Carl Foster, exercise scientist at University of Wisconsin–La Crosse, explains the delicacy and perils of too much training time at heart rates a little or significantly higher than fat max, a zone that he and other physiologists call the "black hole": "We think there's a physiological tripwire. Slip into the black hole for a few minutes—or do an interval or two—and the body reads the whole workout as hard. It cancels the [aerobic session's] recovery effect."

This idea is supported by laboratory research measuring blood lactate levels over the course of a workout, when it's been observed that speeding up even briefly changes blood chemistry for the duration of the workout—the "tripwire" referred to by Dr. Foster. While exercising at fat max or below, blood lactate will be low, typically around 1.5 to 2.0 millimoles per milliliter (mmol/mL). Accumulating this level of lactate in the bloodstream during exercise is completely tolerable and unnoticeable, and you could continue at that pace for long periods. By contrast, anaerobic threshold—also known as the lactate threshold, or redline pace—causes significant and noticeably uncomfortable accumulation of lactate. At threshold, you are producing lactate at the same rate you are able to buffer it; this is identified as 4.0 mmol/mL. A fit athlete can maintain anaerobic threshold pace for around one hour before succumbing to physiological fatigue and being forced to slow down. If you were to speed up beyond threshold and accumulate lactate faster than you can buffer it, you'd be forced to slow down within minutes because of burning, fatigued muscles.

If an athlete accelerates to anaerobic threshold for an interval or two and then returns to fat max pace, blood lactate levels can remain elevated long after he returns to fat max pace—even double the first reading. This effect is most noticeable in novice or intermediate-level athletes. Elite athletes have excellent lactate clearance, so they might be able to get away with doing some short sprints during an endurance session, clear lactate quickly, and carry on in fat-burning dominance. Lactate clearance improves with training, especially when you take the time to build an aerobic base before introducing high-intensity workouts.

BEING PRECISE WITH ANAEROBIC THRESHOLD

Improving your anaerobic threshold involves training at or near a 4 mmol/mL pace with regularity. This will teach your body to buffer lactate accumulation in the bloodstream with maximum efficiency and thereby enable you to sustain a faster race pace.

Precision is important for planning both fat max and anaerobic threshold workouts. You can determine your anaerobic threshold by undergoing a laboratory performance test that measures lactate values in association with heart rate. For example, if you learn that your blood lactate is 4 mmol/mL when exercising at a heart rate of 170 beats per minute, threshold workouts would involve sufficient time spent at heart rates near or at 170 interspersed with rest intervals. You can exercise for long intervals with long rest periods or short intervals with short rest periods, but the key is to bump up against 170 and improve lactate buffering without becoming exhausted. My favorite anaerobic-threshold running session is six times three minutes at anaerobic threshold with thirty-second rest intervals between them.

You can also get a handheld portable blood lactate meter and use it during workouts. By pricking your finger during rest intervals and obtaining real-time blood lactate values, you can calculate your optimal heart rate, speed, recovery intervals, and workout duration. The goal is to stimulate the benefits of training at or near anaerobic threshold but avoid the extra stress and delayed recovery caused by accumulating too much lactate during a workout—e.g., by exceeding your threshold pace and/or doing too many intervals and/or not recovering enough between intervals.

In recent years, a novel training strategy called double threshold has become popular among collegiate and elite distance runners, popularized by the great success of Norwegian Jakob Ingebrigtsen, the world's top middle-distance runner. A double-threshold day would entail two precisely regulated threshold workouts in which the durations are shorter and less stressful than they would be during one long session and in which many hours of recovery separate the sessions. The main sets of these workouts might total twenty to thirty minutes—for example, a morning session of five times one thousand meters at threshold and an evening session of fifteen times four hundred meters at threshold. Don't try this at home! Or go ahead and try double threshold if you are launching off of a base of one-hundred-mile training weeks at mostly aerobic heart rates.

It's so important to be precise with fat max that I don't recommend relying on the talk test or nose breathing to determine when you reach it. If you are a competitive athlete, anaerobic threshold workouts are nothing to fool around with, either—precision is essential. Alas, there will be times when you are without a heart-rate monitor, but be wary of relying on the calculations of a smartwatch. These actually measure pulse rates at the wrist and can be inaccurate enough to compromise the intended benefits of an aerobic training session. Although the best and latest watches from leading brands (Apple, Fitbit, Garmin) can measure with 95 percent or better accuracy, they are not as accurate as a wireless Bluetooth chest strap transmitting to a smartwatch. When in doubt with fat max training, err on the conservative side. You can still obtain outstanding aerobic conditioning benefits when exercising far below fat max, a common practice among elite athletes.

By the way, you never graduate from the need to carefully monitor your heart rate and set limit alarms. There are too many variables influencing your heart rate and that hamper your ability to guess accurately. Fat max pace is so comfortable that you can easily exceed it by allowing your mind to wander during a workout, getting into a lively conversation with a training partner, listening to a favorite song, or encountering a hill, headwind, or challenging terrain, especially in hot temperatures or high altitudes. It's also our natural inclination to try to maintain a specific pace when instead we should really slow down in the latter stages of a workout to compensate for cumulative fatigue and cardiac drift—a term describing your heart rate's tendency to drift upward as a result of increased body temperature, dehydration, and fatigue, even if you are running at a consistent speed. What's more, on many days your pace may be significantly slower than normal at your fat max heart rate because of external stress factors—insufficient sleep, imperfect immune function, a mind ruminating on personal problems, and even the effects of drinking caffeine before your workout. This means you will have to accept a slower pace to achieve an appropriate aerobic training session when you are not 100 percent.

Committing to developing your aerobic system with the correct approach is a huge personal growth exercise and a huge leap forward in the sophistication of your training strategy. You transition from an impatient, impulsive athlete with unregulated competitive urges to someone who cares about optimizing the process and prioritizing long-term development over ego demands. As Eliud Kipchoge said, "Only the disciplined ones are free in life. If you are undisciplined, you are a slave to your moods. You are a slave to your passions." Yes, you have to let go of endorphin addiction and the often unhealthful competitive energy that flows between training partners, but your new approach should give you a huge sense of relief. Training sessions can evolve from mini competitions against the clock and/or your training partners to methodical sessions with a specific metabolic focus. You can relax, likely slow to a walk for at least some and perhaps a lot of your cardio, enjoy the scenery or a social experience with your companions, and still take comfort knowing you are developing your aerobic system optimally.

Why You Have to Go Slow to Go Fast

I hope these insights will help you reject the flawed assumption, held by many endurance athletes, that an optimal training schedule must include a steady dose of runs with a high degree of difficulty, such as interval sessions, hill repeats, tempo runs (in which you hold a specific pace, perhaps simulating race pace), fartlek runs (from a Swedish word meaning "speed play," in which pace varies, often spontaneously), and other stressful, high-glycolytic workouts. For all but elite runners, these fast sessions deliver an incredibly poor return on investment in comparison to slowing down and training predominantly aerobically. This is especially the case when hard efforts are indiscriminate instead of carefully controlled. When you have the patience and restraint to prioritize aerobic conditioning, your fat max pace will eventually become faster, and you can continue longer without becoming fatigued. With a well-conditioned aerobic system, you will preserve precious glycogen so that you will be able to distribute it strategically over the course of an hour of hard effort at anaerobic threshold or over the course of a marathon.

For example, compare the average 4:30 marathoner's 10:18 pace per mile, or a three-hour marathoner's 6:51 pace per mile, to Eliud Kipchoge's historic 1:59 performance—a pace of 4:34 per mile. Extensive anecdotal research conducted by Dr. Phil Maffetone involving both elite and recreational marathon runners suggests that the ideal marathon pace is around fifteen seconds per mile faster than one's fat max one-mile test result. This means that Kipchoge's fat max pace is, in theory, around 4:49 per mile. By comparison, a very fit male distance runner—say, an NCAA Division I cross-country runner—might be able to do a set of six to eight one-mile repeats on the track, digging deep to finish each in 4:49. This is an extremely impressive workout that suggests the potential to run a sub-thirty-minute 10k. However, even if this runner crushes the workout again and again for years—forget about injuries, illness, and fatigue—he will still never be able to ascend to Kipchoge's level of being able to run a 4:49 mile at fat max heart rate and run comfortably for hours at, say, a six-minute-per-mile pace. The collegiate grinder is essentially trying to climb an inverted pyramid instead of building a proper pyramid with aerobic conditioning at the base. You simply cannot struggle and suffer your way to world-class form.

Kipchoge, who started training seriously at age sixteen with his longtime coach, Patrick Sang, took the long route to the top, patiently taking decades to build a phenomenal aerobic base. Initially he was comfortable running perhaps a six-minute mile at fat max pace, then 5:30, then 5:00, and ultimately under five. If you want proof that building an aerobic base drives competitive success, search YouTube for "Kipchoge pace on treadmill" and see a hilarious video from the 2018 Chicago Marathon expo. A giant padded treadmill known as the Tumbleator was set to a speed equal to Kipchoge's 1:59 marathon pace—that's 4:34 per mile, or 1:08 and change for a lap around the 400-meter track in your community. Numerous participants took a crack at staying on the moving belt as long as possible, but many got spit out the back and face-planted onto safety pads within seconds.

The concept that aerobic efficiency is the key to peak performance at fast speeds has been proved true by the world's greatest athletes in every endurance sport since the emergence of the Arthur Lydiard–trained middle-distance runners from New Zealand in the early 1960s. You have probably seen Michael Phelps swim to one of his twenty-three Olympic gold medals and thirty-nine world records. His races lasted from fifty-one seconds to just over four minutes, but he trained for five or six hours a day for two decades to build the massive aerobic engine required to set world records over short distances. The world's top milers typically run around one hundred miles a week—much of that at or below fat max heart rates—to prepare for races lasting less than four minutes.

In fact, endurance champions have been honing aerobic efficiency at comfortable heart rates for more than one hundred years. Consider the anecdote published in *Lore of Running* about the legendary Finnish distance runner Hannes Kolehmainen (1899–1966), four-time Olympic champion and holder of numerous world records. Kolehmainen

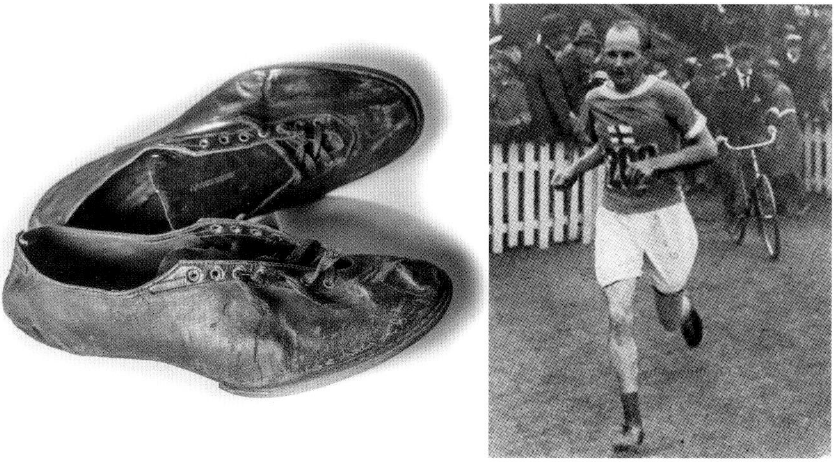

These running shoes, circa 1910, are similar to what Hannes Kolehmainen of Finland, seen above, would have worn during the 1920 Olympics.

was lauded for having "run Finland onto the map of the world" and for being the first of the "Flying Finns": his emergence kick-started a quarter century of Finnish distance-running dominance, highlighted also by the incomparable Paavo Nurmi, who set twenty-two world records and won nine Olympic gold medals. At the 1920 Olympic marathon in Antwerp, Kolehmainen won gold in a new world record time of 2:32. Following is a review of his training log data leading up to the Olympics.

> April 1–7: 108 kilometers [67 miles] of walking, 25 kilometers [15.5 miles] of running. Two days off of training.
> April 8–14: 45 kilometers [28 miles] of walking and 45 kilometers [28 miles] of running. Three days off of training.

Kolehmainen was one of the first athletes to implement high-intensity interval training, laying some hard work atop his walking-driven aerobic base. Kolehmainen, who raced often in the United States and became an American citizen in 1921, probably couldn't run many more miles than he did because of the rudimentary shoes of the day—vastly inferior even to the Onitsuka Tiger Marathon shoes of the 1960s. We're talking streamlined dress shoes with thin leather uppers and a very thin sole made of rigid vulcanized rubber. It's not a stretch to speculate that if Kolehmainen had worn today's energy-return super shoes and lightweight racing apparel, and if he had had the advantage of modern coaching and nutrition—but had maintained the same walking-based training program with lots of rest days—we could subtract ten, fifteen, or twenty minutes from his 1920 marathon time. This means he would qualify for the 2024 United States Olympic Team Trials in the marathon (the entry standard was 2:18).

You may not be an elite athlete, but these examples should be sufficient to persuade you to switch from jogging to walking, at least part of the time, and place more emphasis on walking as a valuable component of your endurance training. What's that you say? You prefer pushing your body hard—trying to hang in there on a figurative 1:59 treadmill? Well, here's what happens when you follow the prevailing instant-gratification, struggle-and-suffer approach to endurance performance: you reduce your fat-burning capacity and instead strengthen your glycolytic energy systems. Of course, during lively boot camp or spin classes, CrossFit workouts, trail runs with faster runners, or Peloton rides at home, you still get an overall athletic conditioning effect, but this is an ill-advised strategy for many reasons.

First, the stress of steady-state, medium-to-difficult workouts will trash your metabolic, immune, endocrine, and cardiovascular systems. Maybe not this week or this month, but you are headed for trouble at some point. This is especially true when you blend your pursuit of exercise endorphins with the many other forms of stress in your life.

Second, you will have a very hard time losing excess body fat. Instead, you'll likely overeat, thanks to the depleting nature of your workouts, and trigger compensatory mechanisms—e.g., general lethargy, low libido, delayed recovery, and suppressed immunity.

Third, you will compromise your athletic potential by working hard without a sufficient aerobic base. Essentially, your grueling workout schedule is like tinkering with a jalopy—your easily fatigued, sugar-burning cardiovascular system—instead of taking the time to build a Ferrari, a robust, fat-burning cardiovascular system.

With an indiscriminate, chronic-cardio approach, you still might be able to run a 3:30 or 4:30 marathon, run a 10k in forty or sixty minutes, or complete a half ironman or ironman triathlon. However, your will most assuredly perform below your true competitive potential. This is especially true when you have limited time to allocate to endurance training and make the flawed conclusion that you must go faster to compensate. In addition, your workouts will often leave you stiff, sore, and fatigued. Statistics suggest that you can count on repeated overuse injuries and minor illnesses. You may even develop psychological issues relating to your immersion in a pattern of self-flagellation amid a culture and peer group that glorifies this type of attitude.

You'll also likely carry excess body fat—especially visceral fat—because you are training your body to operate on stress hormones, sugar, and often caffeine, and you will tend refuel with quick-energy processed carbohydrates. Rev up that jalopy, throw in some cheap gas, bust out a grueling 3:30 or 4:30 marathon, experience massive acute damage to your cardiovascular, endocrine, digestive, and immune systems, then rinse and repeat. Of course, any fitness enthusiast is better off in numerous ways than people who never achieve even a bare minimum of fitness, but once you bank the huge initial benefits from getting active, your returns start to diminish. If you continue with your endurance hobby, you will eventually experience negative returns on your exercise investment. This comes in the form of stubborn belly fat, increased disease risk, compromised general health, and accelerated biological aging.

Secrets of the Elite Endurance Athletes

The website SweatElite.co and other resources have published details of Eliud Kipchoge's training patterns for all interested runners, coaches, and exercise physiologists. He revealed that he trains 82–84 percent of the time at an easy or light intensity, 9–10 percent of the time at moderate intensity, and 7–8 percent of the time at high intensity. The vast majority of his training is at a four- to five-minutes-per-kilometer pace, or 6:26 to 8:03 per mile. This is 29 to 43 percent slower than his world record *marathon* pace!

As Kipchoge says, "I perform at 80 percent on Tuesday, Thursday, and Saturday, and then at 50 percent Monday, Wednesday, Friday, and Sunday." Eliud Kipchoge does thirteen training sessions a week, ten of which are in the easy (for him) category. All told, he logs between 124 and 136 miles each week with extreme consistency. Contrary to tradition, he barely tapers his mileage even before major competitions.

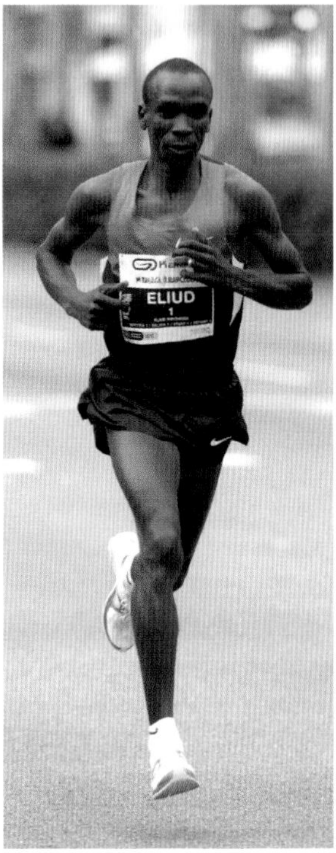

Eliud Kipchoge trains in a relatively less stressful manner than you do—so slow down!

Kipchoge, who was the 2003 world champion at 5,000 meters before focusing on the marathon, has also been remarkably free of major injuries in his two decades at the top of the running world. This is probably because he is always working well within his capacity, even during extremely impressive speed workouts. Overall, his training load is easier—relatively speaking—than that of many typical American collegiate distance runners, whose careers are often burdened by illness, injury, and burnout.

Let's apply this Kipchoge-inspired workout pace to the average 4:30 marathoner running at 10:18 per mile. Going 40 percent slower during easy training sessions, as the greatest endurance runner of all time does, lands the 4:30 marathoner at around seventeen minutes per mile—that's right, walking! Going 29 percent slower than marathon pace during light-to-moderate sessions puts the 4:30 runner at 13:17 per mile, barely faster than the cutoff from walking to jogging. Even hotshot three-hour performers—ranked in the ninety-eighth percentile of all marathoners, mind you—who slow 40 percent from their 6:51 per mile marathon pace would be comfortably trotting along at 11:30 per mile for most of their weekly mileage if they were to honor the Kipchoge approach. Granted, Kipchoge's training camp, in Kaptagat, Kenya, is at an elevation of 8,200 feet, making him an estimated twenty seconds slower per mile than he is at sea level. However, since he's highly adapted to altitude and is also the GOAT, let's respect the aforementioned calculations.

If you're a serious runner chasing a sub-four or sub-three marathon, I imagine you might be feeling stunned and exasperated by these calculations. "How can I possibly improve by walking? Or by shuffling along with the slowest runners in my club?" you might ask. The answer is that you will gradually and reliably improve your aerobic efficiency so that your fat max pace will evolve over time from a brisk walk to a jog-walk to a steady jog when you do it right. Accordingly, you can achieve stunning improvements in performance that are impossible when you insist on tinkering with a jalopy.

Eliud Kipchoge does thirteen training sessions a week, ten of which are in the easy (for him) category.

Kipchoge's approach is consistent with research conducted by Dr. Stephen Seiler, an American exercise physiologist based in Norway who is a leading proponent of the concept of so-called polarized training—going either quite easy or quite hard. Dr. Seiler has studied elite performers in a variety of endurance sports, including running, cycling, triathlon, cross-country skiing, rowing, speed skating, and swimming, and discovered a consistent theme: the vast majority of their workouts are comfortably paced, and a small number of their workouts are conducted at high intensity. For most elite athletes, the distribution is around 80 percent comfortably paced and 20 percent at high intensity.

Notably missing from the formula are the chronic-cardio workouts conducted at medium-to-difficult intensities—too hard to maximize the rate of fat burning but not hard enough to stimulate the benefits of the brief, high-intensity workouts that prepare one for racing. Dr. Seiler offers further support for the effectiveness of polarized training for athletes of all ability levels: "We want to train to signal adaptations at the muscular level without turning on a big stress response. One of the best ways to overtrain an organism is to subject [it] to daily stress that is at the same level. We want to keep a lot of the training under the 'stress radar.'"

This shines a light on a glaring disparity between the way elites train compared to the way amateurs train. Pros are polarized: they go easy or very easy for the vast majority of their total sessions. And when they go hard, they do it correctly—hard enough to stimulate training adaptations but not so hard that they overstress their bodies and delay recovery. By contrast, many amateurs routinely exceed fat max during everyday workouts, driving persistent fatigue and increasing injury risk. Then, when they go hard, they often push themselves too hard—even when running relatively slow times—because their aerobic capacity is so poor. Hey, a new feature film! *Jalopy Versus Ferrari*.

So far, I have largely focused on competitive athletes who should know better, since nearly all of them have at least a basic understanding of endurance training principles, heart-rate monitoring, and exertion zones. But the situation among recreational joggers and gym rats is often worse. With minimal appreciation for heart-rate monitoring and training zones, they have a strong inclination to train at a "medium-to-kinda-hard" exertion rate. This is where you experience a bit of mental strain, shortness of breath, and muscular fatigue and feel like you're getting a "real workout." Unfortunately, these sensations typically kick in well beyond fat max heart rate. At true fat max, perceived exertion feels low to moderate, your muscles are comfortable, and you have sufficient breath to carry on a conversation for the duration of your workout. It's common for new adopters to feel frustration and wonder whether their exertion levels are too low to be effective.

Most mainstream fitness programs are far too stressful for most participants. The same is true in the personal training game, in which many trainers tend to work their clients harder than they should because they want their clients to think they're getting their money's worth. A trainer typically feels much more useful yelling encouragement and working a stopwatch than he does taking a client on a brisk walk through forest trails. Apologies for the blanket condemnation of the fitness industry, but it's time to accept the idea that the struggle-and-suffer ethos is highly destructive, both physically and psychologically. You have to slow down not only to go fast but also to preserve your health.

CALCULATING 80-20 POLARIZATION

The polarized-training concept has been widely misinterpreted and misapplied, because there are many ways to interpret the recommendation to train at a ratio of 20 percent hard and 80 percent easy-to-moderate. The 80-20 concept doesn't mean that 20 percent of your total mileage or total training hours are performed at high-intensity heart rates—this would be ridiculously excessive for athletes of all ability levels. Instead, the idea is that no more than 20 percent of your workouts should include high-intensity effort *of any kind*. This distinction is important because a runner might accumulate only a couple of miles of high-intensity intervals in the course of a workout involving several more miles of low-intensity warm-ups, cooldowns, and recovery interval jogging. A workout with lots of low intensity and a bit of high intensity still counts as a hard session toward the 20 percent quota.

For example, if the aforementioned interval session constitutes one of five workouts in a week, with the other four being comfortably paced, that's an acceptable 80-20 polarization of the five workouts. But let's say the runner instead pursued an 80-20 polarization of total mileage. If he runs thirty miles in a week—four runs of six miles at comfortable pace, and one interval workout of six miles all told—the two miles of actual high-intensity effort during the interval workout is only 6 percent of total volume. The error is to count this workout as "6 percent hard" toward the 80-20 paradigm instead of counting it as a hard session among five weekly sessions—that's "20 percent hard" toward the 80-20 paradigm.

How About a Little Love for Zone 1?

It's become popular in the modern fitness lexicon to define exercise intensity according to five zones, ranked from easy to hard, usually described as follows:

- zone 1 is the easy zone, or the recovery zone;
- zone 2 is the aerobic zone;
- zone 3 is the tempo zone;
- zone 4 is the zone where you reach your anaerobic threshold; and
- zone 5 is the anaerobic zone.

The zones are also defined by the percentage of absolute maximum heart rate achieved within them: for example, in zone 2 you're at

60–70 percent of your maximum heart rate, and in zone 5 you're at 90–100 percent of your maximum heart rate. Zone 2 cardiovascular exercise is a hot new fitness trend, thanks in part to the mainstream medical community's getting on board and emphasizing how important low-level cardiovascular exercise is for enhanced fat metabolism, metabolic flexibility, mitochondrial biogenesis, and an improved insulin response.

With all the emphasis on not exceeding fat max heart rates during cardio sessions, and with the frustration many athletes have with fat max being so slow, it's easy to want to conduct most of your cardio sessions right at fat max—the upper limit of zone 2. While I strongly support the widespread promotion of zone 2 workouts, I want to put in a plug for the wonderful but often underappreciated world of zone 1 cardio. You can still experience fantastic aerobic conditioning benefits while exercising at heart rates well below fat max. This is especially true at times when you need to recover from injury.

Elites in every endurance sport log lots of zone 1 training time in order to minimize the musculoskeletal stress that can result when they work at the limit of their incredibly high aerobic capacity. This goes for Hannes Kolehmainen, constrained by the impact trauma he suffered in his ancient shoes, and Eliud Kipchoge, whose sizzling fat max pace would likely overload his body if he ran it day after day. Hence Kipchoge runs at 50 percent four days a week. Note that I don't mean 50 percent of his pace per mile or 50 percent of his maximum heart rate but rather 50 percent of his *maximum perceived exertion*, which also happens to be around 50 percent slower than his marathon race pace.

Just because your zone 1 might be a medium-speed walk and Kipchoge's is an eight-minute-per-mile pace at high altitude doesn't mean you don't benefit as much as he does from low-level aerobic stimulation. The reason zone 1 works is because it refreshes and rejuvenates the body while still stimulating the aerobic system. Think about a cruise ship outfitted with four giant twelve-cylinder diesel engines. When the four engines are going full-throttle on the open sea, the ship—a floating city with thousands of passengers—can hit a maximum speed of thirty knots (around 34.5 miles per hour). When it's time to navigate through a busy harbor, perhaps only one engine is engaged, running at perhaps half or quarter capacity. However, that engine is still getting a "workout," just as human aerobic enzymes and muscle fibers operating during a zone 1 workout are activated.

The reason zone 1 works is because it refreshes and rejuvenates the body while still stimulating the aerobic system.

Zone 1 workouts can actually speed recovery more than total rest does because you are boosting oxygen delivery, blood circulation, lymphatic function, and immune function without engaging stress mechanisms. By contrast, even a zone 2 session at fat max—something you routinely have no problem with—can be a bit too stressful when you're depleted and trying recover from races or your most challenging workouts.

Another important benefit of zone 1 training is that for many hot-wired, tightly wound endurance freaks, zone 2 sessions often turn out to be conducted at zone 2.3 or zone 2.5. They are characterized by the lack of a heart-rate monitor and/or a lack of the discipline needed to stay below fat max no matter what—typically accompanied by an assortment of rationalizations. Two of my favorites are "It was just for a few hills—they were too steep to stay in zone 2" and "I've been training for years; I can stay below fat max by feel."

In the first example, that's a few hills too many: reference the exercise physiology research revealing that spikes in lactate linger in the bloodstream and compromise fat burning. If you encounter some steep hills during a fat max session, walk them! If you're cycling and hit steep hills that cause your limit alarm to beep every time, install a bigger freewheel cog, a "granny gear." In the second example, you cannot reliably stay below fat max by feel, because there are too many variables involved. If you're reluctant to walk, realize that an estimated 77 to 85 percent of Eliud Kipchoge's training lands in zone 1 and the other 15 percent falls in zones 2 and 3. Ross Tucker, PhD, exercise physiologist and cohost of *The Science of Sport* podcast, who analyzed Kipchoge's training for a 2023 *Runner's World* article, also reminds us that "this is a pattern that you'll see in the schedules of almost all the top performers."

Aerobic Conditioning Is the Foundation for Everyone

All fitness aspirations depend upon the development of an excellent aerobic conditioning base. It's virtually everything in endurance sports, but is also critical in high-intensity sports, ball sports, team sports, and any other form of physical exertion. Even powerlifters, bodybuilders, and pure sprinters require substantial aerobic conditioning—a heart that pumps efficiently, delivers blood and oxygen to working muscles all over the body, and clears waste products.

For example, if a bulky powerlifter or bodybuilder is aerobically deficient and can't regulate her huffing and puffing after only a few sets, the rest of her workout is toast. My goodness—even a golfer hitting a hundred balls on the range and walking a golf course for four hours (typically five to six miles miles in total) requires substantial aerobic conditioning to maintain energy, focus, and precise neuromuscular coordination. I'm not saying a powerlifter's 10k time is going to have a huge influence on her accumulated bench-squat-deadlifting total, but there is no way she can spend long hours in the gym hoisting thousands of pounds of cumulative iron without a strong aerobic base.

CrossFit athletes—who, as many observers legitimately argue, are the most supremely conditioned athletes on earth—offer another important case study in the importance of aerobic conditioning. Winning the CrossFit Games entails performing grueling repeats of assorted complex and explosive exercises that are highly varied and are presented as a surprise to competitors. You might see athletes perform sets of air squats and handstand push-ups while wearing a weighted vest (twenty pounds for men; fourteen pounds for women); execute sets of Olympic lifts, or "muscle-ups," on gymnastic rings, then go on a two-hundred-meter jaunt around a stadium; or run a mile in the weighted vest before performing torturous sets on assorted gym apparatuses. The top contenders are universally ripped, resembling gymnasts who have packed on an extra ten or twenty-five pounds of solid muscle. You don't see the emaciated physique of an endurance athlete at the CrossFit Games—not even in the stands!

An elite CrossFitter needs to have tremendous aerobic conditioning in order to endure those incredibly demanding workouts. For example, Canadian Mat Fraser, who stands five feet seven and weighs 195 pounds—widely recognized as the "fittest man in history" and winner of gold medals in five consecutive CrossFit Games, from 2016 to 2020—trained a reported four to six hours a day six days a week. His superhuman regimen included extensive aerobic exercise, high-intensity intervals, and other metcon (metabolic conditioning) work, including sprinting, hard-core weight lifting, Olympic lifting, and assorted gymnastics-style skill builders such as box jumps, rope climbs, and kettlebell maneuvers.

HINSHAW'S AEROBIC CAPACITY GRAPH

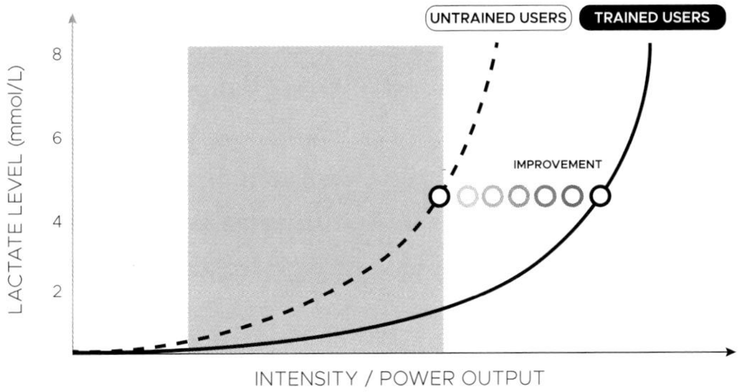

Underpinning Fraser's impressive performances was an outstanding aerobic conditioning base, an advantage that took a while for many CrossFitters to discover. Former Hawaii Ironman runner-up triathlete Chris Hinshaw has risen to prominence by training elite CrossFit athletes in his branded Aerobic Capacity protocols—he's coached thirty-five champions in various CrossFit Games competitive categories. In the 2010s, as Hinshaw immersed himself in CrossFit training, long after his retirement from triathlon, he identified a huge void in the training methodology of elite CrossFitters. They were slamming amazing workouts, but their insufficient aerobic bases were compromising their potential. They lacked the endurance to perform extra reps and sets or deliver repeated explosive efforts on short recovery intervals. They were too aerobically fatigued to do additional anaerobic exercises with stable power and precise technique.

You can experience this phenomenon yourself by mounting a pull-up bar and doing a single set until you can't do any more. How many did you manage? Three? Five? Fourteen? Great job! Next, rest for one minute and try again. You'll likely discover that you can't come close to your first-set performance because your muscles have exhausted their explosive energy capabilities. You may need ten or thirty minutes of rest to deliver an equivalent effort, but you don't get that kind of rest in the CrossFit Games.

In 2014, Hinshaw helped American Rich Froning (five feet nine and 195 pounds), a four-time (2011–2014) CrossFit Games champion—perhaps the co-GOAT of CrossFit alongside Mat Fraser—improve his mile time from six minutes to 5:41 in twelve weeks "by focusing on his weakness." According to Hinshaw, this was Froning's aerobic capacity. As suggested by Hinshaw's aerobic capacity graph (page 175), improving your aerobic capacity will enable you to produce less lactate at all intensity levels and generate more power output at the key anaerobic threshold marker of 4mmol/L. The "Trained Users" slope reveals an ability to buffer acid accumulation in the muscles instead of succumb to the dreaded burn. Here's how Hinshaw describes the concept:

> High-intensity training will develop your ability to deliver solid performances up to 2–3 minutes. However, any inefficiencies within your aerobic energy system will begin restricting performances as you extend beyond three minutes. The primary limiting factor is the ability to move and absorb oxygen. Yes, speed is still critical to success. However, to build capacity, nothing is more important than your ability to utilize oxygen.

VO2 Max: Correlating Cardiovascular Fitness with Longevity

Beginning in the 2010s, a laboratory cardiovascular performance test called VO2 max rose to prominence in the mainstream medical, fitness, and biohacking communities as an excellent way to measure general cardiovascular health, disease risk, and longevity potential. It's great to see the integration of performance-oriented metrics into wellness and medicine. However, like many aspects of exercise science that have been co-opted for mainstream fitness promotion and biohacking, VO2 max might be drifting into the "overrated" category. In essence, a low VO2 max is a huge red flag of impending demise for the unfit; improving it through cardiovascular exercise is the most urgent of health objectives. But for those who are fit or super fit, VO2 max is less important than you might think.

There are numerous performance metrics that you can track from now through the rest of your life that are just as significant as VO2 max but are either less quantifiable or less glamorized. I'd say choosing a few quantifiable fitness challenges that are of most interest to you and repeating tests for years to come is a fantastic strategy—as good as any high-tech test result. How fast can you swim across the lake at your summer cabin? How long does it take you to climb to the top of your favorite hiking trail or to climb twenty flights of stairs in your office building? How fast can you run a mile? How many times can you deadlift two hundred pounds? You get the picture.

Note that there is extensive research correlating grip strength, push-up competency, squat competency, and mile-run time as excellent predictors of longevity. A study of sixty-six thousand participants conducted by the Cooper Institute and University of Texas Southwestern Medical Center drew a strong correlation between one's time in the mile run at age fifty and one's chances of reaching the age of eighty-five in good health. Males running under eight minutes and females running under nine minutes are in the superior category, while males slower than twelve minutes and females slower than thirteen minutes fall into the unfit/high-risk category. Dr. Jarett Berry, a cardiologist at the UT Southwestern Medical Center, in Dallas, says about the study data, "If you are fit in midlife, you double your chance of surviving to 85." If you are unfit, researchers contend that you will take eight years off your projected lifespan. I will suggest other ways to track full-body fitness and longevity prospects in chapter 9.

Ah, yes, back to today's media darling—VO2 max. This is a measurement of the maximum volume of oxygen in milliliters one can consume per minute per kilogram of body weight, identified while exercising at near maximum intensity. A VO2 max score is usually presented as, for example: "53 mL/min/kg." Most cardiologists, as well as respected sources such as the Mayo Clinic, are now touting VO2 max as a cardiovascular marker superior to anything found in blood work, EKGs, and other routine screenings.

VO2 max is a cardiovascular marker superior to anything found in blood work, EKGs, and other routine screenings.

I say VO2 max emerged in the 2010s, but competitive endurance athletes have been testing VO2 max in sophisticated sports performance laboratories for decades as a way to predict competitive potential. Someone who can process a high volume of oxygen in relation to his body weight theoretically could climb high mountains in the Tour de France along with the leaders or hang with the lead pack in a marathon. A VO2 max test entails getting on a specially equipped treadmill or stationary bike and running or pedaling to the brink of exhaustion while breathing into a mask with tubes connected to a "metabolic cart" machine. The cart tracks the rate of oxygen utilization during respiration. As you continue to escalate effort (via a treadmill speeding up or increasing wattage output on a stationary bike) until you can go no more, the highest value is recorded. You can get a VO2 max test usually for around $100 to $150 at many fitness clubs, athletic training centers, sports performance physical therapy clinics, and cutting-edge wellness centers. Sorry, but you should ignore the extremely inaccurate VO2 max estimates served up by smartwatches and internet calculators.

People who build a high VO2 max in their youth and preserve it throughout life have excellent longevity prospects. Those who have a poor VO2 max are at the highest risk of all-cause mortality, especially heart disease, diabetes, depression, dementia, and breast, lung, and gastrointestinal cancers. The Cleveland Clinic and the American Heart Association contend that a VO2 max of 32 mL/min/kg is the bare minimum passing grade for cardiovascular and general health. If you are below that, you can't even climb a set of stairs comfortably.

A VO2 max of 18 mL/min/kg represents a huge mortality risk. This is the score of someone who gets winded while getting up from the sofa to walk across the room and can barely live independently. Falling below 18, as do patients in the final days of hospice, for example, suggests an imminent failure of the cardiovascular and respiratory systems, a harbinger of death by "natural causes."

VO2 MAX PREDICTS LONGEVITY

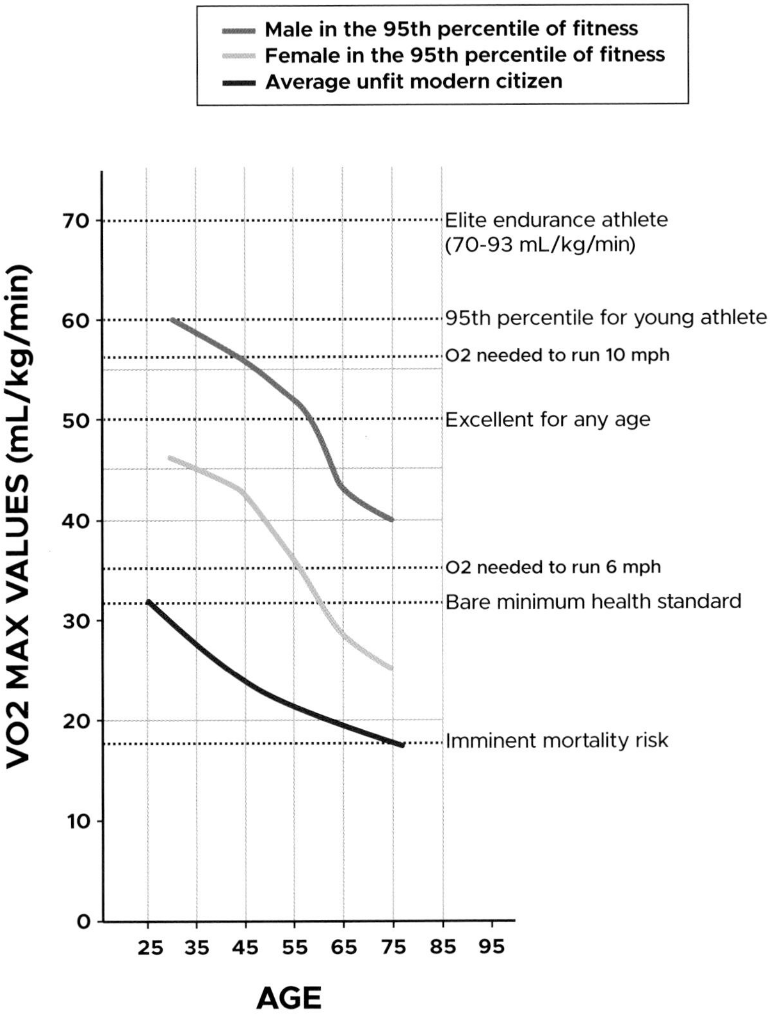

VO2 max is a great longevity metric, but so is getting fit, period.

Frank Booth, PhD, a professor at the University of Missouri's Dalton Cardiovascular Research Center and an expert in physical fitness and its influence on aging, contends that a low VO2 max is directly associated with chronic disease—but researchers are not sure exactly why. Booth asserts that "you want to fight like hell to keep your VO2 max from falling if you want to keep your health span" and explains that one's rate of VO2 max decline can be used to estimate life expectancy. In *Lore of Running*, Tim Noakes highlights three studies predicting that athletes with high VO2 max values in their youth (50–60 mL/min/kg at age twenty) could live for one hundred to 125 years if they continued to train at an ambitious level.

While cessation of training resulting from a variety of factors, including, injury, disease, and/or loss of interest, typically intervene to limit the potential of fit people to become centenarians or supercentenarians, it's encouraging to realize that bumping up your VO2 max at any age and fighting to maintain it over the years is the essence of aging gracefully. In fact the American Heart Association states that increasing VO2 max by 3.5 mL/min/kg will produce a 10–25 percent improvement in longevity.

Today, average VO2 max scores are 30–35 for males and 25–30 for females. Females are typically 15–30 percent lower than males, who generally have stronger hearts, more muscle and less fat, and higher hemoglobin counts—see the ninety-fifth-percentile values for males and females on the VO2 max values graph (page 179). That's right: most people today are overfat, unfit, and flirting with flunking the VO2 max baseline standard of 32. A VO2 max above 50 is considered excellent, indicative of a young, highly athletic individual or an elite athlete. Elite endurance athletes typically test above 70, and a handful of champions have tested in the 90s. VO2 max declines substantially with age, even for fit folks. Hence in your thirties, 60 mL/min/kg for males and 46 for females puts you in the ninety-fifth percentile. In your forties, it's 56 for males and 43 for females; in your fifties, it's 51 for males and 36 for females; in your sixties, it's 43 for males and 29 for females; and in your seventies, it's 40 for males and 25 for females.

Precise workout protocols designed to raise VO2 max have become popular—for example, four hard efforts of four minutes each at around 85–90 percent of absolute maximum heart rate with a four-minute rest interval between each effort. By contrast, the typical HIIT workout features shorter work efforts and shorter rest intervals—e.g., the popular Tabata protocol calls for twenty seconds of work followed by ten seconds of rest, repeated for eight rounds. But the longer work efforts, usually between three and eight minutes each, and longer rest intervals in a VO2 max session allow you to repeatedly work up to near your maximum oxygen consumption.

Most VO2 max workout recommendations are sensible and validated by science, but I prefer that you don't think of VO2 max in a vacuum. All manner of cardiovascular training, from easy to all-out, will contribute to improving your VO2 max. If anyone tells you otherwise, turn and walk away—and keep walking all the way to a higher VO2 max. It is a *robust aerobic base* that helps you absorb and assimilate the extremely challenging, anaerobically oriented VO2 max workouts without falling apart. This big-picture insight often gets lost in the shuffle when research gets co-opted for magazine cover stories ("Killer four-by-four sessions to boost VO2 max!").

Understand that you desperately need an adequate VO2 max to avoid an early demise, but once you get healthy and reasonably fit, your VO2 max score has minimal impact on your athletic performance or longevity. Extensive research reveals that one's VO2 max is hugely influenced by genetics and is minimally trainable. That is, once you elevate your VO2 max beyond the high-risk category and into the fit category—perhaps through both getting fit and dropping excess body fat, since the value is calculated in milliliters per kilogram of body weight—you will have difficulty increasing it even through vigorous training.

For example, running economy (see page 76) is as important as or more important than VO2 max in predicting competitive potential. So are a whole bunch of other factors, such as training methodology, mindset, diet, lifestyle, and recovery strategies. When we watch Tour de France cyclists climbing the mountains or marathoners running in the Olympics, they certainly have VO2 max scores ranging from 70 to 90, but the finishing order will have no relationship to those numbers.

What About Speedwork?

Wait, Mark: Isn't regular speedwork necessary to achieve a competitive edge in endurance events? Indeed, it's important to occasionally practice running at your desired race pace or faster, but only by building a phenomenal aerobic engine can you absorb and benefit from the small percentage of your workouts that should be conducted at high intensity. There are no shortcuts to peak endurance performance—you can't just jump into high-intensity training sessions with faster runners and try to hang with them unless you develop a base that will absorb and benefit from these workouts. Here's a reminder from Arthur Lydiard: "The fundamental principle of training is simple, which may be why it needs repeating so often: it is to develop enough stamina to enable you to maintain the necessary speed for the full distance at which you plan to compete."

Only by building a phenomenal aerobic engine can you absorb and benefit from the small percentage of your workouts that should be conducted at high intensity.

Furthermore, deriving quick and significant fitness benefits from high-intensity training is only possible if you conduct those sessions correctly. Because of their stressful nature, there is a high risk of injury and exhaustion. Even when endurance athletes build a sufficient base and introduce speed sessions, they routinely screw them up by pushing too hard. Jakob Ingebrigtsen explains that he never exceeds 87 percent of his capacity—his anaerobic threshold—during workouts. The intense muscle burn and extreme fatigue that come from exceeding anaerobic threshold and giving near-maximum efforts are saved exclusively for races on the pro circuit. However, Ingebrigtsen does double-threshold days twice a week. Similarly, Eliud Kipchoge rarely exceeds 80 percent of his capacity, lower than Ingebrigtsen because of the much longer duration of his focal event.

If you like to incorporate challenging sessions such as intervals and hill repeats into your training schedule, or if you like to do high-intensity workouts in a group setting, you are exceeding your anaerobic threshold more often than the greatest middle-distance runner on the planet does. Remember: anaerobic threshold is the pace of a one-hour maximum effort. So when you're doing hill repeats or track intervals lasting two to five minutes at threshold, you should feel only mild strain. After all, it's a pace you can hold for an entire hour. Granted, you're going to feel pretty tired after a properly conducted threshold session, but I don't want you collapsing at the side of the track or wobbling back down the hill after your last rep. These are signs that you have gone over the edge and are swimming in a pool of lactate.

Don't you dare play the amateur card right now and say, "Well, I have to go faster if I want to make the most of my limited training time." This rationale does not hold water. In fact, the opposite rationale is more logical: you might consider polarizing your training even further by maintaining a 90-10 ratio. Elite athletes have certain genetic preispositions, are supremely well conditioned, and have decades of high-volume aerobic exercise under their belts. They have vastly more capacity than a recreational runner does to push their bodies hard and absorb and benefit from the work. For example, Kipchoge—despite being one of the wealthiest and most famous citizens in his country—lives a spartan life in a dormitory with his teammates and takes a two-hour nap every day!

A properly conducted high-intensity session should entail a consistent quality of effort on each repetition.

Let's analyze a typical too-stressful high-intensity session conducted by an earnest amateur runner, such as eight 400-meter runs at 1:30 each (see page 189). The runner may not exceed anaerobic threshold on the first four reps, but the last four may start to get ugly. This commonly happens when runners try to maintain their pace instead of deliver a similar effort throughout the reps. A properly conducted high-intensity session should entail a consistent quality of effort on each repetition. For example, the runner might strive to conduct each rep at a certain heart rate or a subjective degree of difficulty of 88 percent. If the athlete maintains this 88 percent rate, completes six reps at around 1:30, then finishes the seventh rep in 1:35, this is a sign that sufficient fatigue has accumulated to warrant ending the session. The consistent quality of effort has slipped. Similarly, if the athlete doggedly insists on arriving at 1:30 for each rep, that seventh rep might require a 92 percent effort—again, a loss of consistency resulting from cumulative fatigue.

Unfortunately, this obsession with meeting predetermined interval times and reps seems to be the prevailing approach to high-intensity training. This is typically influenced by the advice given in coach-guided group workouts or even in internet articles and YouTube videos. But going a little too hard, doing a few too many reps, and taking insufficient recovery intervals can easily become destructive. When a runner digs deep to arrive in 1:30 on those seventh and eighth reps, this prompts acid accumulation in the muscles, disassembling and deamination of cellular proteins, overproduction of stress hormones, delayed recovery time, and immune and hormone suppression. This is especially true when these workouts become a pattern, as they do when you go for the perfect attendance award at your local running club's Tuesday night track workout.

Remember: it's quality over quantity when it comes to speedwork. And by quality I don't mean improving your interval times from last week but delivering a consistent quality of effort. Go ahead and set objectives for times, reps, and rest intervals, but apply an intuitive element to be sure that you don't overextend yourself. Buy a portable blood lactate meter, which costs around $200, or track variations in heart-rate patterns during the session. For example, if your heart rate is more elevated at the end of your two-minute rest interval than it was on previous reps, fatigue is accumulating. Sure, you can complete more reps by slowing down or taking a longer rest interval, but it's best to be conservative and terminate the session when your consistency falls off. Log the details of your high-intensity workouts so you can learn from experience and design sessions that are appropriate for your present fitness level.

I urge you to save digging deep for races. Granted, learning to maintain your pace amid fatigue is obviously a critical part of competitive success, but you don't have to suffer royally to get good at this. Here's how to reject the "no pain, no gain" rationale: first, the brain does not need to be trained to suffer. It needs no more prompting than the excitement of a race environment and the buildup in your mind toward the valiant effort required on the big day. Instead of suffering repeatedly during workouts in the name of race preparation, you will set up peak performance when you nurture your health every day, carefully regulate your competitive intensity, and prepare strategically for your big competitions. Think about a lost backcountry skier who survived for eight days in the snowy wilderness, digging a cave for shelter and rationing her last two energy bars. Had the survivor "trained" for the ordeal by foolishly sleeping out in the elements and shivering away two nights a week, her survival chances would be worse than if she had saved her energy for the time when maximum effort was most needed.

Second, your anaerobic muscle fibers adapt best to occasional workouts featuring brief, explosive efforts followed by extensive recovery. The anaerobic system responds very poorly to excess volume—meaning workouts that are too frequent, too strenuous, and have too many work reps and/or too-short rest intervals. Unfortunately, this is the template for almost all HIIT-style workouts. An efficient aerobic system—which responds well to high volume and low intensity—helps nourish and rejuvenate the muscle fibers.

Many athletes ignore the important role of the aerobic system in supporting anaerobic metabolism. As you increase exercise intensity beyond fat max and approach anaerobic threshold, lactate is produced mainly in the fast-twitch muscle fibers. Clearing that lactate before you succumb to the burn is mainly the responsibility of the adjacent slow-twitch fibers, because they have much more mitochondrial density as well as the necessary lactate-specific transporters and enzymes. Of course, it's necessary to occasionally train at or near anaerobic threshold in order to increase the quantity of your glycolytic fast-twitch muscle fibers and improve their ability to transport lactate over to the slow-twitch fibers for eventual clearance. However, anaerobic threshold training is only worthwhile when it's supported by a robust aerobic system—otherwise you're back in the greasy garage tinkering with a jalopy.

For all the competitive runners scheming to implement Jakob Ingebrigtsen's double-threshold training protocol and reap the benefits, it's important to get some perspective on what supports such a challenging regimen. Jakob started training seriously at age six, following in the footsteps of his world-class older brothers Henrik (European 1,500-meter champion and fifth in the Olympics in 2012—when Jakob was twelve) and Filip (European 1,500-meter champion in 2016). On the five-season reality TV show *Team Ingebrigtsen* (formerly on YouTube; replaced by *Ingebrigtsen: Born to Run* on Amazon Prime), were able to witness the steady progression of the young athlete over a decade of footage. Early seasons showed young Jakob training fervently and winning races at age eleven, and the final season culminated in 2021 with Jakob winning Olympic 1,500-meter gold in Tokyo at age twenty-one. Jakob explains that he occasionally ran as much as seventy-five to ninety miles a week between the ages of nine and eleven: he has been running at least eighty-seven miles a week since the age of thirteen. Now he routinely runs more than one hundred miles a week as a pro and claims to have not missed a scheduled workout since childhood.

It follows that it is important to build an outstanding conditioning base through the practice of periodization before introducing high-intensity workouts. Periodization means that you should dedicate blocks of your annual calendar to different types of fitness stimulation. Notably, the vast majority of elite endurance athletes begin their competitive seasons with an aerobic base-building period, featuring lots of volume and minimal high-intensity exercise. Once a sufficient aerobic base is established, high-intensity sessions can be conducted with increasing frequency in order to generate rapid and significant boosts in fitness.

HOW TO INTEGRATE HIGH-INTENSITY WORKOUTS INTO YOUR TRAINING REGIMEN

High-intensity workouts must be integrated into your routine with great caution and restraint.

First, you must have completed a successful base period as evidenced by steady improvement in maximum aerobic function test results.

Second, you must feel 100 percent healthy, rested, and energized any time you attempt a high-intensity workout. If your muscles or central nervous system are fatigued and you attempt to go fast, you will literally be training your muscles and central nervous system to go slow. This is because a fatigued mind and body will expertly try to protect you from injury by generating less vertical force production, less overall energy output, and associated degradations in technique—such as an overstride instead of a midfoot strike—which then become "learned" by the central nervous system. Even if you have so much as a scratchy throat or a sore hamstring, you must take it easy and wait until all systems are go again.

Third, your periods of emphasizing high-intensity workouts, and the corresponding reduction in total volume, should last a maximum of six weeks, followed by a small rest period, followed by a small aerobic base-building period. These microperiods will help you absorb and benefit from periods of high-intensity workouts with less risk of breakdown and burnout.

Finally, your high-intensity sessions must be designed to prompt fitness benefits without exhaustion. You must select the distance, rest interval, speed, and number of reps that you can complete with a consistent quality of effort and precise technique. For example, instead of eight 400-meter runs of 1:30 each, a runner might instead strive to do six 400-meter runs in 1:33—an 85 percent degree of difficulty. Always be willing to adjust your workout on the fly when you slip from consistent quality of effort.

The Maximum Aerobic Function (MAF) Test

As you work through your initial frustrations and get accustomed to training at a slower pace, it can be helpful to get quantifiable proof that you are improving your fat-burning efficiency and elevating your competitive potential by performing a simple performance test known as the maximum aerobic function, or MAF, test. Yep, it's an acronym and also an homage to the creator of the test, Dr. Phil Maffetone. The MAF test entails timing yourself over a specific distance or course while staying as close as possible to fat max heart rate.

First choose the activity of your highest competency and competitive interest. Then design a course or test protocol that takes around ten to twelve minutes to complete. For example, a runner could perform a test of one to two miles on a 400-meter track, treadmill, or pedestrian path. A cyclist could climb from the bottom of a hill to the top or pedal a stationary bike for two to four miles, and a rower could complete one thousand to two thousand meters on a machine at the gym—all while striving to stay as close as possible to fat max heart rate for the duration of the test. Record your finishing time and repeat the same test (same course, same conditions, same heart rate) once every three to four weeks. For runners, the pace might be a brisk walk, slow jog, steady jog, or 4:49 mile (!), depending on aerobic ability.

A MAF test entails timing yourself over a specific distance or course while staying as close as possible to fat max heart rate.

Marathon aspirants can run a one-mile MAF test, then calculate their recommended marathon pace at fifteen seconds per mile faster than that, per Dr. Maffetone's recommendation. Remember that most running tracks are 400 meters and that a mile is 1,609 meters. So you must run nine meters past the finish line on your final lap to obtain your MAF mile time. Elite long-distance athletes can perform MAF tests lasting up to thirty minutes; professional cyclists and triathletes often pedal long climbs at fat max, or anaerobic threshold, and track their performance over the season with repeated tests.

Although a MAF test is not strenuous, because you are only going at fat max pace, you should only conduct the test when you feel fully rested. You want to deliver an impressive result that reveals your true fitness progress. During your extensive warm-up before each test, make sure your body feels energetic and your heart rate seems appropriate to the level of effort. If you feel sluggish or notice your heart rate higher than expected during warm-up, save the test for another day. Also try to make sure the conditions are consistent—avoid testing under extreme weather conditions. This is why cycling uphill or on a stationary bike is better than cycling on a flat course, where wind can influence test results.

On test day, warm up thoroughly, then commence the test by starting your timer and gracefully accelerating to reach your fat max heart rate. Try your best to stabilize your heart rate at your fat max number for the duration of the test, knowing it will surely dance around the exact number. Aim to be slightly under rather than slightly over. For example, if your fax max heart rate is 138 beats per minute, you might strive to keep your heart rate between 135 and 138. Expect to slow down in the latter stages of the test to keep your heart rate in check.

A faster fat max pace translates directly into a faster race pace. But unlike race results, MAF test results can't be improved by pushing harder and digging deeper. You are beholden to the heart rate beeper alarm, perhaps frustratingly so, but your results are deeply revealing of your true level of aerobic conditioning and consequently your competitive potential. If you deliver a couple of slower-than-usual MAF test results in a row, this is almost always an indicator of overtraining and/or overstress patterns in daily life—or an obvious sign of deconditioning after an illness or break from training. This is why you should only attempt the test when you feel great and can perform at a level representative of weeks of successful aerobic conditioning.

DATE	COURSE	AVERAGE HEART RATE	TIME
January 8	8 laps 400-meter track	139	16:41
February 4	8 laps 400-meter track	141	16:01
March 12	8 laps 400-meter track	140	15:54
April 4	8 laps 400-meter track	138	15:28
May 18	8 laps 400-meter track	139	15:14

Regularly performing the MAF test is especially helpful for the type As out there who have difficulty slowing down and managing competitive intensity. If you experience doubts or frustrations about having to continually answer to the beeper alarm, faster MAF test results will give you unassailable validation that your training is working. You will grow to appreciate the big-picture objective of steadily and patiently

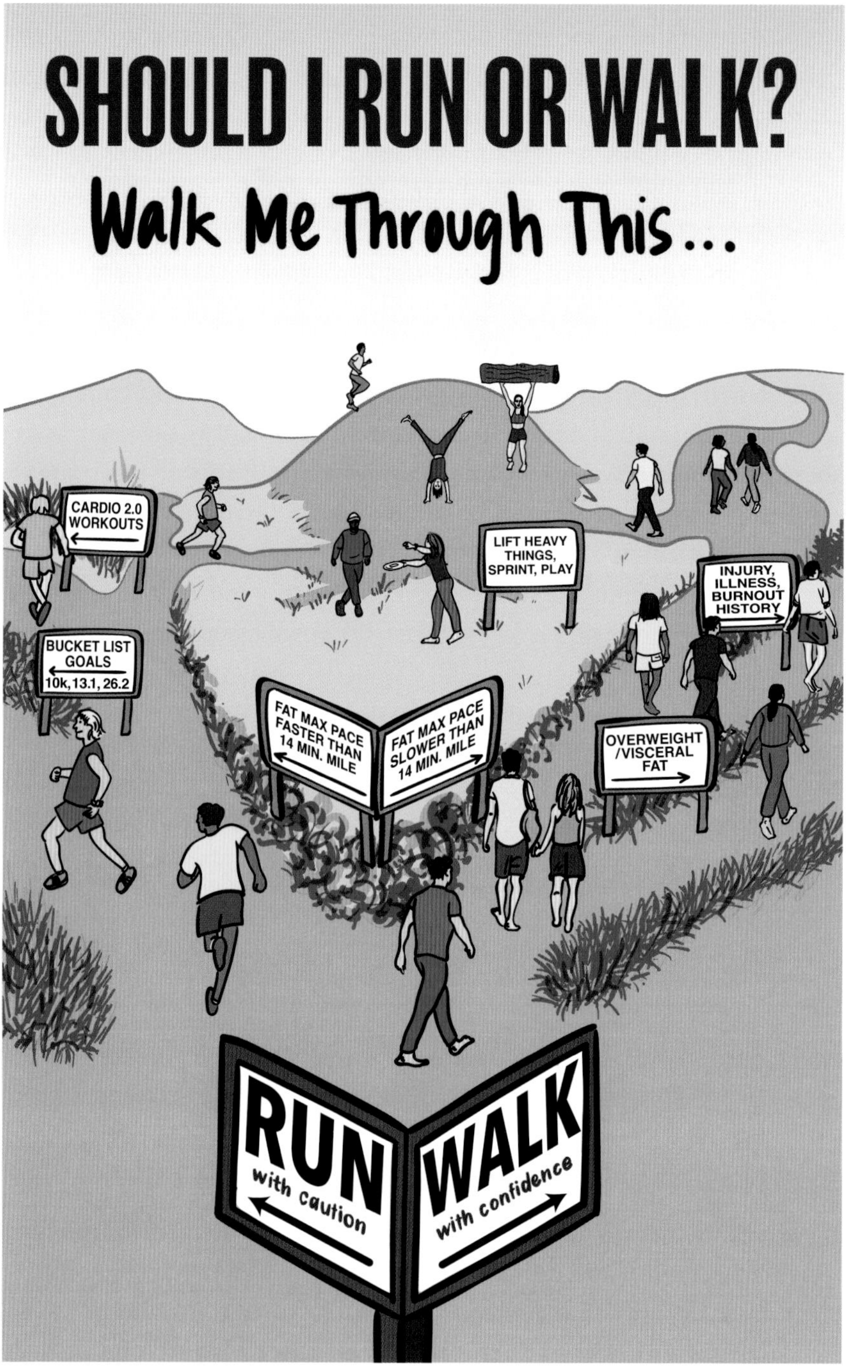

The road to aerobic development occurs at or below fat max heart rate. Avoid the pitfalls and detours caused by chronic cardio.

improving aerobic function without the interruptions caused by high-stress workouts that require extensive recovery and that increase the risk of setbacks such as illness and injury.

The chart on page 189 shows some hypothetical test results of a runner who performs the MAF test repeatedly and shows steady improvement. Keep a similar log for yourself as you integrate regular MAF tests into your training program.

Navigating the Obstacles

Even if you have demonstrated the ability to perform well in the 5k, 10k, half-marathon, or marathon—and/or you are able to jog instead of walk at fat max heart rate—you are going to want to reduce your jogging and do more walking if any of the following road hazards apply.

Overfat and Injured

If you qualify as overfat, with a waist circumference of more than double your height and/or if you've had recurring overuse injuries over the past few years, you must take drastic action. I suggest ways to optimize diet, sleep, and stress management in my other books, including *The Primal Blueprint*, but for now it's time to slow your cardio down to a walk. This will minimize stress hormone production and improve fat metabolism. If you have competency in strength training or sprinting, you can include these types of workouts to speed your progress. Just no chronic cardio!

Crappy Diet

Diet can be a big factor in inferior MAF test results. A high intake of processed carbs, for example, can interfere with your fat-burning capacity—both during exercise and as you go about your everyday life.

General Health and Wellness

If you're battling a chronic illness, especially those in the fatigue and autoimmune categories; or if you have an inordinate amount of life stress or mental health challenges such as anxiety and depression; if you regularly use recreational drugs or prescription drugs, have poor dietary habits, travel frequently through time zones, work extremely long hours, suffer from major sleep disturbances (e.g., you're caring for an infant or doing shift work); or if you experience other significant disturbances to your daily energy, hormonal, and metabolic levels, you must urgently reduce your overall exercise stress. This means practicing low-level aerobic conditioning and avoiding high-stress workouts.

Slower MAF Test Results

If you notice a plateau or a worsening of your MAF test results over time, you'll want to lower your MAF heart rate by five or ten beats for at least a month—then continue at that lower fat max rate until you notice an improvement in test results. There are only two reasons for a decline in aerobic performance: detraining or overly stressful life and exercise patterns. If detraining is the cause, it's going to be quite obvious. Time to get back into the exercise groove and rebuild your aerobic conditioning.

It's common to reach a plateau or experience a regression when you're training regularly. Remember: only do a MAF test when you feel fully rested and energized. But I'm not talking about a slow test result on a bad day. I'm talking about a clear pattern of slow test results and/or feeling slow, sluggish, and generally less peppy during workouts. And hey, if you can't reliably find a good day on which to conduct a proper MAF test every three to four weeks, then this itself might be indicative of overly stressful training patterns.

CHAPTER 7
The Genetic Imperative to Walk

Let's set endurance performance goals aside for a moment and recognize that walking is the quintessential human form of locomotion and the foundation of a healthful, active lifestyle. Walking helps boost digestion and the assimilation of nutrients; it is directly associated with improved sleep quality; it helps trigger parasympathetic nervous system activity and thus improves stress management; it improves glucose regulation; it helps boost the production of anabolic hormones such as testosterone, human growth hormone, sex hormone–binding globulin, insulin-like growth factor 1, and DHEA; and it generally promotes homeostasis.

Walking makes you feel alert and energized instead of fatigued, hungry, and depleted. It helps regulate mood, appetite, and alertness all day long—no crash-and-burn effects, as there are in the hours after strenuous workouts. Walking hones metabolic flexibility, so you can lose excess body fat the right way and keep it off forever. Chronic cardio often does the opposite, promoting carbohydrate dependency and flipping the genetic switches for muscle loss, bone loss, and fat storage. Walking makes you supple, mobile and flexible—unlike chronic cardio, which makes you creaky, achy, stiff, and sore. You are highly unlikely to develop a stress fracture, tendinitis, IT band syndrome, chondromalacia ("runner's knee"), shin splints, or plantar fasciitis—even from extensive walking—but you can virtually guarantee that this carnage will happen to you, and happen over and over again, if you run. Walking is in fact the primary way to recover from any type of overuse or acute injury as well as from illness and surgery. Yet these benefits rarely receive the attention lavished on the benefits of getting buffed, toned, and sculpted by bestselling, highly strenuous fitness regimens.

The health benefits of walking are legion. They accrue with short, frequent walks as well as with long walks and hikes. Any time you have a few minutes to spare, walking is a fantastic way to generate an immediate boost in energy, mood, musculoskeletal health, and cognitive performance. Making small shifts in daily routines and habits that enable you to take more daily steps can deliver a phenomenal range of physical and cognitive benefits, especially in the following areas.

Brain and Cognition

The connection between walking and brain health is tremendous. Walking boosts the production of an important protein called brain-derived neurotrophic factor, or BDNF. BDNF has been shown to help improve neuron firing, build new neurons, increase blood circulation and oxygen delivery, help prevent cognitive decline, alleviate symptoms of depression and anxiety, and improve neuroplasticity, the brain's ability to form new connections and pathways. Harvard psychiatrist John J. Ratey, MD, calls BDNF "Miracle-Gro for the brain." Furthermore, a brief morning stroll is a reliable way to optimize your circadian rhythm and boost mood-elevating hormones such as dopamine, serotonin, and norepinephrine. This tees you up for a happy, productive day and sets the stage for the hormonal processes that promote restful sleep at night.

When walking becomes a lifelong habit, the hippocampus and other areas of your brain grow thicker, a sign of improved memory formation and consolidation and improved resistance to cognitive decline. A widely publicized 2017 study conducted at UCLA, which compared the MRI scans of active and inactive people over the age of sixty, revealed that active folks have bigger, better brains than inactive folks. Study subjects who walked more than 1.8 miles a day have faster brain processing speed, better working memory for quick decisions, and better memory consolidation than inactive folks. The bilateral hippocampal volume in the active group was 12 percent more than that of the less active group. In his book *The Real Happy Pill*, Swedish researcher Dr. Anders Hansen reports that just taking a daily walk can reduce your risk of dementia by 40 percent.

The popular notion that walking helps with creative thinking and problem-solving has been strongly borne out by research. A prominent Stanford University study revealed that walking can increase creative output by an astonishing 60 percent. Walking stimulates something called divergent thinking, which allows you to ponder numerous scenarios and solutions in a free-flowing manner. Researchers speculate that walking challenges executive function with the dual task of walking and thinking, which may spur a boost in creativity by "relaxing inhibitory competition among memories and allowing ideas with low levels of activation to push through." I can confidently say that I've done some of my best "writing" on long hikes. Reflecting on my projects from a distance has stimulated fresh ideas and perspectives that I jump on as soon as I return to the keyboard.

Mental Health

Walking helps alleviate depression symptoms and contributes to improved quality of life scores. A three-phase study published by the American Psychological Association showed that a twelve-minute walk delivered a boost in happiness, energy, focus, and self-confidence in comparison to sitting, even when participants weren't interested in walking and had no expectation of such an effect. Walking in nature has particularly potent mental health benefits, as evidenced by the increasing popularity of forest bathing in Japan and even in the United States. Strolling through nature has been proved to prompt a reduction in stress hormones, boost immune function, alleviate depressive symptoms, and curb rumination, which is considered destructive behavior. Doctors are now prescribing forest bathing as a legitimate treatment for a variety of mental and physical health conditions.

Fat Metabolism

Walking trains your body to efficiently burn free fatty acids for fuel. It's low-intensity, so it uses fat as its predominant energy source, but it is far more metabolically demanding than sitting. Metabolic stimulation from walking and other low-level, purely aerobic activities helps you burn fat twenty-four hours a day and stabilizes mood, energy levels, blood glucose, and appetite. A Harvard University study revealed that an hour a day of brisk walking minimizes the influence of obesity-promoting genes. Studies conducted at the University of Exeter showed that a mere fifteen-minute stroll can reduce both cravings and the intake of chocolate and other sweets.

Immune Function

Regular walking increases blood circulation, delivers anti-inflammatory benefits, counters the inflammatory effects of sitting, and strengthens your antibodies. Just a few minutes of walking increases the number of immune cells in your leukocytes and boosts white blood cell production, making you more resilient against cold and flu. One study of a thousand subjects showed a 43 percent reduction in sick days among those who walked a minimum of twenty minutes a day five days a week.

Disease Prevention

Assorted studies reveal that everyday walking can greatly reduce the risk of heart disease and strokes. It can also minimize hospitalizations and the duration of hospital stays, lower blood pressure and resting heart rate, and reduce diabetes risk. A six-year study conducted at the University of North Carolina–Chapel Hill involving more than sixteen thousand women ages sixty and up revealed a 32 percent decrease in disease risk among subjects who walked at least two thousand steps a day. Every increase of one thousand steps a day was associated with a 28 percent decrease in mortality risk. Interestingly, the health and disease prevention benefits of walking seem to plateau at 4,500 steps a day. This suggests that we should focus on finding small opportunities to increase daily walking and not get discouraged about falling short of the arbitrary ten-thousand-step edict (see page 199).

Musculoskeletal Function

Walking strengthens muscles, bones, joints, and connective tissue. This reduces the risk of falling, which is the leading cause of injury and death in Americans over the age of sixty-five. Walking also builds a foundation that enables you to engage in brief, explosive high-intensity exercise that might otherwise be too difficult for unfit individuals to attempt. Regular walking also helps alleviate arthritis pain and reduces the likelihood of developing arthritis by keeping joints and connective tissue well lubricated. Walking with minimalist footwear and using proper form can help you reorganize faulty biomechanics and become more efficient. This can help you naturally and safely alleviate chronic conditions such as foot and low back pain.

Mitochondrial Function

Walking may not give you the immediate sense that you're on your way to awesome fitness, but it's an incredibly effective way to increase the number of oxidative enzymes inside your mitochondria. Exercising below fat max heart rate still provides sufficient oxygen to stimulate lots of mitochondria, strengthening them in the process. The oxidative enzymes in your mitochondria improve the metabolic function of your skeletal muscles, boosting fat and carbohydrate metabolism and improving the rate of adenosine triphosphate energy production. Having abundant oxidative enzymes improves performance and provides greater protection against oxidative stress at all exercise intensities—recall the description of the ways in which your aerobic system can nurture the anaerobic system on pages 147 and 151.

Unlike low-level aerobic exercise, which involves plenty of oxygen and lots of mitochondria, high-intensity exercise will burn glucose without the need to involve mitochondria—this is known as anaerobic metabolism. You're in a hurry (literally!), so you just need some energy—lots of energy—quickly, and you can't go to the trouble to burn energy cleanly and efficiently. Remember the contrasting campfires—the glowing logs of aerobic metabolism and the twigs and newspaper of anaerobic metabolism. When you go anaerobic, you generate ATP more quickly, but you also generate more free radicals, lactic acid, and elevated ammonia levels in the blood because of the disassembling and deamination of cellular proteins. This is why it takes longer to recover from a sprint workout than a walk.

Well-functioning mitochondria can help manage the free-radical load resulting from intense exercise by spreading the burden to lots of other mitochondria. Understand that the cellular stress of high-intensity exercise also stimulates mitochondrial biogenesis in its aftermath. However, it does so by lighting up completely different message-signaling pathways from the ones aerobic activity activates. Both low- and high-intensity exercise turn on a "master switch" called PgC1α, which triggers a favorable rise in mitochondrial density and oxidative enzyme activity. So we have an urgent need to engage in both low-intensity cardio and high-intensity strength and sprint workouts for maximum mitochondrial health.

Your exercise patterns are a key driver of mitochondrial health, but diet and other lifestyle factors also exert a big influence. If an unfit, inactive person eats too many carbohydrates, this promotes a pattern of bypassing mitochondria and burning mostly sugar—like an inefficient power plant that burns coal and spews smoke. The same thing happens when you engage in chronic cardio, which can damage mitochondria and promote sugar burning even after you've finished one of those depleting workouts. In these cases, mitochondria can atrophy or become dysfunctional. This makes you prone to oxidative damage not only from exercise stress but also from all forms of life stress.

By contrast, a healthy aerobic system turns you into a high-production solar power plant made up of capillaries and mitochondria. It enables mitochondrial biogenesis to occur from anaerobic activity, too. That's right: walking supports your performance and recovery from explosive activity such as sprinting and lifting weights as well as endurance performance at high intensities.

Sitting Is the New . . . Path to More Sitting, Inflammation, Obesity, Musculoskeletal Dysfunction, and Stupidity

A lack of walking and everyday movement in general is one of the most serious and obvious health problems of modern life. As author Rebecca Solnit writes in her book *Wanderlust*, "Walking as a cultural activity, as a pleasure, as travel, as a way of getting around, is fading, and with it goes an ancient and profound relationship between body, world, and imagination." We are significantly less physically active than our parents' and grandparents' generations were: consider Amish farmers still operating in a traditional manner today: they walk nearly four times more than their high-tech counterparts. Doctors and fitness gurus urge us to take a minimum of ten thousand steps daily—around five miles—a lofty guideline that most Americans fall well short of. Interestingly, this widely promoted edict has been revealed to be both arbitrary and completely unsubstantiated by research. The idea that one should take ten thousand steps a day was concocted by a Japanese pedometer company in 1964 as part of an advertising campaign. It seems the Japanese character for the number 10,000 resembles the lower body of a striding human; hence the device was called the ten-thousand-step meter.

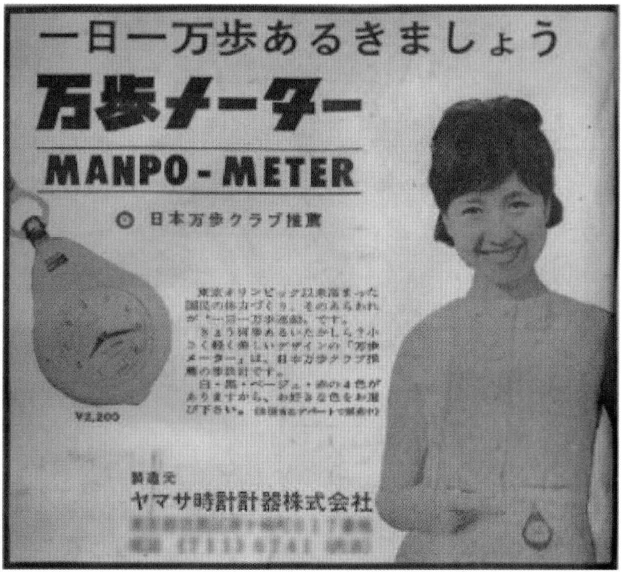

The recommendation to take ten thousand steps a day is arbitrary, originating from a 1964 Japanese advertising campaign for a pedometer.

While residents of pedestrian-friendly nations such as Australia and Switzerland routinely do reach the lofty ten-thousand-steps-daily count, Americans take only half that number of steps, qualifying them as a clinically sedentary population. While the ten-thousand-step public service message is well intentioned, many folks are so deficient that setting such a high bar may have the opposite effect—intimidating those individuals and discouraging efforts at more frequent movement.

Walking doesn't have to be a strenuous, time-consuming endeavor that you squeeze into an already busy schedule. One prominent study revealed that the health benefits of walking in short stints throughout the day and taking a lengthy daily walk are similar—as long as the steps are a daily habit. Dr. Haitham Ahmed of the Cleveland Clinic says, "Even just going up the stairs instead of using the elevator or going on short walks throughout the day will increase your step count and also add cumulative aerobic exercise. This has tremendous benefits over the long term." Dr. Thomas Frieden, former director of the Centers for Disease Control and Prevention, contends that "physical activity is the closest thing we have to a wonder drug."

Walking and other forms of general everyday movement are more conducive to longevity and disease prevention than adhering to a strict fitness regimen.

Indeed, many other health experts now contend that walking and other forms of general everyday movement are more conducive to longevity and disease prevention than adhering to a strict fitness regimen. Of course, when you stay fit, you enjoy the best of both worlds—an acceptable baseline level of activity combined with the massive benefits of a workout regimen, such as increasing muscle mass, increasing VO2 max, enhancing aerobic fitness, and enjoying the many social and psychoemotional benefits of a fitness lifestyle. While it might seem illogical that merely getting up and walking around the block can score longevity points in the same manner as hitting it hard at the gym and logging impressive road miles, it is nevertheless true. Walking is an absolute human necessity, regardless of how fit you are. Furthermore, devoted fitness enthusiasts who live otherwise sedentary lifestyles are are not immune to the cellular dysfunction and metabolic disease patterns driven by inactivity. This phenomenon is known as active couch potato syndrome.

A 2022 Finnish study classified 3,702 participants in four categories based on activity levels. These were (1) active couch potatoes, people who work out regularly but have the least light activity time and the most sedentary time—more than ten hours a day; (2) sedentary light movers, who don't work out but do more light activities and have less sedentary time than active couch potatoes; (3) sedentary exercisers, who work out regularly but log less light activity time than sedentary light movers; and (4) movers, who work out regularly, move the most, and sit the least. Of course the latter had the best cardiometabolic health markers, but guess who had the worst? Yep—the active couch potatoes. But before people in the other sedentary categories pat themselves on the back, let's acknowledge that virtually all of us in the modern world are at elevated risk of disease and dysfunction resulting from insufficient daily movement. Furthermore, fitness freaks may not gloat: research clearly indicates that you cannot escape these risks by running for thirty or even sixty miles a week or by hitting the gym every morning for a group class or a circuit of weight machines.

Think about it: even people with the most impressive dedication to fitness and athletic training are working out for perhaps ten or, in extreme cases, twenty or more hours a week. With 168 hours in a week, and sleep ideally occupying around fifty-six of those hours, we are talking about more than one hundred hours in which we have the chance to support health with movement or compromise it with stillness.

How many people do you know—athletic or otherwise—who are doing a stellar job at this today? James Levine, MD, PhD, a Mayo Clinic researcher, international expert on obesity, and author of *Get Up! Why Your Chair Is Killing You and What You Can Do About It*, reports that the average Westerner working in an office environment sits for some thirteen hours a day, including commuting, working, and leisure time; sleeps for eight hours; and moves only for three. The 2018 Nielsen Total Audience Report revealed that "American adults spend over 11 hours per day listening to, watching, reading, or generally interacting with media." The Kaiser Family Foundation reported in 2010 that youth between the ages of eight and eighteen consume entertainment media for seven hours and thirty-eight minutes a day and that they multitask to the extent that they accumulate ten hours and forty-five minutes of total screen time daily. This includes the hotshots on varsity soccer and swim teams who practice two to three hours a day.

I've said that endurance training is not natural and can easily be overly stressful and health-destructive, but it's also important to acknowledge that stillness is not natural, either, and further, that it is highly health-destructive. The mandate to move more frequently might be especially applicable to devoted fitness enthusiasts because many seem to give themselves free passes to a life of leisure and inactivity when they're not pursuing their impressive workout regimens. Chronic-cardio enthusiasts have long been fond of cashing in on those free passes. It's been a celebrated aspect of running culture for decades to throw down your Sunday morning twenty-miler, then relax with beer, chips, and guacamole and watch the NFL the rest of the day. The "lazy athlete" phenomenon not just intentional and celebratory. The inclination to be lazy in daily life is also driven by hormone signaling and subconscious survival programming at the genetic level. Overexercising drives laziness and overeating as the body attempts to survive what it perceives to be a life-or-death situation: expending excess energy in daily activities.

What's the big deal about sitting in front of a screen all day, especially if we dutifully put in our miles and our gym sessions? The answer is that prolonged periods of stillness have been shown to inhibit cognitive function, metabolism, and regulation of energy and mood. For example, sitting for just twenty minutes has been shown to generate a significant decrease in glucose tolerance and an increase in insulin resistance. If you don't get up and move, you may soon crave quick-energy processed carbohydrates, especially if you drifted a little—or a lot—over your fat max heart rate during that twenty-miler. Also, sitting for hours during a typical workday has been found to prompt a 50 percent reduction in the enzyme activity that converts triglycerides, the stored form of fat, into free fatty acids that the body can burn for energy.

Sitting also interferes with leptin signaling between the brain and the digestive system. Leptin is a key hormone that regulates appetite, satiety, fat metabolism, and reproductive functions. Along with insulin, it's considered a "master hormone" for wide-ranging metabolic and hormonal function. Leptin exerts a strong influence on other appetite hormones such as ghrelin, which triggers hunger, and CCK, which conveys a sense of satiety and influences the speed of digestion. Leptin also influences the production and distribution of sex hormones and is involved in the processes that increase bone density. Compromised leptin signaling causes us to eat more food, be less active, and store more fat. When stillness becomes a habit, you experience chemical changes in your brain that beget further inactivity and increased inflammatory processes throughout the body. These reactions to stillness are your body's futile, confused, and misguided efforts to achieve the energy stabilization that naturally results from activity in daily life. For example, increased inflammatory processes burn energy, but this is an unhealthful way to allocate the body's resources, unlike the aforementioned wide-ranging health benefits of burning energy through walking.

Prolonged periods of stillness have been shown to inhibit cognitive function, metabolism, and regulation of energy and mood.

The diminished cognitive function caused by prolonged stillness occurs because the aforementioned rapid-onset metabolic disturbances trigger a reduction in blood flow and oxygen delivery to the brain as well as impaired neurotransmitter signaling, which can create mood disturbances and depression. Research on the concept of sustained attention reveals that we can only sustain around twenty minutes of intense focus and peak cognitive performance until we require a break to zone out. If you don't stop what you're doing, get up, and move around a bit every twenty minutes, "breaks" will be automatically happen anyway in the form of diminished concentration, focus, and willpower. You'll jump from working on your important PowerPoint presentation to scrolling on social media, answering text messages, or watching entertaining YouTube videos.

It's also extremely beneficial to give your eyes a break from sustained focus on a fixed-distance screen, which essentially puts your ocular muscles into spasm, especially if you're wearing prescription glasses. Over time, this will accelerate visual decline and make you more reliant upon ever-stronger prescription lenses. So during your break time, make a concerted effort to gaze at distant objects, ideally while outdoors looking at the horizon—or at least looking out a window at the horizon. Shift your gaze from long distance to objects at medium distance and short distance, then back to long distance. Also alternate between precise focus on a single object and a more relaxed gaze that incorporates your peripheral vision.

If hours of unbroken desk work and screen time become a habit, you can experience long-term damage to the brain's temporal lobes, which are responsible for memory. Research has confirmed a direct link between inactivity and diminished brain functioning as well as an elevated risk of dementia. The group in the UCLA study who failed to accumulate a minimum daily step count had thinner hippocampi, slower processing speeds, inferior working memory for quick decisions, and inferior memory consolidation compared to their active counterparts.

Sitting Is a Pain in the Butt, Too

Beyond the metabolic and cognitive drawbacks, prolonged sitting is obviously highly destructive to your fitness pursuits and overall musculoskeletal and cardiovascular health. Hip flexors and hamstrings shorten and tighten. Gluteal muscles are deactivated, making your balance and gait unstable during exercise. The lack of engagement of abdominal core muscles promotes an assortment of postural imbalances and puts excessive strain on the spine and back. By contrast, core muscles are constantly activated when standing, walking, squatting—the default resting position for humans throughout history and for the majority of the global population today—and performing all manner of physical work.

As Katy Bowman explains in her book *Move Your DNA*,

> Cells are always responding to mechanical input via a process called mechanotransduction. When individual cells are unmoved or under-moved, they adapt to repetitive positioning by changing their cellular makeup and literally becoming sticky and stiff. Even those

> who are superfit can have certain muscles and joints with reduced range of motion and an actual hardening of arterial walls in certain areas; for example, sitting in a chair all day with bent knees.

It's indeed possible to possess excellent cardiovascular fitness and poor cardiovascular health at the same time. Witness the alarming number of elite and serious amateur endurance athletes who have developed serious heart problems or even suffered from sudden death by heart attack. Just because you can engorge your heart and specific muscles with blood as you execute repetitive athletic maneuvers such as running thirteen miles doesn't mean you won't develop stiff cells, joints, and connective tissue and weak, dysfunctional muscles from sedentary lifestyle patterns.

But when you give your cells optimal, evolutionarily honed inputs such as walking frequently every day, regularly loading the muscles with resistance training, and occasionally performing brief, explosive sprints, you experience an assortment of benefits from mechanotransduction. Bones, joints, tendons, and muscles become strong, supple, and fluid. You send signals for increased protein synthesis, recover more quickly from workouts, become more resilient to all forms of life stress, and reduce your risk of cardiovascular disease and dysfunction. Perhaps most interesting of all, your patterns of movement beget more movement—naturally, spontaneously, and intuitively. They say there are no secrets to losing weight and keeping it off, but this insight qualifies as a secret. Make a concerted effort to move every day, and it becomes easier to move naturally. This is validated by Newton's first law: An object in motion stays in motion, and an object at rest stays at rest.

Movement Makes Us Human

The idea that our genes crave movement is a fundamental tenet of evolutionary biology. We have a genetic imperative to be engaged in near-constant low-intensity movement throughout the day in order to be healthy. This has been hardwired in us through two million years of evolutionary selection pressure. Moving supports the complex and synchronous interactions between organs and systems throughout the body that make us healthy, strong, resilient, and adaptable to all manner of stress. For perspective, consider the contrasting genetic imperative of *Panthera leo*—the lion—who has evolved to sleep or rest for an average of twenty-one hours a day. This conservation of energy, especially during the heat of the day, since lions have poor cooling mechanisms, allows these apex predators to launch powerful, explosive, and brief all-out attacks on prey when the time is right. After a big feast, lions are known to crash out for twenty-four hours. The lion sleeping her days away and feasting occasionally is a lion living her best life.

But living *our* best life entails making a concerted effort to put one foot in front of the other so we can minimize the negative effects of commuting, office work, and leisure-time screen entertainment. Go ahead and pursue goals such as five thousand or ten thousand steps a day if you like, but I also urge to you to make a fundamental shift in your beliefs and behavior patterns and regard walking as much more than a fitness to-do list item: rather, it is a big part of what makes you a healthy human.

Regard walking as much more than a fitness to-do list item: rather, it is a big part of what makes you a healthy human.

If you're an endurance runner, you can take comfort knowing that walking can be an integral and valuable component of your training, just as Kipchoge's leisurely eight-minute miles are for him. If you've been too intimidated to join your pals in pursuit of running goals such as the annual half-marathon or marathon in your city, now you can confidently make a foray into the scene. Ditto if you're one of the many frustrated and often-injured runners who are on the verge of giving up or have already given up on the sport. Instead of heading out the door and right into the fast lane toward burnout and injury, you can instead safely build a robust aerobic base with extensive walking. Then you carefully increase your running competency by going "long" once a week. You might start with just a few miles and escalate sensibly over time until you can run for an hour or even two hours. As you have learned, it's best to stay below fat max heart rate on these runs—whatever pace that correlates to (yeah, it might be walking). However, if you're getting swept into running culture and insist on keeping pace with others, it's okay to exceed fat max once in a while. The big problems of chronic cardio are driven by exceeding fat max routinely for a bit or a lot during most workouts.

If you're intimidated by the hassle or additional time burden of trying to accumulate a certain step count, especially if you're a hard-core runner who likes to cash in your sedentary-time passes, you can take comfort knowing that sprinkling in even the shortest breaks adds up to tremendous success over time. Let's be clear that you cannot bypass this genetic imperative by crushing a 7:00 a.m. interval workout and then being chained to your desk the rest of the day. Nor can you bypass it by biohacking your butt off with cold-water plunges, red-light panels, intermittent fasting, ketogenic eating, or a cupboard full of performance supplements. If you want a fighting chance at being healthy and avoiding the prevailing disease patterns of modern life, you have to JFW—just f*cking walk.

Frequent low-level movement prompts the genetic signals for optimal metabolic, immune, cognitive, and hormonal function in the Homo sapiens species. This is validated by research involving the Hadza peoples in Tanzania, one of the last remaining hunter-gatherer societies on earth—around 1,300 strong. The Hadza walk 3.7 to nine miles each day. They track animals, gather and prepare food, transport water and supplies, build shelters and tend to camps, make tools and fires, and engage in leisure-time play, dance, and other active endeavors. We're talking nineteen thousand steps a day for the males and thirteen thousand for females. By contrast, "sitting is the new smoking" research reveals that prolonged periods of stillness trigger the genetic switches for chronic system-wide inflammation—yep, the same condition caused by excessive exercise, processed foods, and overly stressful lifestyles.

Herman Pontzer, PhD, evolutionary anthropologist at Duke University, author of the book *Burn*, and one of the world's leading experts on energy expenditure in humans and other primates, explains that stillness leaves our cells confused and agitated so that the energy we are designed to burn through basic movement and exercise gets reallocated into overactive inflammatory processes and stress reactivity. This assertion is supported by the groundbreaking premise advanced in Dr. Pontzer's book that humans burn around the same number of calories every day regardless of activity level. This idea, known as the constrained total energy expenditure model, replaces the flawed foundational premise of the fitness industry—the additive energy expenditure model—in which we calculate our basal metabolic rate and count on the extra calories burned during workouts to help us lose weight.

Dr. Pontzer and his team's groundbreaking 2017 research among the Hadza delivered a surprising and shocking conclusion: a highly active Hadza adult burns no more energy than the average desk-working, TV-watching modern citizen. As Dr. Pontzer explained, "The similarity in [total energy expenditure, or TEE—the amount of calories we burn in day] among Hadza hunter-gatherers and Westerners suggests that even dramatic differences in lifestyle may have a negligible effect on TEE." The only adjustments are for body mass and muscle mass: obviously, a large-framed, muscular person will burn proportionally more calories than a small, light, less muscular person will.

Stillness leaves our cells confused and agitated so that the energy we are designed to burn through basic movement and exercise gets reallocated into overactive inflammatory processes and stress reactivity.

How can it possibly be that we burn as many calories by sitting on the subway and in the office as the Hadza do on their hunting excursions? First, the ravenous human brain burns 20 percent of our daily calories. The liver and heart have high burn rates, too. The thermic effect of food accounts for around 10 percent of our total caloric expenditure. That is, if you consume one thousand calories, it takes one hundred calories to digest that food. When it comes to protein, the thermic effect can be as much as 25 percent.

Exercise obviously burns extra calories, but we engage in a variety of compensations to keep us under the TEE ceiling. For example, a Tour de France cyclist is so energy-efficient that pedaling for one hundred miles doesn't require nearly as many calories as a recreational rider setting out to pedal one hundred miles. The less fit you are, the more energy it takes to climb a flight of stairs or walk your dog around the block. We must also acknowledge that if we are insufficiently active, triggering systemic inflammation around the clock is also metabolically expensive. These insights should be sufficient for you to acknowledge once and for all that calorie counting for weight loss is complete folly, and you are better off focusing your efforts on being more active.

Dr. Pontzer uses a firefighter analogy to describe the adverse compensation mechanisms triggered by sedentary patterns. We want the fire department—our innate and adaptive immune systems and inflammatory mechanisms—to be ready at all times to battle pathogens, infections, and acute injury and illness. However, we don't want the crew hanging around our house every day, rushing up our staircases and bashing in our doors for sport because they're bored by a lack of actual emergency calls. Overactive immune and inflammatory mechanisms, i.e., bored firefighters blowing off steam, are what drive autoimmune conditions, neurodegenerative diseases, and assorted other inflammation-driven diseases and dysfunctions.

I realize it's tough to wrap your head around the concept that those of you who log fifty miles a week and those of you who just walk the dog around the block share a TEE ceiling. Consider Dr. Pontzer's explanation: "Reproduction, repair, growth, and locomotion are a zero-sum game." If you locomote to excess with chronic cardio, you will automatically turn down the other dials in order to limit your total energy expenditure. These compensations can manifest themselves as delayed recovery, increased injury frequency, reduced libido, a slightly colder body temperature, and a reduced dopamine response, meaning less motivational or celebratory energy.

Elite female athletes with very low body fat offer an extreme example of the zero-sum game. Their arduous training regimens, especially when combined with restrictive dieting, can cause body fat levels to fall under a safe threshold and prompt amenorrhea—the cessation of menstruation. Whether or not a female athlete is interested in fertility at a given time, we must acknowledge that reproductive fitness is the most prominent genetic and biological imperative of humans. Our evolutionary purpose—the essence of our existence—is to survive the forces of selection pressure (namely, starvation and predator danger) long enough to be able to reproduce. Everything else, including the pursuit of longevity, can be accurately classified as secondary. Females and males who overtrain to the point of diminished libido and impaired reproductive function are unhealthy by the most simple and profound evolutionary measure.

You have a species-specific imperative to move that's just as important as your imperative to sleep.

Making Like Thoreau

Let's pause at this juncture for an important commercial: it's essential that you grok the need to walk—to understand thoroughly and intuitively that you have a species-specific imperative to move that's just as important as your imperative to sleep. No, you won't experience life-threatening symptoms and eventually death if you don't walk for a week, as will happen with sleep deprivation, but you'll compromise your pursuit of health, vitality, and longevity—just as you will by smoking, eating junk food, and engaging in other adverse lifestyle practices.

Obviously, few among us will volunteer to ditch the sedentary aspects of modern life for an existence inspired by Henry David Thoreau, who famously walked the talk: "I think that I cannot preserve my health and spirits, unless I spend four hours a day at least—and it is commonly more than that—sauntering through the woods and over the hills and fields, absolutely free from all worldly engagements." If your schedule is a bit too full to squeeze in daily four-hour jaunts over hills and fields, it's comforting to realize that correcting the problems associated with a stillness-dominant lifestyle is much more doable and less time-intensive than you might imagine—it's certainly easier than adhering to a serious workout regimen.

However, because we are so deeply dependent on comfort, convenience, and modern transportation for our daily routines, we are obligated to go out of our way to orchestrate artificial walking opportunities. Kelly Starrett, leading sports physical therapist and bestselling author of *Built to Move* and *Becoming a Supple Leopard*, would park his car a mile away from the elementary school his daughters attended just so he and wife, Juliet, could walk with them every morning—missing the traffic jam at the drop-off line to boot. The Starretts also initiated a campaign to get standing desks into their daughters' elementary school classrooms and formed a charity called Stand Up Kids to get fifteen thousand kids standing in classes throughout America.

Even brief breaks from prolonged periods of stillness can deliver huge metabolic, hormonal, and cognitive benefits. This means getting up and moving for just a minute or two after every twenty minutes of deep cognitive focus in front of a screen—ideally, outdoors in the sunlight, fresh air, and open space. This also means getting out for a walk after dinner: one Mayo Clinic study revealed that a leisurely (one mile per hour) fifteen-minute postprandial stroll cuts the typical two-hour postmeal glucose spike in half. And it means that if you own a dog, you sure as heck should honor your commitment to caring for the animal by getting out for at least a couple of short walks each day—regardless of weather or your own motivation levels.

Dr. James Levine cites research suggesting that performing an activity as simple as standing up at your desk instead of sitting increases caloric expenditure by 10 percent, while taking frequent movement breaks during the day can add up to an additional thousand calories burned or more. Because of the TEE ceiling, this extra thousand calories a day is not going to help you lose two pounds of body fat a week for months on end. Instead, being more active in this manner might prompt a reduction in sitting-induced inflammation and send the body signals to burn fat instead of store it. A 2022 meta-analysis published in *Sports Medicine* revealed that intermittent light-intensity walking throughout the day lowered blood glucose levels by 17 percent and that walking for as little as two minutes after a meal can help control blood sugar.

THE REAL SECRETS OF THE BLUE ZONES

You've likely heard of the blue zones—places around the globe where researchers have identified pockets of long-lived populations and analyzed the reasons for the residents' longevity. Often we hear that a plant-based diet is a big factor, but blue zones advocates have been roundly criticized for cherry-picking and misrepresenting this assertion. Dr. Paul Saladino, author of *The Carnivore Code*, calls the plant-based angle propaganda, citing evidence that well-sourced animal products are a centerpiece of blue zone diets and that some researchers have admitted to editorializing about plant-based lifestyles. If you come across completely unsubstantiated assertions from blue zones researchers such as "A cup of beans a day could add two to three years to your life" and "It's very clear that the more meat you eat, the earlier you die," that's your cue to run screaming in the other direction. And by the way, Hong Kong residents have the world's highest meat consumption per capita as well as the world's longest life expectancy.

Dr. Saladino and others further argue that blue zone longevity could be most strongly influenced by other factors. For example, blue zone residents likely have favorable genetic attributes in the form of SNPs—single nucleotide polymorphisms. SNPs are variants in DNA sequences that affect gene expression, so folks like the Okinawans—global exemplars of longevity well before the blue zones were identified—likely possess advantageous SNPs. Granted, genetic blessings might help blue zone residents make the most of their many positive lifestyle behaviors, such as eating natural, nutritious, unprocessed foods (Okinawans eat more meat than the Japanese average, incidentally) and being active and social.

The true magic of the five societies originally profiled by blue zone research—located in Sardinia, Italy; Okinawa, Japan; the Nicoya Peninsula, in Costa Rica; Ikaria, Greece; and Loma Linda, California—are that their lifestyles are centered on extensive everyday movement and strong social connections. The blue zones demographers developed a Power 9 list that they describe as a "cross-cultural distillation of best practices . . . a shorthand for the Blue Zones approach." First on the list is "move naturally," which means that people in blue zones live "in environments that constantly nudge them into moving." Blue zones folks have gardens, walk to errands and social occasions, and either eschew or have no access to modern transportation.

A 2020 study conducted by the National Institutes of Health and the Centers for Disease Control and Prevention validated the importance of walking for longevity. The study, published in the

Journal of the American Medical Association, revealed that people who take more than eight thousand steps a day reduced all-cause mortality by a stunning 51 percent compared to people who take fewer than four thousand steps a day. Taking twelve thousand steps a day produced a 65 percent lower risk. A movement-based lifestyle stands in stark contrast to standard Western lifestyles and the assorted influences that promote stillness as well as social isolation.

Let's hark back to the commentary in part 1 and answer a few rhetorical questions.

- Is walking most appropriate for skinny, superfit, competitive types and inappropriate for most everyone else? Nope: walking is the quintessential human activity, accessible to nearly all of us from the moment we take our first steps as toddlers.
- Does walking trigger compensatory mechanisms and lead to overeating, fat storage, and bone and muscle loss? Nope: in fact walking signals the body to activate its mechanisms for fat reduction and improved fat metabolism.
- Does walking prompt poor technique and increased injury risk if you wear elevated, cushioned shoes? Nope: the risk of injury from walking is inconsequential—indeed, walking is the way to *recover* from overuse injuries. You don't need cushioned shoes for walking, and you can quickly and safely transition to walking in minimalist footwear. This transition will improve foot strength, mobility, and overall efficiency and reduce the injury risk and the chronic foot pain that millions of people suffer from daily.
- Will you increase cardiovascular-disease risk factors by walking too much? Nope: quite the opposite. Walking improves cardiovascular health and reduces disease risk factors.
- Does walking suppress immune function, promote chronic inflammation, compromise gut health, and damage mitochondria? Nope: walking boosts immune and digestive function, strengthens anti-inflammatory processes, and stimulates mitochondrial biogenesis.

- Do you add to your overall life stress by walking? Nope: in fact walking is a fantastic way to alleviate emotional stress, spark creativity, refresh cognitive performance after prolonged periods of focus, trigger parasympathetic nervous system activity, and improve recovery from strenuous workouts or days at the office.
- Is there a registry for people who walk too much and trash their health, as there is for obligate runners? Nope: but there is an impressive list of historical figures and modern cultural leaders who tout walking as a centerpiece of healthful, balanced living and a catalyst for creative energy. Among them are historical figures such as Henry David Thoreau, Friedrich Nietzsche, Albert Einstein, Charles Darwin, Virginia Woolf, Beethoven, Aristotle, Socrates, and John Muir as well as modern notables such as writer Bill Bryson, musician Art Garfunkel (who walked completely across the continental United States in short stints between 1983 and 1997 and has walked across Japan and Europe), Madonna, Heidi Klum, Julia Roberts, and Brooke Shields.
- Does walking interfere with aerobic development and make you a sugar burner? Nope: walking is the essence of aerobic development and delivers excellent results—even if you are superfit and think walking is too easy to improve your aerobic conditioning.
- Is walking the antidote to the stressful and destructive effects of running? That's a little harsh, but the answer is yes.

While walking is perhaps the simplest and most easily accessible way to start, you can also increase your general everyday level of activity by by engaging in formal movement practices such as yoga, Pilates, and tai chi. Other options include anytime-anywhere calisthenics, body-weight resistance exercises—e.g., rattling off some deep squats or logging some plank time while binge-watching a Netflix series—and a morning stretching-flexibility-mobility sequence (search YouTube for "Brad Kearns Morning Routine" for inspiration). Even self-myofascial release (foam rolling) can count toward your movement objective. Integrating this stuff into your daily routine is easy and fun and delivers an instant payoff, reinvigorating mind and body after periods of stillness. You also don't have to hassle the often-challenging logistics of carving out time or getting to a separate venue for a formal workout.

Walking Your Way to Health, Then Fitness

If you are overfat or unhealthy in any way, you most certainly should be walking, not running. Sorry: this is not up for debate. Attempting endurance running—that means anything over a mile or two, per exercise physiology—when you are overweight, overfat, or lack aerobic fitness is unequivocally too stressful to provide meaningful health benefits and will most likely be mildly to significantly destructive to your health. If you have excess visceral fat—a red flag for deficient general health and too much overall life stress—it's time to slow down and get your act together. This might mean getting more sleep, extricating yourself from dysfunctional relationships or jobs, avoiding processed food (including the performance drinks, bars, and gels that fuel your ill-advised endurance runs at chronic-cardio heart rates), and slowing from a jog to a walk.

Granted, I know you may still be able to run a marathon in 4:30 or 3:30, even if you're overfat, unhealthy, immobile, weak, and chronically injured. But whatever accomplishments poorly adapted individuals are able to achieve, we must acknowledge that they are by definition mediocre. Well, not mediocre in comparison to the efforts of the average citizen, who has a 29 VO2 max and who gets winded climbing stairs, but mediocre for the amount of time, energy, heart, and soul dedicated to the endeavor. Remember: mediocrity in something as daunting as a marathon is only made possible by elevated, cushioned shoes and perhaps by the comfortable lifestyles that enable people to spend an excessive amount of energy on workouts instead of toiling on a farm or a factory assembly line.

On the flip side, I'll graciously accept arguments from accomplished runners who have favorable waist-to-height ratios and claim that their passion for running enriches their lives and improves both their fitness and their health. This includes those who have no interest in methodical process, finish times, or the pursuit of excellence but who nevertheless enjoy their time sweating on the road. If it's truly working for you, good on ya. And when I say "truly working," I mean that it brings joy, vitality, health, fitness, excellent blood work, little or no visceral fat, a connection with nature, a sense of adventure and accomplishment, increased confidence, social enrichment, and the like. I don't mean that it works for you on a perverse, dysfunctional level, providing a steady stream of endorphin hits to the point of addiction. Or that it enables you to accumulate free passes and consume indulgent treats and sit around all day after your workout.

If you are overfat or unhealthy in any way, you most certainly should be walking, not running. Sorry: this is not up for debate.

Jogging, even at a slow pace, will quickly prompt an overfat person's heart rate to exceed the aerobic limit and drift into sugar burning—just what one does not want when one is fighting the belly-fat battle. For reference, when I say "slow pace," I'm talking twelve, thirteen, or fourteen minutes per mile. Exercise physiology gait analysis reveals that most people naturally transition from a brisk walking gait to a slow jogging gait at around 4.3 miles per hour—that's a 13:57 mile. If your running pace is close to—or, heaven forbid, slower than—fourteen minutes per mile, slowing down to a walk will reduce impact trauma, and your risk of overuse injury will go from extreme (as it is for all runners, at all speeds) to almost nil. Think about it: most people cannot run significantly faster than they can walk. So why court injury, discomfort, and adverse metabolic consequences for a marginal increase in speed?

I get it: you'd rather jog than walk for the exhilaration, the feel of a good sweat, the sense of accomplishment, and to satisfy some ego demands. I get it when you explain that you still feel "comfortable" when jogging at slightly to significantly anaerobic heart rates, because true discomfort doesn't kick in until you approach anaerobic threshold, marked by labored breathing, a slight burning sensation caused by acid accumulation in the muscles, and a heart rate that's typically twenty to thirty beats above your fat max.

This is the point where we must reject the marketing hype promoting running shoes, the running lifestyle, and inherently health-compromising events such as running 26.2 miles on paved roads and training for an ironman triathlon around a life packed with work and family responsibilities. Essentially, the chronic-cardio crowd is in training to become sugar-burning, sugar-chomping, inflamed, fatigued, overstressed organisms that remain overfat, since weekly mileage logged under a chronic-cardio approach leads directly to the inhalation of Ben & Jerry's pints. I guarantee you that among the 15 percent of the population who were obese in 1974, none of them was out there running. But today there are a great many folks who are carrying excess baggage on the roads and trails.

Running Is Catabolic; Walking Is Anabolic

At all times, your body is engaged in processes that can be described as either anabolic or catabolic. Anabolic processes are involved in the repair and rejuvenation of molecules, and catabolic processes are involved in the breakdown of molecules. Despite the way the terms are often used, it's not that anabolic is good and catabolic is bad; rather, we need to achieve a harmonious balance between the two. Humans actually switch back and forth between anabolic and catabolic processes all day long. This is the essence of the homeostatic drive of all organisms.

Biochemically, the word "anabolic" refers to the assembly of raw materials, such as amino acids, fatty acids, micronutrients, macronutrients, and cellular material, into more complex molecules—replenishing, repairing, and building muscles, organs, and connective tissues. For example, most people recognize that building muscle is an anabolic process, but forming a scab over a wound and eventually sealing it with new skin is also anabolic. Anabolic hormones include testosterone, estrogen, human growth hormone, and insulin, which is responsible for delivering nutrients to cells in order to replenish energy.

The word "catabolic," biochemically, refers to the process of disassembling large, complex molecules and converting them into energy—for example, breaking down ingested carbohydrates or stored glycogen into glucose and breaking down stored triglycerides into free fatty acids and/or ketones. The fight-or-flight response is catabolic—it "liquidates your assets," converting amino acids into glucose (e.g., in the process of gluconeogenesis) for immediate energy needs. Catabolic hormones include cortisol, the various adrenaline-like chemicals, and glucagon, insulin's counterregulatory hormone, which is responsible for liberating energy from storage.

It's not that anabolic is good and catabolic is bad; rather, we need to achieve a harmonious balance between the two.

You'll recall that adenosine triphosphate, or ATP—produced via catabolic reactions in the Krebs cycle, a.k.a. the citric acid cycle—is the energy "currency" stored in cells throughout the body. Well, ATP is also the necessary fuel for anabolic processes. Hence, the Krebs cycle is amphibolic—both catabolic and anabolic. In fact, the anabolic process of synthesizing complex molecules is fueled by energy created through catabolic processes.

Humans can manage catabolic and anabolic processes concurrently and gracefully. For example, it's possible to simultaneously build muscle (an anabolic process) and reduce excess body fat (a catabolic process) by practicing effective eating and exercise habits. It's when overloads and imbalances occur that we run into problems. An anabolic imbalance might be marked by producing too much insulin and storing excess body fat. A person with such an imbalance needs to get out there and burn more calories—trigger more catabolic processes. A catabolic imbalance is marked by overproduction of stress hormones, frequent injuries, and suppressed immune function. A person with this kind of imbalance needs to burn less energy and get more sleep—i.e., nurture more anabolic processes.

By now, it should be clear that chronic cardio is out-of-balance catabolic: you generate an overwhelming number of free radicals, break down muscle tissue, traumatize and inflame connective tissue, and break down lots of fats and carbohydrates to fuel your incessant medium-to-difficult workouts. In a desperate attempt to regain homeostatic balance, the body will often trigger compensatory anabolic processes to excess—overeating, laziness, and fat storage.

Interestingly, although all activity and calorie burning is catabolic, strength training and sprinting are widely characterized as anabolic because they send the necessary signals to initiate anabolic activity afterward. These exercises generate fewer free radicals because the workouts don't last that long. Instead of promoting catabolic imbalances, they prompt an appropriately brief catabolic fight-or-flight response. Consequently, before too much catabolism has occurred, high-intensity workouts send strong genetic signals for anabolic processes to repair and rejuvenate cells and muscle fibers depleted by explosive effort. Similarly, the protein smoothie you drink after a high-intensity workout must be metabolized into amino acids (catabolic), but then the presence of these amino acids causes anabolic building and repairing of lean muscle tissue.

Sleep, like the Krebs cycle, is amphibolic. The body is undergoing lots of anabolic repair and rejuvenation, but you are also burning through available energy stores so that you awaken in a catabolic state until you get your first dose of protein in the morning. Overall, you manufacture and secrete the highest amounts of anabolic hormones such as testosterone and human growth hormone at night. You also rejuvenate the immune system, refresh the sodium-potassium pumps that fire brain neurons, heal injuries, cuts, and other tissue damage, and generally flip on the genetic switches for restoration and rejuvenation with minimal catabolic activity.

Walking can also be characterized as anabolic—technically, an activity that triggers anabolic processes. It is minimally catabolic while prompting anabolic intracellular signaling and mitochondrial biogenesis. With a good foundation of extensive walking and excellent sleep and stress management habits, along with a nutritious diet involving adequate protein consumption, you are poised to flip the big switches for anabolism in the form of high-intensity exercise. If naysayers want to argue that walking is not literally anabolic, we can certainly rephrase this and assert that *not* walking is catabolic. Remember Dr. Pontzer's observation that stillness leaves our cells confused and agitated so that the energy we are designed to burn through basic movement and exercise gets reallocated into highly catabolic overactive inflammatory processes and stress reactivity.

Professor Sisson's Evolutionary Anthropology 2.0

I'm not sayin' that the illustrious evolutionary anthropologists who endorse the endurance running hypothesis are wrong, but as it does in many aspects of science, interpretation can make a huge difference. I am, therefore, going to take exception to the smug assertion that humans prevailed on the food chain because they were able to expertly wear down big game on the hot African savannah after many miles of running. Although we possess the genetic ability to perform such heroic feats under life-or-death pressure, it's preposterous to suggest that this was our go-to way of life. The essence of selection pressure is for a species to conserve energy at all costs in service to the ultimate goals of survival and reproduction. Our hunter-gatherer ancestors intelligently did the bare minimum necessary to survive—nothing more. They didn't know what tomorrow held, so the risks of overextending themselves with epic endurance feats were too great. Furthermore, there was no survival benefit to stockpiling extra hunting bounty or amassing more material possessions than they could carry with them.

Our innate capacity for endurance exercise is impressive, but the human brain takes center stage in our evolutionary journey. The fossil record confirms that our earliest hominin ancestors—dating back six or seven million years—were foragers. Around two million years ago, the first Homo erectus groups were classified as opportunistic scavengers. After the apex predators of the day finished feasting on their kill, our ancestors would drag the leftovers to a safe place and use rudimentary stone tools to harvest the flesh and crack open bones for marrow. They gradually improved their hunting skills with help from the discovery of fire, around one million years ago. There is evidence that around five hundred thousand years ago, we crafted wooden spears and were able to take down big game. We lived as hunter-gatherers for eons until signs of agriculture appeared around ten thousand years ago, when we learned how to cultivate and store grain and, later, livestock. Agriculture enabled humans to become civilized, live in one place and increase population density. The specialization of labor agriculture gave rise to continues with the inexorable technological progress we are experiencing today.

For the past two million years, our ancestors had no consistent need or selection pressure to run long distances on the regular. Instead, they used their brains to walk, hide, climb, sprint, jog, and crawl as they excelled in scavenging and persistence hunting. By the time the first modern Homo sapiens appeared, around two hundred thousand years ago, in East Africa, they were able to deploy quite sophisticated weapons and techniques. This included engaging in deft teamwork and communication to collectively outwit physically superior beasts. Yes, they were still persistence hunters, and the most gifted of them would, like the Greek hemerodromoi, surely threw down some impressive endurance performances now and then (as did the San hunters in *The Great Dance*), but it's undisputed that they weren't doing chronic cardio like a modern mileage junkie. Hence our glorious history of population explosion, successful migration to every corner of the globe, and ascent to the top of the animal kingdom is characterized by getting progressively smarter, not fitter. Oh, and by walking virtually everywhere.

Our glorious history of population explosion, successful migration to every corner of the globe, and ascent to the top of the animal kingdom is characterized by getting progressively smarter, not fitter. Oh, and by walking virtually everywhere.

As I explain and complain about our misappropriation of the endurance running hypothesis into modern fitness-industry marketing hype, I want to remind you of its anthropological validity. Our capacity for endurance, which is vastly superior to that of our ape cousins and all other animals, is attributable to numerous amazing physical attributes, including

- a narrow, upright frame, ideal for bipedal locomotion and evaporative cooling;
- springlike lower extremities;
- huge, powerful glutes;
- short toes with a nonopposable big toe;
- efficient sweat mechanisms;
- short forearms and independent movement of the upper and lower extremities, allowing us to counterbalance running forces with arm swing;
- comparatively large vertebrae and discs for superior shock absorption;
- "decoupled" shoulders and a nuchal ligament, allowing the body to rotate and the head to remain stable during running;
- large surface areas in the hip, knee, and ankle joints for superior shock absorption;
- feet that have incredibly intricate functionality—each one has thirty-three joints as well as a longitudinal arch for excellent shock absorption and propulsion; and
- a strong connection between the pelvis and spine, creating stability.

These attributes evolved under withering selection pressure for a reason: to allow us to capitalize on our fantastically superior brainpower and prevail in survival-of-the-fittest conditions. Please—compare and contrast this history lesson and glorious human evolutionary victory with the utter stupidity of the modern zealots overtraining to the point of stress fractures and arrhythmias. I can't think of a more embarrassing example of misinterpreting and misappropriating our genetic gifts than running oneself into a stress fracture.

In leveraging our brains and our endurance, we were able to persistence-hunt by walking, jogging a bit, sprinting occasionally, and working together. Our hunter-gatherer ancestors could easily spend all day trying to outsmart or outlast a beast at comfortable heart rates, but if they were faced with the prospect of running at an aggressive pace for a long distance—shifting into glycolytic metabolism—this could spell big trouble. Run out of glycogen chasing a beast at anaerobic threshold for too long in the heat, and you become exhausted yourself. If you are lucky enough to bag the beast, at least you get to eat it. But fail in your mission, and your sorry, fatigued, glycogen-depleted butt is now vulnerable to becoming some other beast's dinner. That's a lot worse than today's penalties of an overuse injury or adding some belly fat. Our ancestors were too smart to chase prey for an hour at anaerobic threshold. Besides, any worthwhile prey could easily dash to freedom by running for just a few minutes at speeds vastly superior to that of the fleetest human. Our ancestors most certainly chose strategies other than the Kipchoge 1:59 marathon protocol, or we wouldn't be here today.

The endurance running hypothesis might be better described as the "walking-sprinting-jogging-hiding-climbing-crawling-collaborating-strategizing hypothesis."

The endurance running hypothesis might be better described as the "walking-sprinting-jogging-hiding-climbing-crawling-collaborating-strategizing hypothesis." If you disagree with me, please explain how we got here when so many predators can smoke us six ways to Sunday in the wild. There is no way we led the human evolutionary success story with endurance running.

I contend that the flourishing of the modern running boom and the dreamy "born to run" ideal is a product of modern consumerism constructs: grain-based, high-carbohydrate diets—quite unhealthful, but they do restock glycogen so that you, unlike our ancestors, can run daily, carbo-load, and run again; elevated, cushioned running shoes, enabling the poorly adapted to pound the pavement and the elites to pound the pavement for more miles; and brazenly misappropriated insights about our natural running prowess, inspired by unique populations such as the Tarahumara and the genetic freaks who dedicate their lives to training for Olympic medals and ultramarathon titles. Granted, it's unlikely that any reputable institution will award me a PhD in evolutionary anthropology for these arguments, but I'll defend my thesis against anyone for longer than it takes for today's average marathoner to complete his course.

There is a huge disconnect between the endurance running hypothesis and the way we live today because we are no longer highly active, highly adaptable hunter-gatherers. Influenced by decades of marketing hype, we are trying to exploit our natural endurance gifts in spite of the fact that we've spent too much time on the sidelines. Christopher McDougall tried to deliver words of caution in *Born to Run*, but the message was kinda ignored amid the excitement of discovering, as the titillating subtitle says, *A Hidden Tribe, Superathletes, and the Greatest Race the World Has Never Seen.* In the book, McDougall unwittingly offers support for my walking-sprinting-jogging expertly strategizing man hypothesis, writing that "we're designed for persistence hunting, which is a mix of running and walking."

While celebrating our evolved attributes for running, McDougall also points out that the running boom has led us astray by encouraging bad form (enabled by cushioned shoes) and overly stressful training patterns: "The sense of distance running being crazy is something new to late-twentieth-century America," he remarked to a *New York Times* reporter. "It's only recently that running has become associated with pain and injury." Indeed, it's not McDougall's fault that gung-ho endurance enthusiasts read the book, dropped $125 on some three-millimeter-thin Vibram shoes, and took off in pursuit of ultramarathon finisher medals with woefully dysfunctional feet, poor general fitness, excess visceral fat, unregulated competitive intensity, and a habit of popping too many Advils and energy gels from their fanny packs.

Mount Everest and Endurance Running

The high-cost, high-tech, gizmo-obsessed, carbon-plated, moisture-wicking, biohacking shortcut approach to endurance running reminds me of the mockery that summiting Mount Everest has become today. What was once rightfully considered one of the greatest feats of human endurance has now largely become a joke—a bucket-list item for wealthy, often ill-prepared Westerners—a chance to wave one's flag (or one's expedition sponsor's flag) at the summit and capture an

Instagram moment in the most foolhardy, unsportsmanlike, eco-destructive, and culturally disrespectful approach imaginable.

Since 1953, when Sir Edmund Hillary and Tenzing Norgay first climbed to the top of the 29,032-foot peak in Nepal—the highest point on earth—the endeavor has become increasingly exploited and commercialized. Today, most climbers pay around $60,000 to join an expedition comprising an experienced leader and climbing guides; a support team for communications, meals, and medical care; and extensive labor support from the local Sherpa peoples. Sherpas carry your crap the entire way, make camp for you at several points up the mountain, feed you meals, install a route to the summit with climbing ropes and ladders, and last but not least ply you with a steady supply of oxygen bottles to neutralize the brutal effects of high altitude.

You don't have to qualify for an expedition, as you do in order to race the Hawaii Ironman World Championship. You just have to write a big check. While the majority of climbers are experienced, it's also common for astonishingly unprepared folks to take a crack at it. Get this: a journalist from Los Angeles was assigned to cover an expedition group that was also chronicled in a Discovery Channel television series (2006–2009) called *Everest: Beyond the Limit*. The journalist was stationed at the Everest base camp (elevation 17,598 feet) to observe and interview team members as they made their customary repeat ascents to increasingly high elevations and returns to base camp for gradual altitude acclimation in advance of an eventual summit push.

Base camp is a tent city filled with as many as 1,500 people during peak climbing season, a mix of climbers on summit teams, scientists, doctors, journalists, and hundreds of Sherpa laborers. Some forty thousand lookie-loo trekkers also make the eighty-mile hike from Lukla, Nepal, to base camp to check out the scene each season. The journalist's main protagonist was a motorcycle dude from Los Angeles with no climbing experience, a leg previously shattered in a motorcycle accident and pieced together with hardware, and an incredibly stubborn, delusional, adventurous bent. Think leather-clad urban motorcycle dude parking his Harley, throwing on a parka and an oxygen tank, and trying to climb Mount Everest. He almost got himself and his Sherpas killed with his dangerously slow pace and refusal to turn around after numerous checkpoint deadlines had passed despite several direct orders turned impassioned pleas from the expedition leader. Indeed, everyone's life is on a time clock on Everest. Linger for too long at the highest altitudes and most exposed terrain, and you can die at the hands of a sudden weather shift, a single misstep, or prolonged lack of sufficient oxygen, leading to fatal exhaustion. Hence elevations above twenty-six thousand feet are referred to as the "death zone." Up that high, even if you're breathing bottled oxygen, the brain, heart, lungs, and muscles function so poorly that it's impossible to conduct a rescue operation, and death is imminent unless you can descend under your own power.

Clearly undeterred by chronicling a farce with life-and-death consequences, the journalist was so inspired by her protagonist's grit that she decided to attempt Everest the following year, despite having no high-altitude mountaineering experience. Hiking for two weeks in the Himalayas to base camp is an impressive achievement but not quite résumé fodder for a summit candidate. Expedition leaders grew concerned early on when the journalist put her crampons on backwards. When the time came for the leader to gently inform her that she would not be selected for the cream-of-the-crop summit team, she shed tears and repeatedly begged for a spot.

Another character on the Discovery Channel program showed up at base camp fresh off a succession of thirty knee surgeries. Wouldn't you know it? His flimsy joint became dislocated on the steep slopes, and we watch him writhing in pain in the snow while directing two fellow climbers to yank his leg and pop his knee back into place. After a complicated rescue to get him down to the nearest camp, he, too, begged his leader for another crack at the summit. Beyond the limit indeed—the limit of common sense.

Today, an excessive number of Everest permits are granted by greedy government agencies, meaning that there are too many people on the mountain to ensure safe and orderly climbing. Instead, massive traffic jams typically form on the summit routes, because the weather window for summit attempts is only around three weeks a year—and within that, there are perhaps only a handful of optimal days. That's when numerous teams are compelled to head for the top. These traffic jams significantly increase the perils of an already extremely dangerous endeavor because they force climbers to spend extra time in the death zone.

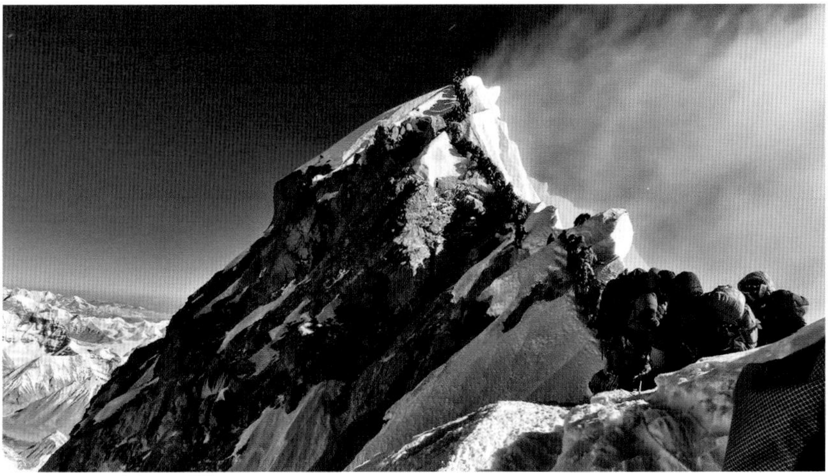

This traffic jam on Mount Everest is a powerful visual reminder of the bastardization of what was once one of the greatest human achievements of all time.

Critics of today's big-business mountaineering point out that the economically disadvantaged Sherpa are being exploited and endangered. They take huge risks on the mountain, in borderline inhumane working conditions, and have no job security. The best Sherpas earn enough to be considered successful in their society, around $15,000 to $20,000 in a climbing season, but it's still a pittance by Western standards. The mountain is a giant garbage dump, too, with literally thousands of discarded oxygen bottles and hundreds of dead bodies strewn along the route; it's too physically strenuous for anyone to remove them safely. The death rate on Mount Everest is around 6 percent, making one wonder why anyone would attempt anything with such poor odds. Since the mysterious disappearance of British climbers George Mallory and Andrew Irvine, in 1924, the first Westerners to attempt Everest, some 340 people died on the mountain in the ensuing one hundred years—including around 130 Sherpas. The popular book and feature film *Into Thin Air* chronicled an unexpected blizzard in May of 1996 that claimed eight lives in a single day, including a couple of the world's most experienced guides.

Interestingly, and perversely, 80 percent of Everest deaths occur on the descent, because climbers expend too much energy and/or spend too much time in the death zone to be able to make it back to base camp. I'm compelled to make a harsh comparison here to the runner who blows through all the warning signs and comes up with a stress fracture: "What were ya thinking?!" On Everest, many seem to forget that the goal is not simply to reach the top of the world but to summit and return to base camp safely. Similarly, the runner's goal should not be to finish a certain race or hit a certain weekly mileage target but to achieve these goals safely and sensibly—without stress fractures.

The runner's goal should not be to finish a certain race or hit a certain weekly mileage target but to achieve these goals safely and sensibly.

My apologies to all dilettante mountaineers who've successfully summited high peaks, but if you're using supplemental bottled oxygen to do so, you're bastardizing the accomplishment. Of the more than six thousand people who've summited Everest, only 219 have done so without using supplemental oxygen. Among them are mountaineering legends Reinhold Messner of Italy and Ed Viesturs of the United States, two of only nineteen people in history to climb all fourteen of the world's eight-thousand-meter peaks without oxygen. Climbing while breathing oxygen from a backpack tank at a rate of two to three liters per minute effectively lowers one's altitude by around five thousand feet. When one is stopped at the top taking photos, the summit feels only half as high with your mask on. Don't get me wrong: it's an incredibly difficult endurance feat to climb Everest, even with oxygen, but we might all wonder: What's the point? As Ed Viesturs noted, "Ninety-nine percent of the people who have climbed Everest would not have climbed Everest without the use of supplemental oxygen. In respect for a 29,000-foot mountain, I try to climb it under its terms. It's not as intriguing if I 'bring the mountain down.'"

Now for the coup de grâce: What's the point of training for a half-marathon or marathon if it's gonna get you injured, fat, and tired?

Might the coveted medal be a less extreme example of the flag-waving summit photo achieved by using supplemental oxygen, exploiting disadvantaged Sherpas, and taking unfathomable risks with potentially devastating consequences? Couldn't you devoted endurance enthusiasts instead resolve to safely and effectively develop an aerobic conditioning base that will allow you to pursue appropriate goals that support health and longevity instead of compromise it? For aspiring Everest climbers, why not marvel at the likes of Messner and Viesturs, who bagged the high peaks in the most honorable, sportsmanlike, and sustainable manner while you endeavor to climb the highest peak in your county or state? For aspiring marathoners, why not let Kipchoge and Sifan Hassan push the limits of human endurance while you enjoy long walks in nature until further notice? Hey—do what you're gonna do, and don't let me stop you from living a brave, adventurous, exciting life. But as you absorb the extreme tales of folly on Everest, consider the satisfaction, contentment, and personal growth to be had from pursuing the most lifestyle-appropriate goals in a safe, sensible, healthy, and respectful manner.

How to Up Your Walking Game

The following suggestions can help you build new walking habits that feel natural, comfortable, and easy to maintain for a lifetime.

Morning Stroll

Resolve to make locomotion your very first act of the day—before you reach for your phone, pour a cup of coffee, or wonder whether you have enough motivation to get out the door. Make the walk short enough to be considered a no-brainer—in the same category as using the bathroom upon awakening. Even if your walk is only five minutes, make a sincere commitment to it. Never skip a day without an unimpeachable reason: this creates momentum, and small behavior changes can gracefully inspire escalating commitments over time. A legit five-minute daily walking habit might just evolve into a seventeen-minute neighborhood loop every day. Lasting habit change requires wiring new neural networks in the brain. You might get to the point where you can't even imagine your morning without a walk.

Taking baby steps requires very little willpower and psychic effort, yet it yields the biggest long-term payoff. And it entails little risk of backsliding.

You'll also be able to train your circadian rhythms if you expose your eyes to direct natural light as soon as you awaken—exactly what our genes have come to expect for two million years. Morning light exposure prompts a boost of energizing, mood-elevating hormones such as cortisol and serotonin. You'll also trigger a concurrent suppression of adenosine and melatonin, both of which can make you feel groggy when they linger in the bloodstream in the morning.

Note that it doesn't have to be sunny for you to experience the benefits of morning light, but you do have to get outdoors so the light isn't filtered through a window. Virtually all glass blocks important UVB rays and inhibits vitamin D production. Even if it's cloudy or rainy, you'll get plenty of natural light exposure and benefit from the positive hormonal effects. With sufficient light exposure in the morning and throughout the day, your circadian rhythms will be poised to initiate hormonal processes that promote winding down and eventual sleepiness in the evening.

It doesn't have to be sunny for you to experience the benefits of morning light, but you do have to get outdoors so the light isn't filtered through a window.

Caffeine acts as a stimulant in large part because it blocks the receptors for adenosine in brain neurons, but natural light can be even more effective than caffeine. Sunlight will help suppress adenosine while prompting a desirable natural spike in cortisol. In fact caffeine's tendency to spike cortisol can be inappropriate when cortisol is already naturally elevated—i.e., in the morning. When caffeine's effects wear off, you can potentially experience an energy dip and develop a dependence on caffeine to get you going again: for example, you might get a headache when you miss your morning cup. It's best to get direct light exposure first thing in the morning and wait one to two hours before drinking your first cup of coffee. This will help you leverage the natural hormonal benefits of light exposure and let you enjoy your coffee with minimal adverse effects.

Canine Companionship

Someone important, fiercely loyal, and deeply appreciative is counting on you. Dog owners, honor yourself and your original commitment to care for an animal by getting out for a morning walk with your canine companion. Dogs love routine, and experts contend that dogs require three outings a day for optimal health. Leash up at the same time every day, and, as if on cue, your dog will come to expect an outing with great anticipation and excitement. This, in turn, gives you the most fantastic accountability partner imaginable.

If occasions arise when you're feeling crunched for time, unmotivated, fatigued, distracted by screen stimulation, or facing inclement weather, gaze into your dog's eyes and explain the reason why you can't make it today. Seriously, try this technique: it can be a highly effective strategy to help change your mind and get you out the door, especially if your dog is inclined to pace around, moan, and scrape on the door at the appointed time. Revel in your dog's joy in the outdoor experience regardless of mud, rain, sleet, snow, and other challenges. Whatever hesitations and trepidations you harbor will be washed away in exuberant canine energy. If you don't have a dog, consider walking a friend's dog, fostering a dog from a local shelter, or signing up as a provider on dog-walking apps such as Rover and Wag!. Do whatever it takes to turn a daily stroll—or three—into a habit.

Orchestrated Obligatory Walking

Most of our natural opportunities to walk have been eliminated by modern comforts and conveniences. Hence we are compelled to orchestrate opportunities to be active—even if it seems silly at first.

- When you enter large parking lots at the mall, supermarket, or big-box store, park in the farthest spot from the entrance and hoof it the rest of the way. You'll save on door dings, too.
- Exit the subway one stop prior to your usual stop and enjoy strolling the extra blocks to your office or home.

- Stop at a park on your commute home, complete a lap, then resume your commute.
- If you work or live in a tall building, make a habit of taking the stairs for the final five, ten, or even twenty floors to your destination. If you live or work in a low-rise, swear off the elevator and make the stairs mandatory—both on the way up *and* on the way down. Descending stairs is great for preserving balance and bone density.
- Incentives are allowed! How about a walk to the local bakery or ice cream store for a treat? Or a walk to another celebratory destination? It's a great way to impress upon kids that effort can be celebrated with reward.

Walking at Work

Expand your idea of what's possible, and make a point of moving more and sitting less during your workday. Resolve to get up and move for a minute or two after every twenty minutes of focused attention, and take longer breaks every two hours—at least five minutes. You'll return to your desk with more energy and brainpower, guaranteed.

Granted, it's often tough to break the flow when you are engrossed in a challenging task or working closely with others. It's also tough to motivate yourself to get up when you have been sitting for a long time, because your resolve and willpower are waning. Consider establishing a series of prompts to set yourself up for success. For example:

- Set alarms that will appear on your screen.
- Post a written reminder to move that's in your visual field all day long.
- Leave important items in your car so you will be forced to retrieve them at some point during the day.
- Take mobile phone calls and join virtual meetings while walking. Even if you have to move really slowly to concentrate and minimize ambient noise, it's vastly superior to being chained to your desk.
- Hold in-person meetings on the move whenever possible, or at least walk to an outdoor seating area.

- If you're in a management position, lead by example: move around the office frequently and being seen doing so. Establish a policy of taking frequent breaks from the screen so it becomes part of team culture. Take a cue from entrepreneur Arianna Huffington, author of *The Sleep Revolution*, who famously used to nap in a glass-walled office in plain view of fellow employees. Her installation of designated napping rooms in the corporate offices of the *Huffington Post* paved the way for many more forward-thinking companies to do the same.

Recovery Walks

Gentle movement can speed your recovery from illness and injury faster than complete rest can. Walking and other low-level activities—e.g., yoga and maintaining an easy pace on a stationary bike, rowing machine, or step machine—have been shown to trigger a boost in parasympathetic nervous system activity, increase heart-rate variability, improve oxygen delivery, boost blood circulation, boost lymphatic function, speed the removal of waste products from fatigued muscles, and generate anti-inflammatory benefits.

Make a special effort to increase movement at times when you feel stiff, sore, or fatigued. Take longer walks the day after your most strenuous workouts. Draw inspiration from Tour de France cyclists, who pedal at a comfortable pace for two or three hours on their precious two official rest days during the grueling, three-week-long tour. Cycling lore says that easy pedaling can alleviate muscle soreness, speed the removal of waste products, protect against cramping, and prevent legs from feeling heavy upon return to racing. These ideas have now been validated by science.

Even acute injuries that have been traditionally treated with rest and immobilization are now treated with walking and mobility exercises. Forward-thinking physical therapy and rehabilitation experts are abandoning the treatment protocol of RICE (rest, ice, compression, and elevation) in favor of ECM (elevate, compress, and move). During the initial twenty-four-hour acute phase, icing an injury is still recommended, because it can inhibit the acute inflammatory response in a desirable manner. After that, elevation and compression enhance the function of the circulatory and lymphatic systems and keep the inflammatory response under control. Movement—now the gold standard for injury healing—increases blood flow, oxygen delivery, and mobility of injured joints and tissue. Obviously, walking on a sprained ankle can feel unpleasant, but this type of light activity can often speed healing and prevent atrophy better than total rest can.

Stress Management

Try walking as a therapeutic practice when you are experiencing an emotional disturbance of any kind. It will spur an instant change in blood chemistry, making you feel calmer, less stressed, less emotional, and more energized. These benefits are especially evident when you walk in nature. Granted, you will probably not have the urge to take a stroll when you are experiencing a negative emotional charge, so this is another situation in which making a deliberate choice is essential. You're still allowed to be angry, sad, and frustrated; just do it on the move.

After-Dinner Stroll

Research shows that a short, comfortably paced walk after meals can have a profound impact on glucose regulation. Exercising your muscles will pull glucose out of the bloodstream that might otherwise linger there and necessitate an insulin spike. Postprandial glucose spikes typically peak around an hour after eating, so be sure to get moving within that one-hour time window. Studies conducted by researchers in New Zealand suggest that the effects are most noticeable after the evening meal, because this is when people typically become inactive. Even a ten-minute after-dinner stroll has been shown to lower blood glucose by 22 percent among diabetics. Keep the effort light, because vigorous exercise after a meal can interfere with the digestive process. But casual walking aids digestion by stimulating peristalsis, the movement of material through the digestive system.

Before-Bedtime Stroll

Consider making a brief stroll part of your evening wind-down ritual before going to bed. Perhaps you can establish a rule to walk for a bit immediately after you finish your screen engagement for the evening.

Getting outdoors into fresh evening air, cooler temperatures, and a dark environment triggers important hormonal processes that promote sleepiness and a smooth transition to a good night's sleep. The same circadian benefits apply to canines, so grab that leash and take at least a short stroll no matter what.

Move to Miami

Just kidding—sort of. But I did experience a profound revelation about the importance of walking in 2018, when my wife, Carrie, and I moved to Miami's South Beach neighborhood after three decades of living in Malibu, California. While Malibu provides the opportunity for a beach lifestyle amid the urban sprawl of Los Angeles, it is one of the most unwalkable towns on the planet. On the long, skinny strip of coastline up against a mountain range that is Malibu, the hectic, busy Pacific Coast Highway is the sole means of access to shopping centers, restaurants, and public beaches. PCH, as it's known, is extremely dangerous and entirely unfit for pedestrians; tragic accidents are commonplace. We enjoyed great hiking in the mountainous trails above Malibu and great walks on the beach, but driving, not walking, was the essence of our daily lives.

Our high-density high-rise in South Beach offers a completely different experience. Carrie and I walk everywhere, to the tune of at least five miles each day, not counting our designated workouts and dedicated walking outings. I rarely drive unless I'm headed out of town or catching a rideshare home after walking to the supermarket. I feel more connected to my community than I ever did during my car-centric decades in Malibu. I also notice that I can process emotions and complex work challenges better when I'm on the move. And it seems like I have a higher baseline of cardiovascular fitness, better posture, more flexibility, fewer aches and pains, and better core stability from which to launch all my other workouts. I know this is all thanks to my daily walking habit, because things change quickly when I'm traveling and out of my typical daily routine. If your community is not particularly walkable, you will have to make an effort to create safe walking opportunities—perhaps you can drive to a park or hiking trail. In most cases, only minor adjustments to your schedule will be needed.

CHAPTER 8
Natural Foot Functionality and Human Locomotion

FOOT FUNCTIONALITY IS ONE OF THE MOST critical aspects of musculoskeletal health and overall fitness, because almost all complex kinetic-chain activity in the body is initiated from and anchored by the feet. We are highly reliant upon their intricate and incredibly dense network of nerve endings, muscles, tendons, ligaments, fascia, and fifty-two bones—around a quarter of the body's total—to interact with the ground and allow us to stand, walk, run, jump, squat, bend, extend, throw a ball, kick a ball, swing a club or a racquet, do chores around the house on in the yard, and perform all manner of physical labor and complex fitness and athletic activities.

Our feet help us absorb impact gracefully, balance moving body weight, harness elastic energy, and generate forward, upward, and side-to-side rotational kinetic energy. The fact that we are bipedal and not quadrupedal adds another layer of complexity and elegance to our foot functionality. We need to be precisely balanced on two small contact points with the ground at all times—otherwise we would topple over. We take standing, walking, and running for granted, but watch an infant struggling to stand or walk for the first time and you will realize that human locomotion is a miracle. It's all about the feet for any feat you try to complete!

As you learned in Chapter 3, we have badly neglected this elegantly evolved and extremely important part of our anatomy under the guise of fashion, comfort, and performance. The results of this neglect are glaring: the American Podiatric Medical Association reports that 83 percent of Americans complain of chronic foot pain. Reflect on that for a moment: today, you're an outlier if you *don't* have foot pain.

My goal for you is to minimize the damage and destruction caused by shoes by getting your feet as strong and functional as you can. This means spending as much time as possible barefoot or in minimalist shoes. This also means coming up with creative ways to focus on and activate your feet, such as putting a pebble mat under your stand-up desk, walking backwards on an inclined treadmill wearing only socks or minimalist shoes, sprinting barefoot in the sand, going out of your way to walk on rough terrain, and generally finding other ways to let your feet be feet.

The safest and most effective way to strengthen your feet is to simply walk around barefoot or in minimalist shoes.

For example, on a recent vacation to Hawaii, I went out intending to walk along the beach. But instead of remaining in the sand, I was drawn to the extremely rough and uneven lava flow along the coastline. It was a great joy and revelation to navigate the challenging terrain in my minimalist shoes. As I traversed the obstacle course–like surface, I thought, Why don't we schedule ourselves for a "foot day" at the gym, the same way we have focused "leg days" and "back, bi's, and tri's" days? My lava adventure wasn't much for cardio stimulation, but it helped hone important balancing skills and was a supremely beneficial foot-conditioning session.

You can certainly augment your progress toward barefoot competency by sitting down and doing foot circles and toe pointers, or doing sets on the calf machine at the gym, but the safest and most effective way to strengthen your feet is to simply walk around barefoot or in minimalist shoes. This helps your feet and the muscles throughout your lower body become stronger and more functional without any impact trauma. It's like building an aerobic base for your feet.

The great news is that transitioning to a barefoot-oriented lifestyle—with walking as the centerpiece—is within reach of everyone.

Becoming barefoot-competent will reduce your risk of chronic pain and injury and improve your movement technique, posture, balance, speed, endurance, and kinesthetic awareness. These benefits can help unfit people improve their general fitness and mobility and can help both recreational and elite athletes reduce injury risk and improve performance. Don't worry: the idea is not to suddenly swap your current shoes for minimalist models—this can increase risk of injury in poorly adapted feet. For example, endurance running in minimalist shoes might not ever be advisable unless you have excellent foot functionality and are extremely fit and highly adapted for running. And indeed, running itself may not be advisable if you don't have sufficient aerobic conditioning.

Why Bare Feet Are Better Than Running Shoes

In chapter 3, you learned that shoes enable technique errors, an increase in impact trauma, and an inappropriate dispersion of impact forces into the lower extremities. Interestingly, when running barefoot or in minimalist shoes on a hard surface, even a novice will intuitively execute a correct midfoot landing under a balanced center of gravity because the impact trauma caused by an inefficient landing is immediately obvious and punishing. Daniel Lieberman's research at Harvard (see page 68) revealed the mind-blowing insight that impact forces when we run barefoot are similar whether the surface is hard or soft. Our bodies have the incredible kinesthetic ability to figure out the most efficient, least jarring running style. After a few strides running barefoot on a hard surface, we feel the vibration through our bones and soft tissues and make intuitive adjustments on the fly. Through principles called preactivation and muscle tuning, we calibrate to a hard surface or a lack of cushioned footwear by increasing the stiffness of our muscles and connective tissues and increasing the bend in our ankles and knees during impact. Hey, who needs dirt trails or woodchip paths? Just run barefoot down the sidewalk!

Wait: You mean evolution is superior to modern shoe technology? Yes! The foot is able to efficiently absorb an impact load of several times your body weight better than any shoe. This may seem impossible to believe, but it's an unassailable fact of biomechanics and human physiology. Note that I didn't say, "Your foot, right now, is better than any shoe," because modern citizens have destroyed their foot functionality by encasing their feet in shoes for years and decades. The resulting atrophy and dysfunction means you are mostly likely maladapted to run even a short distance in bare feet or minimalist shoes.

Impact forces when we run barefoot are similar whether the surface is hard or soft.

However, for validation of the amazing functionality of the human foot, we can look to highly adapted athletes such as the legendary Ethiopian two-time Olympic marathon champion Abebe Bikila. In 1960, he broke the marathon world record with a time of two hours and fifteen minutes—still an Olympic-caliber time today—running barefoot through the streets of Rome. In the 1980s, a teenage female prodigy named Zola Budd broke middle-distance world records in South Africa and competed in the 3,000-meter finals at the 1984 Olympics running barefoot. One of the reasons cited for the dominant performance of East African distance runners from the Great Rift Valley, including Kenya and Ethiopia, is that they grew up going barefoot and ran back and forth to school daily.

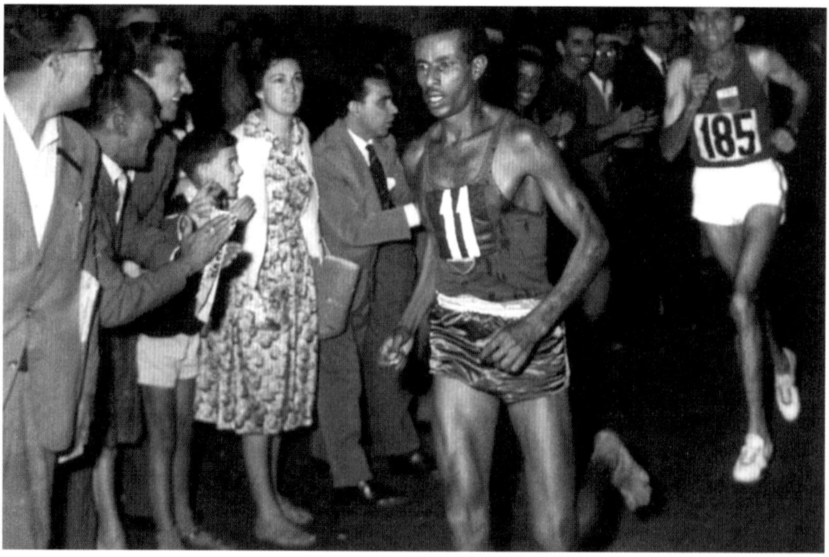

Before "Just do it," Abebe Bikila just did it—without shoes.

A FUTURE OF BAREFOOT WORLD RECORDS? DON'T LAUGH!

Abebe Bikila and Zola Budd gained a huge performance advantage over their shod opponents by becoming adapted for barefoot running. How? First, they were swinging much lighter lower limbs—unweighted by shoes. Ounces really count, especially over long distances and at high speeds. Numerous studies suggest that an elite marathon runner can save one minute per hundred grams of subtracted shoe weight. This gave Bikila a theoretical two-minute advantage over a rival wearing an approximately eight-ounce racing flat like the Onitsuka Tiger Marathon. Second, a barefoot runner doesn't sacrifice any elastic kinetic energy by compressing a shoe sole. Instead, the foot, particularly because of the dorsiflexion and takeoff from the big toe, is allowed to generate maximum vertical force per stride.

The incredibly light weight and energy-return resiliency of super shoes are the main reasons for their advantage, but it's important to note they are still mechanically inferior to a bare foot on a surface with excellent traction, such as a modern all-weather running track. The advantage is theoretical, of course, because an athlete has to be highly adapted in order to run barefoot without becoming fatigued by repeated unprotected impact. In his 2014 book, *1:59*, Dr. Phil Maffetone made the audacious prediction that elite marathoners would continue to improve and one day break the unthinkable two-hour barrier. Eliud Kipchoge proved Dr. Maffetone right surprisingly quickly with his 1:59 just five years later. Some skeptics discount Kipchoge's performance, since it wasn't in a "real" competition. Instead, he used a rotation pack of pacers and pacing lights on an automobile racetrack for his solo attempt against the clock. In the 2023 Chicago Marathon, the late Kelvin Kiptum set the official record at 2:00.35, so a "ratified" 1:59 seems imminent.

While Dr. Maffetone could not anticipate the stunning improvement in shoe technology that Nike debuted in 2016, he did propose that an elite runner who could adapt to racing barefoot, perhaps from a lifetime of barefoot living, would experience a 4 percent improvement in running economy.

Understanding Human Locomotion

In exercise physiology, walking and running are considered two distinct gait modes—just as a horse can walk, trot, canter, or gallop. Walking and running have similar neural patterns but some fundamental technique differences. Chief among them is that when you walk, you always have one leg on the ground to support your body weight, whereas when you run, there is a "flight phase" during which both feet are in the air.

In addition,

- when you walk, the correct landing is on the heel; a midfoot landing is correct for jogging, running, and sprinting;
- running requires more muscle activation, oxygen consumption, balance, stride length, and range of joint motion—and generates more vertical force—than walking;
- when you run, the amount of time you spend connected to the ground lessens by 35 percent compared to walking, and you spend less time in the air as well;
- running generates at least 50 percent more impact forces than walking, and the percentage increases as speed increases.

Overall, running is characterized by high peak forces and short ground-contact times; walking is characterized by low peak forces and long ground-contact times. But they are similar in that ground-contact time for both walking and running is around 50–60 percent of the total time required to take a stride. We instinctively adopt a gait that results in the most efficient oxygen consumption and energy production for a particular speed. Hence we will naturally proceed through slow walking, then brisk walking (up to around fourteen minutes per mile), then jogging (faster than fourteen minutes per mile), then faster running, and finally sprinting. Clearly, running demands much more energy and generates much more impact load than walking and is thus vastly more difficult to execute with good technique.

Because of the high risk of injury associated with running, you should only run when you can use correct technique and preserve it for the duration of your run. I cannot overemphasize the importance of developing the foot functionality, musculoskeletal resilience, and aerobic capacity necessary to execute the correct running stride. When you insist on running without sufficient aerobic capacity, you not only train your body to burn sugar and invite fatigue, you also, almost certainly, will quickly exhibit poor technique.

Even if you are able to conjure memories of your high school track days and take off down the road with decent technique, your lack of aerobic capacity will quickly cause your form to degrade when fatigue sets in. Recall the various technique flaws exhibited by poorly conditioned runners: heel-striking, overstriding, a hip-drop pattern, inefficiently slow cadence, insufficient forward lean of the trunk and/or ankles, poor glute activation, and poor hip extension. This means you must dedicate extensive time to walking in order to increase aerobic capacity and improve foot functionality. After you build a strong base and strong feet by walking—even short walks help—you will eventually be able to start jogging safely and comfortably for sustained periods.

Correct Locomotion Technique

The technique lesson starts with assuming good standing posture:

- a straight and elongated spine from the head through the tailbone;
- head and shoulders in vertical alignment with the spine;
- torso, hips, knees, and feet facing forward;
- a balanced center of gravity, with your weight loaded onto your heels; and
- a slight engagement of the abdominals to achieve a slightly anteverted (downward-pointing) pelvis and prevent loose (protruding) abdominals and excessive arching of the lower back.

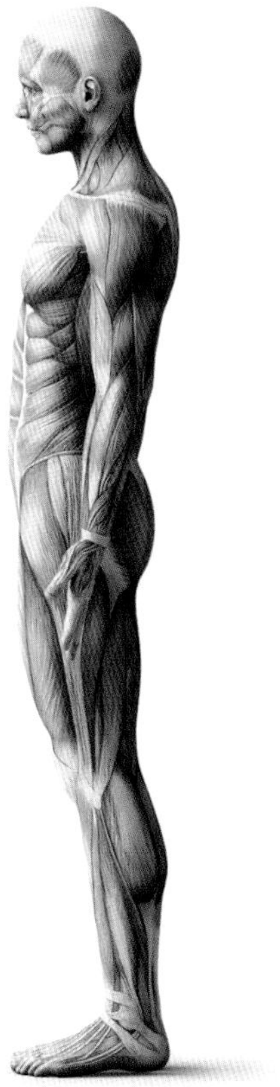

Correct posture—loading your body weight over your heels—is impossible in elevated, cushioned shoes.

From this standing posture, you commence the walking stride by stepping forward and landing gently on the heel. The heel's weight-bearing role in standing and walking is the reason the calcaneus, or heel bone, is so dense and cross-reinforced; it serves as the foundation for all other tarsal and metatarsal bones of the foot. When you heel-strike while walking, the extra fat pad on the heel will absorb some of the landing force.

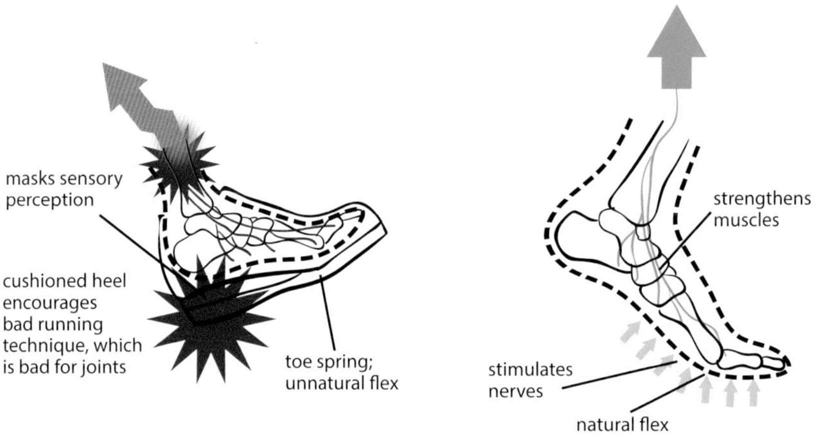

Unlike the heel strike of walking, the optimal human running gait entails striking the ground in the forefoot, or midfoot, area, emphasizing the outer edge of the foot. The ankle is plantar-flexed (pointed) at impact and will dorsiflex (straighten) during the landing to minimize the force of your body weight striking the ground. At foot strike, the center of gravity is balanced—feet, knees, and shoulders are aligned and almost perpendicular to the ground over the landed midfoot—see page 69. During the walking gait, you roll from your heel strike to this same balance point—with center of gravity over the midfoot—that happens at running footstrike. Then the toes splay wide, a phenomenon known as toe abduction, and grab the ground to provide balance and start harnessing energy for forward propulsion.

As you land, you will quickly move your body weight over your foot as it rolls onto your arch, which flattens and tightens. This is known as the windlass mechanism. Windlass is a sailing term describing the tightening of a rope or cable; during the running stride, the windlass mechanism helps support moving body weight. The windlass mechanism causes the foot to roll inward in what's called pronation. Pronation allows the plantar fascia and the complementary muscles in the arch area to act as natural shock absorbers as well as begin the process of harnessing the elastic energy needed for takeoff. The extra fat under the midfoot also helps with impact absorption.

Contrary to running-shoe marketing precepts, pronation is a normal and appropriate element of the human running gait. Remember: shoes cannot limit pronation anyway. Search YouTube for "Running myth: pronation is bad" and you'll see an example of what is widely derided as overpronation by Eliud Kipchoge—who was on his way to setting world records.

When you heel-strike while walking, the extra fat pad on the heel will absorb some of the landing force.

Concurrently to the arch flattening and tightening, the Achilles tendon and heel will drop toward the ground to further absorb impact and start coiling energy through the foot and calf muscles for an explosive takeoff. At final landing, your entire foot touches the ground briefly—including the heel, very gently. The bones of the midfoot, including the talonavicular and calcaneocuboid as well as the ankle, are built for flexibility, shock absorption, and elastic energy storage. The extra fat under the midfoot also helps with impact absorption. Your center of gravity loads over your foot when it's flat on the ground—shortly after it touches down. At this point, the foot, knee, hip, and shoulders are aligned and perpendicular to the ground. Force is generated vertically—directly into the ground underneath you—on each stride.

For takeoff, the big toe plays an important role. It dorsiflexes, harnesses elastic energy, provides balance for moving body weight, and triggers the activation of the powerful glute muscles. The weight of your entire body moves over the big toe during the running stride, making this single joint one of the most critical body parts of the human species. When the big toe is weak, rigid, and functioning poorly—in part because of atrophy and in part because of being constrained in a shoe—it causes a chain reaction of dysfunction and inappropriate load on other joints and connective tissue. At takeoff, the incredibly strong and coiled Achilles tendon rises from the ground, and a forceful launch occurs from kinetic energy stored in the toes (they go from dorsiflexed to plantar-flexed, a.k.a. pointed, at takeoff), metatarsals, longitudinal arch, Achilles, calf muscles, and, notably, in the glutes, thanks largely to the big toe's triggering them to fire.

Once airborne, the ankle and toes will quickly return to a dorsiflexed position in preparation for the next foot strike. That is, unless you have crappy, shuffling running form—in which case you'll drag your limp toes and ankle, a.k.a. lazy foot, into position for another energy-inefficient heel-first, braking, overstriding landing. The next time you run, think about maintaining "strong feet"—try to actively dorsiflex the ankle and keep the big toe high as soon as your foot leaves the ground.

In both walking and running, the arms will swing naturally in coordination with your leg movements. This means the left arm swings forward in tandem with the right leg swinging forward and vice versa. The arm swing helps the body stay in balance so the counterbalanced leg swing can generate forward propulsion. When you're running, arms can bend to around a ninety-degree angle on the forward swing and get to nearly straight during the downswing and backswing. Keeping the arms nearly straight while walking is the most efficient. The stride pattern is then repeated with strides of ideal length to keep your center of gravity balanced over the landing foot.

VERTICAL FORCE PRODUCTION DRIVES RUNNING SPEED

Sprinters obsess about vertical force production because it is the essence of running fast. This is actually true at any speed. Head over to YouTube and search for "Usain Bolt slow motion." Notice how Bolt's legs strike the ground powerfully underneath his center of gravity—he generated nearly one thousand pounds of force with each stride en route to his 9.58 100-meter world record in 2009. His stride length was an incredible eight feet.

Then watch a video of Eliud Kipchoge running a marathon and focus on his foot strike. He, too, strikes the ground with significant force, running at an astonishingly fast pace to achieve an explosive takeoff and a stride length of six feet three inches. A study of three hundred finishers of the 2020 Mumbai Marathon revealed that the average stride length of a three-hour marathoner is four feet three inches, whereas marathoners running slower than four hours have an average stride length of three feet three inches.

The physics students in the crowd might ask, "If Bolt is striking the ground with one thousand pounds of vertical force, why doesn't he launch into the sky?" The answer is that the gravitational pull of the earth immediately acts upon that vertical force. Instead of launching him into the sky, each of Bolt's powerful strides sends him eight feet farther down the track for the next landing. Gravity, not wind resistance, is the biggest obstacle to increasing running speed.

Recall the commentary in chapter 3, and you'll realize that every single element in the aforementioned step-by-step human gait sequence is severely compromised when you wear elevated, cushioned shoes. Amid the atrophy and dysfunction caused by shoes, you are compelled to make technique compensations that ingrain further inefficiencies and injuries. Witness the die-hard runners who eventually become hunched over to a forty-five-degree angle and can barely lift their feet off the ground. Don't believe me? Search YouTube for "Nike—Just Do It (1988)—Very First Commercial" and behold the Nike commercial that launched one of the most iconic advertising campaigns of all time. It features the late San Francisco running legend Walt Stack at age eighty waddling across the Golden Gate Bridge. Every day for twenty-seven years, Stack, recognized by many motorists and pedestrians, ran the same seventeen-mile route, crossing the bridge and returning to Sausalito. It's still a great achievement for an eighty-year-old to cover seventeen miles every day, and it's safer for the cardiovascular system to waddle instead of push into the high-heart-rate zones. However, at that point, why not slow down to a walk and enjoy the scenery?

HOW TO IMMEDIATELY IMPLEMENT CORRECT RUNNING TECHNIQUE

Here's a quick exercise that will help you immediately experience what it feels like to run with correct form, absorb shock optimally, and become springier and more propulsive.

Find a smooth stretch of pavement or a hard indoor surface such as a basketball court or long hallway. Then remove your shoes and run some strides at a decent pace. You will notice that you instinctively land lightly and gracefully on the midfoot, with a balanced center of gravity and a harnessing of elastic energy for an explosive takeoff. As Daniel Lieberman discovered, you will instinctively bend your knees and ankles so you can gracefully absorb impact on the hard surface. He asserts that running barefoot is within reach of anyone: "Most people today think barefoot running is dangerous and hurts, [but] you can run barefoot on the world's hardest surfaces without the slightest discomfort and pain. All you need are a few calluses to avoid roughing up the skin of the foot."

This exercise allows you to get a glimpse of your natural ability to absorb impact optimally. Obviously, it's not a great idea to log a bunch of barefoot sidewalk running miles out of the blue. However, even if you're a novice and untrained in correct running mechanics, you can quickly improve your technique by introducing short bits of running on a forgiving surface such as grass or turf or a rubber track. Ideally, you would do these bursts when barefoot or in minimalist shoes, but you can wear your typical cushioned shoes at first.

Overall, the best strategy is to build your aerobic capacity by walking (with correct technique) and then carefully sprinkle in some running in short bursts, focusing intently on correct technique. Be sure to remain under fat max heart rate at all times. This might entail setting out for a brisk walk, running for thirty to sixty seconds, then returning to a walk before your heart rate beeper alarm sounds or your form is compromised. Spend at least an equivalent amount of time walking, then try another brief running stint. I don't see many people on the paths and trails following such a system, but it is vastly superior to huffing and puffing along at steady state with crappy form, an elevated heart rate, and excess impact trauma.

In truth, the only reason to maintain a steady-state pace during a training session is to simulate race conditions, where pace precision is necessary for peak performance. Most recreational runners don't care about race performance; if they do enter organized events, their main goal is to simply finish. Feel free to experiment with varying the pace of your training sessions, especially alternating between walking and jogging to minimize workout stress.

Building a Barefoot Base

Making a smooth transition to a barefoot-inspired lifestyle after years and decades of reliance on elevated, cushioned shoes can be a big challenge. It's critical to proceed with patience and caution by gradually integrating time spent in bare feet with walking in the most minimalist type of shoe possible—one with a zero drop, a flexible sole, minimal padding, and, ideally, articulated toes. Walking will make your feet stronger and more resilient without the impact trauma and risks associated with complex activities that you are ill-prepared for. As you build a barefoot base, you can start to further integrate minimalist shoes into your routine: wear them at gym classes and during strength training sessions; on long walks and hikes; and eventually for more challenging activities such as rugged hiking (really!), running, jumping, short sprints, and even side-to-side sports such as pickleball, Ultimate Frisbee, and CrossFit.

Following is a tiered, step-by-step protocol to help you transition safely. Choose an appropriate starting point based on your present fitness and foot functionality, proceed at your own pace, and monitor yourself carefully for soreness, stiffness, and minor new aches and pains that will require you to back off and recover.

Let Your Feet Be Feet

Strive to make barefoot the norm in your home. Go barefoot in other safe environments, too, such as the beach, a manicured grass or turf field, or an appropriate indoor space. As you pitter-patter around your house with your feet liberated, tune into the concept of proprioception and notice how incredibly sensitive and reactive your feet are to the ground. Try standing on one foot for a bit and notice how the delicate small muscles of your foot activate gracefully to help balance your body weight. These are innate human skills that you have suppressed and atrophied through the prolonged use of bulky shoes. Consider using toe separators to train your toes to separate, which will speed your progress.

Walking in Daily Life

Any devotion to walking is a step in the right direction, so I'm not going to criticize you too harshly for walking in regular shoes. However, the musculoskeletal benefits of walking are vastly enhanced if you do it in minimalist shoes. Also, try to wear minimalist shoes for everyday shopping, errands, and outside activities—and even in the workplace, if possible.

Walking for Fitness

In tandem with cultivating a walking-oriented lifestyle, integrate longer-distance walks in minimalist shoes into your exercise routine.

As I wrote in chapter 6, these walking outings can replace some of your running workouts to your great benefit. Novices can start with a ten-minute walk, while people with more fitness or barefoot experience can start with a thirty-minute walk. See how your feet feel the next day and the day after—sometimes it takes as long as forty-eight hours to experience postactivity muscle soreness. If you experience any stiffness or soreness in the heel, arch, toes, or calf muscles after your introductory walks, wait until symptoms clear before you try another walking outing.

Foot Exercises

Spending a few minutes a day doing foot exercises will speed your progress and help you avoid setbacks. I don't want to overwhelm you with another fitness assignment on your already packed to-do list, so please just familiarize yourself with the exercises and sprinkle them in when you are relaxing in front of screen entertainment or even working at your desk. A few minutes a day makes a huge difference over time. I recommend doing a few simple foot-mobility exercises, such as foot circles and isometric holds, before getting out of bed in the morning.

Gym Workouts

Wear your minimalist shoes—or even go barefoot if possible—for low- or no-impact gym workouts. These include strength training; step, barre, and other aerobics or metabolic-conditioning classes; and home-based workouts. Minimalist shoes are extremely beneficial when you apply force into the ground to perform squats and dead lifts or do anything that requires balance or impact absorption, such as box jumps and working with TRX straps.

Hiking

After you get some experience walking in minimalist shoes, take them off-road for an introductory trail hike. You can start modestly, with an outing of medium duration on comfortable terrain, but you should soon be well prepared for a challenging hike on rough terrain. You will quickly discover that minimalist shoes are vastly more comfortable and functional than sturdy, high-top hiking shoes with a thick, rigid sole. A classic hiking shoe destroys your proprioception and disconnects your feet from the kinetic chain. You become like a robot stomping over whatever is in your path. A sturdy hiking shoe or boot will protect you from debris and toe stubs for sure, but after hours on the trail, your entire lower body may feel the effects of inappropriately dispersed impact trauma.

What's more, your risk of tripping, stumbling, twisting your ankle, and misstepping and falling is not reduced one iota in a hiking boot. In fact, risk increases the further disconnected you become from groundfeel—the ability of your foot to sense the terrain underneath. This is also true for high-top basketball shoes—no less risk of ankle sprain. One study of more than six hundred college intramural basketball players published in the *American Journal of Sports Medicine* revealed no difference in the rate of ankle sprains among players wearing high-tops, low-tops, and the gimmicky 1990s-era high-tops with inflatable air chambers. Despite extensive research, it has never been proved that any shoe can provide enough ankle support to prevent injury.

Ankle taping or bracing remains a popular practice in sports training. It has long been said to protect an existing injury from further damage and possibly reduce the risk of future injury. However, emerging research suggests that the protective benefits (e.g., preventing sprains) might not result from the fact that the shoe restricts the ankle's range of motion. Instead, the benefits of taping or applying an ankle brace may be attributed to the placebo effect. The athlete feels more confident when the joint is taped; she also may note an increase in proprioception as the ankle mobilizes against the constraints of the tape or brace.

Medium-Impact Activity

As you build your competence in minimalist shoes, you can progress to workouts that entail significant side-to-side movements, such as CrossFit and boot camp–style classes. You can also introduce low- and medium-impact running and jumping drills, which are best done in minimalist shoes that promote correct technique. Hill repeats, stair climbing, and sled pushing are also safe ways to perform high-intensity efforts in minimalist shoes. Monitor yourself carefully for post-workout soreness, and never attempt anything challenging unless your feet feel great at the outset.

High-Impact Activity

While many minimalist shoe enthusiasts may not ever want to attempt high-impact activities in minimalist shoes, there are many accomplished athletes who demonstrate that anything is possible when one has the patience and discipline to become highly barefoot-adapted. Check out YouTube channels such as Peluva, the Foot Collective, and the Barefoot Sprinter for informative content about taking things to the next level. When you are able to successfully build your competency with the tiered recommendations in this section, minimalist shoes can potentially become your preferred choice for activities such as extreme hiking, short-distance jogging, pickleball, solo basketball practice, and even high-intensity wind sprints—five- to seven-second accelerations to near full speed followed by a graceful deceleration—and even longer sprints. Remember, the majority of benefits come when you go barefoot as often as possible and walk as often as possible in minimalist shoes. When you develop excellent foot functionality, you will be better adapted to whatever type of specialized shoes you choose, whether for sport, work, or fashion.

Transitioning for Runners

Running-shoe choices have always been strongly driven by personal preference. If you are enjoying a smooth, injury-free experience, with uninterrupted improvement and excellent competitive results, hey—keep doing what you're doing and wearing the shoes you're wearing. But if you're sick and tired of recurring overuse injuries and are sold on the benefits of a barefoot-inspired lifestyle, you can implement a strategic approach to reducing your reliance on elevated, cushioned shoes.

But let me first reiterate the importance of exercising at or below fat max heart rate during the majority of your endurance training. This likely means that walking will become more prominent in your regimen. You can easily walk in minimalist shoes and improve foot functionality and aerobic capacity without the risk of injury or overtraining.

Second, let me reiterate the importance of running with correct form—executing a midfoot landing underneath a balanced center of gravity with a straight and elongated spine and avoiding the common flaws of heel-striking, overstriding, and hip drop during your stride. If you cannot exhibit and maintain correct form, you shouldn't run—just as you shouldn't squat or deadlift with crappy form. Alternating between walking and jogging is a great way to preserve good technique without having cumulative fatigue turn you into a shuffler.

Third, it's important to dedicate sufficient time to mobility exercises, flexibility exercises, dynamic stretching, static stretching, and rehab and prehab exercises that will help you correct the biomechanical and musculoskeletal deficiencies, weaknesses, and imbalances caused by sedentary behavior. For example, sitting for long periods can shorten and weaken hamstrings and hip flexors and deactivate the glutes so they are less functional when running. If you have struggled with overuse injuries, you should seek expert guidance and develop a customized exercise routine that addresses your specific issues. Dr. Kelly Starrett contends that runners should devote 25 percent of their total training time to mobility and injury-prevention exercises.

Now let me advise you how to make a safe and sensible transition to a minimalist running experience. Consider where your current shoes fall on the continuum from super-cushioned to minimalist, then consider a gradual integration of some minimalist shoes into your rotation. For example, a longtime big-shoe user might introduce a pair of Nike Frees for a small percentage of her weekly mileage. Nike Free has a very flexible sole, plenty of cushion, and a drop of four to six millimeters from heel to toe. When you acquire any new running shoe, start by running just a mile or two at recovery pace on a soft surface such as grass, turf, an all-weather running track, or a dirt road or trail. If you experience any stiffness or soreness afterward, wait until the soreness clears completely, then attempt another session of less distance or slower pace. Complete three to six short jogs before increasing your distance or trying a harder surface.

Strive to progress to running 10 percent of your weekly mileage in your new minimalist shoes. With success, you can consider running a greater percentage of your mileage in them and/or introducing an even more minimalist model, looking for shoes with less vertical drop and less cushioning. With more progress and adaptation, you can consider introducing one of the many zero-drop running-shoe models, which still offer significant protection and lateral stability suitable for trail running.

This mission—should you choose to accept it—is best driven by personal preference and subject to ongoing favorable results. It might seem like too much hassle or too much risk to depart from your favorite shoe models, but it's important to acknowledge that overuse injuries are driven by poor foot functionality and increased impact trauma caused by the poor form that is enabled by cushioned shoes. It's essential to strive to improve your form and achieve graceful midfoot landings in whatever shoe you are wearing. Interestingly, when you start executing midfoot landings in your elevated, cushioned shoe, you realize that you don't really need the extra heel elevation or cushion. You can make progress by improving your technique and integrating minimalist footwear.

CHAPTER 9
Broad-Based Fitness for Longevity

It's time to establish an effective, enjoyable fitness program that builds aerobic competency, VO2 max scores, muscular strength and endurance, and explosive speed and power. These are the attributes that support broad-based fitness competency as well as general health, vitality, and longevity. This type of fitness is a refreshing and empowering alternative to blindly pounding the pavement in a chronic-cardio model that most certainly compromises your health, vitality, and longevity in return for running in a straight line for long distances.

As you have—I hope—become convinced by this time, walking is the essential foundation from which you launch all other types of fitness endeavors. Even the most brief, explosive athletic efforts are nurtured by the aerobic system. So the more you can walk and are generally active in daily life, the more you will develop your aerobic base and the better you will be able to perform and recover from lifting heavy weights in the gym, sprinting on the track, skiing down a mountain, hiking up a mountain, working the kitchen in pickleball, running around with the kids on the soccer field, and anything else athletic you aspire to do.

It's perfectly fine to go for a run once in a while at whatever pace you choose. You see, the damage, destruction, and dysfunction I wrote about in the previous chapters are predominantly driven by chronically overly stressful catabolic patterns. If you have an excellent aerobic foundation from a history of extensive cardio or a generally walking-friendly lifestyle, these occasional peak-performance running efforts can go quite well. Show up at your town's annual turkey trot or Fourth of July 10k and run your heart out—fat max beeper alarms be damned. Same for putting the hammer down a couple of times a month at that lively Saturday morning group trail run or Friday night rock-and-roll spin class or challenging four-hour hike in the rainforest on your vacation to Costa Rica. Even if you have suboptimal fitness and overall activity levels, it's okay to depart from your comfort zone, challenge yourself with an occasional endurance effort, and stimulate a fitness breakthrough. Granted, major efforts might leave you feeling a little sore and beat up for a few days, so you have to take extra care to rest and recover. What I want you to end once and for all is the indiscriminate application of inappropriate chronic stress to an already hectic, high-stress modern life. Your heart-rate monitor is going to be your most trusted guide on this journey, followed by common sense.

The following sections will cover the four pillars of full-body fitness: aerobic conditioning, lifting heavy things, sprinting once in a while, and playing.

Aerobic Conditioning

These days, health and fitness have become a bit too complicated for my old-school liking—what with all the technology attempting to quantify every possible aspect of your workouts and overall life. That said, competitive athletes can certainly benefit from precise tracking of performance and recovery variables, especially because they are often pushing the limits of their capacity. But for most recreational enthusiasts, a casual, intuitive approach to training can be empowering, doable, and easy to adhere to.

Building an aerobic conditioning base starts with increasing all forms of general everyday movement. Remember: any type of exercise stimulates the aerobic system, and even brief efforts can yield tremendous benefits over time. Taking quick walking breaks away from desk work, walking the dog as a daily ritual, taking the stairs instead of the elevator, and engaging in formal movement practices such as yoga, tai chi, and calisthenics all contribute to your aerobic conditioning base.

Even with devoted efforts toward increasing general everyday movement, the many sedentary influences in modern life compel us to also include structured steady-state cardiovascular workouts if we want to optimize aerobic conditioning. I've long recommended that you strive to accumulate two to five hours a week of low-level cardiovascular exercise at or below fat max heart rate as a bare-minimum safeguard against the many hazards of insufficient daily movement. Accumulating a handful of hours of cardio each week is easily obtainable for anyone wishing to lead a healthful lifestyle and minimize risk of disease and injury—including falling.

I'm going to characterize the pillar of aerobic conditioning as "all manner of everyday movement and exercise."

Furthermore, because exercising at aerobic heart rates is comfortable, enjoyable, and minimally stressful to the hormonal, immune, musculoskeletal, and metabolic systems of the body, benefits continue to accrue the more low-level cardio you do. For example, walking five miles every day delivers massive benefits with none of the downside risks covered in part 1. Ditto for spending a month trekking the Camino de Santiago, in Spain, or the 211-mile John Muir Trail, in the Sierra Nevada mountains of California. It's all about maintaining a fat-burning pace and avoiding chronic patterns that are depleting and destructive.

It's also important to appreciate the reality that all forms of movement and exercise stimulate the aerobic system, not just traditional steady-state cardio (walking, jogging, cycling, machines, and so on). This includes resistance training as well as brief, explosive sprint efforts, because the cardiovascular system is stimulated by all kinds of muscular demand. Consequently, I'm going to characterize the pillar of aerobic conditioning as "all manner of everyday movement and exercise"—not repeated and potentially excessive bouts of steady-state cardio pegged at the zone 2 limit in pursuit of an A-plus grade in cardio class.

Powerlifters and sprinters are getting excellent aerobic stimulation during their workouts, which consist of lots of warm-ups, drills, brief bursts of explosive effort, and frequent rest breaks. Similarly, the aerobic system is engaged from the time you get out of your car and start walking to the gym for your basketball game. You do your dynamic stretches, dribbling and shooting drills, and play hard as the aerobic system answers to these demands. Even when you sit on the bench during breaks, your aerobic system is working to help you recover from the bursts of anaerobic effort on the court. Your heart rate is likely to be least double its resting level for the whole two-hour period, until you get back in your car to drive home. Sure, pegging your heart rate at fat max, or the upper limit of zone 2, will deliver excellent aerobic benefits, but upper-limit zone 2 and fat max workouts should be only a portion of your overall aerobic conditioning program.

BUT MARK, WHEN CAN I GET PERMISSION TO RUN?

If you're excitedly nodding your head and agreeing that walking will be your bread and butter forevermore, that's great. However, I realize that if you have an extensive history of and passion for endurance running, it's not easy to extinguish that drive. I know how you love to get out there and feel the wind in your face, get a nice sweat going, escape the confines of indoor life, explore your natural environment, and feel the exhilaration of a job well done. I just want you to devise a workable plan with specific guidelines and metrics that will allow you progress according to your aerobic competency. I want you to actually enjoy endurance exercise and avoid the many pitfalls and negative consequences of following the running boom to breakdown, burnout, illness, and injury.

The plan entails conducting almost all your cardio at or below fat max heart rate. Your MAF test results will dictate whether you'll be walking, walking briskly, or jogging slowly during aerobic training sessions. If you do things right, you can expect to progress to a faster gait pattern over time while still performing at fat max heart rate. This is why it's important to repeat the MAF test every three to four weeks to track your progress and identify any problems. Typically, a regression in MAF test results is driven by overtraining.

Remember: the watch doesn't lie, so your pace will be constrained by the beeper alarm at fat max heart rate. Pace per mile—an obsession for many runners, especially those outfitted with high-tech GPS watches—is irrelevant to the goals of conducting an aerobic workout. Whether you're hiking up a steep hill, running downhill with a tailwind, exercising at high altitude, or running in ninety-degree heat, high winds, or pouring rain, your heart rate will reflect the degree of difficulty of the site and weather conditions. Your assignment is to conduct an aerobic workout by honoring the beeper alarm on your watch and nothing else. Your mood, the speed of your training partners, your urge to get some instant gratification by busting out a challenging effort after a tough day at the office, and the fact that the hill is so steep you have to walk—none of that matters. Do whatever it takes to stay aerobic.

If your athletic goals are endurance-oriented, you'll want to spend a few months focusing on building a strict aerobic base, with all your workouts conducted at or below fat max heart rate. If your goals involve broad-based fitness competency, team or ball sports, or high-intensity activities, you can still do your sport-specific training while taking care to conduct all your cardio at or below fat max heart rate. Remember: there's nothing that says you have to bump right up against your fat max every time you conduct an aerobic session. You can get tremendous aerobic benefits with minimal downside risk by exercising ten, twenty, or even forty beats below your fat max—yes, that includes tons of walking!

Lift Heavy Things

Readers of my other books will recognize "lift heavy things" as my Primal Blueprint Law number 4. Regularly subjecting your muscles to resistance load while performing full-body movements is one of the ten fundamental elements of modern health inspired by our ancestral past. Emerging science is validating the idea that maintaining muscle mass and muscle strength throughout life is one of the key factors to aging gracefully and minimizing disease risk. Dr. Gabrielle Lyon, family physician, podcaster, and author of *Forever Strong*, promotes a concept called muscle-centric medicine. The premise is that when you build and maintain muscle mass and strength, it implies that you are physically fit and protected against the diseases of accelerated aging. You work hard, have good blood chemistry, insulin sensitivity, and blood pressure; and have good hormonal, neurotransmitter, mitochondrial, immune, and cardiovascular function. Being strong makes you less likely to accumulate visceral fat or excess subcutaneous fat—although it's still possible to do so if you eat a crappy diet.

Focusing on muscle contrasts with our longtime obsession with tracking body fat and body weight for metabolic health. Our skeletal muscles make up 30–40 percent of our body mass, and, like visceral fat, are classified as endocrine organs for their ability to produce and release signaling proteins. In contrast to the health-destructive effects of cytokines, released by visceral fat, myokines, released by muscles, deliver an assortment of antiaging and general health benefits, including increasing glucose uptake, boosting fat metabolism, improving inflammatory balance in the body, exerting beneficial effects on mood and motor learning, and protecting against cognitive decline. Muscles serve as "glucose sinks" because they soak up glucose in the bloodstream and store that glucose as glycogen. Regularly emptying your glycogen stores through exercise and replenishing them with nutritious carbohydrates helps stabilize blood glucose levels, improve insulin sensitivity, and protect against the modern epidemic of insulin resistance.

Skeletal muscles make up 30–40 percent of our body mass, and, like visceral fat, are classified as endocrine organs.

Preserving muscle mass and strength throughout life is one of the most profound longevity boosters ever discovered. Being strong gives you a high level of organ reserve—the capacity of your organs to perform beyond baseline levels. When you challenge the muscles to perform, you also challenge the heart, lungs, liver, and other organs to become stronger and more efficient—think of the low resting rate and high stroke volume of a fit heart. Organ reserve comes in handy when your health and survival are challenged by illness, injury, surgery, or the inevitable atrophy associated with chronological aging.

Being strong also helps you maintain and even improve balance and motor control. These attributes help prevent falling, which the US Centers for Disease Control and Prevention cites as the number one cause of injury-related death in Americans over the age of sixty-five. Interestingly, senior citizens have the ability to make faster incremental gains in strength and power than any other age group. In just weeks of devoted high-intensity workouts, seniors can attain strength benchmarks and sex hormone levels that are similar to those of unfit people who are decades younger.

Numerous studies reveal a powerful correlation between high-intensity training and health span. This term describes the portion of your life in which you are in good health, in contrast to plain old lifespan, which counts years without regard to your level of physical or cognitive functionality. Physical fitness attributes that predict health span include grip strength, squat competency, push-up competency, mile-run time, MAF test time, and many more. The reason you see that contraption with the squeeze handle attached to a readout meter in many doctors' offices is because grip strength is easy to measure in a clinical setting and has proved to be an extremely reliable indicator of one's general rate of aging. Insufficient grip strength has been found to be a more accurate predictor of mortality risk than blood pressure. It is also an independent risk factor for type 2 diabetes, an indication of other functional limitations such as poor walking speed, and even a risk factor for depression. The Honolulu Heart Program, a study of six thousand Japanese participants between the ages of forty-five and sixty-eight, discovered that grip strength, even in midlife, accurately predicted mortality risk twenty-five years later.

In a study in Brazil of two thousand subjects between the ages of fifty-one and eighty, researchers were able to predict mortality risk with great accuracy based on a subject's competency in performing a basic squat. Compared to those who attained basic competency, those who were incompetent were five times more likely to die in the ensuing six years, and those who had minor difficulty squatting were twice as likely to die. A British study of 324 identical twins revealed a profound link between leg strength and cognitive health. Participants, whose average age was fifty-five to start, performed leg-strength tests and a battery of cognitive assessments at the beginning of the study, then underwent the same cognitive tests ten years later. Those who were stronger in the first assessment had significantly less age-related cognitive decline a decade later. The lead researcher, Dr. Claire Steves, said, "It's compelling to see such differences in cognition and brain structure in identical twins, who had different leg power 10 years before."

Unfortunately, we are not doing a good job staying strong as we age. Instead, we are experiencing accelerated aging driven strongly by the conditions of sarcopenia and dynapenia—the age-related loss of muscle mass, strength, power, and speed. Sarcopenia and dynapenia play a central role in the metabolic patterns that contribute to the so-called four horsemen of chronic disease identified by Dr. Peter Attia: heart disease, metabolic disease, cancer, and cognitive disease. Strange as it may seem, losing muscle and becoming frail can indeed influence your risk of cognitive decline. For example, researchers sometimes call Alzheimer's disease type 3 diabetes because it is marked by dysfunctional glucose metabolism in the brain.

It's urgent to fight back against sarcopenia and dynapenia by regularly putting your muscles under resistance load via whatever type of strength-training activities you enjoy the most and will adhere to for a lifetime. It's simply not enough to stay aerobically fit with a routine of jogging or walking. Sure, you'll be vastly better off than an inactive person by every measure, but you will only experience a small number of the many benefits of becoming truly strong. There are many seniors who get out and walk every day in the name of health—a mile, five miles, or what have you. This is a laudable habit and good promoter of health span, but without resistance exercise and high-intensity sprinting, the walk will become slower and shorter over the years, with likely more aches and pains and greater risk of falling from a simple misstep. I discuss the topics of strength training and sprinting in detail in my book *The Primal Blueprint* and in my comprehensive online Primal Fitness Expert Certification course, at PrimalHealthCoach.com.

For our purposes here, I want to introduce you to the world of strength training in a simple, nonintimidating manner. Whatever your age or current level of fitness or mobility, you can get stronger in far less time and with less complexity than fitness industry marketing hype leads you to believe. You can get a fantastic full-body strength workout by using a handful of easy-to-learn machines at your local gym or just by working with simple equipment at home, including mini bands, stretch tubing, dumbbells, and kettlebells. Heck, you can get strong and even superstrong by doing only body-weight exercises—what I call the primal essential movements: sit-ups, pull-ups, squats, and planks. When you start to experience the life-changing benefits of getting stronger, including transforming your physique in a way that endurance training never will, you will likely become more devoted to it over time.

Granted, you are going to have to evolve beyond an endurance-obsessed training mentality and embrace a new paradigm of what it means to be fit. Many people who are deep into the endurance scene lack the energy for or interest in strength training. But even if you care mainly or only about endurance performance, neglecting strength training is a huge mistake, because getting stronger has a direct correlation to endurance performance.

If you want to live a long, healthy, active, energetic life, it's simply not enough to become an endurance machine and hit your weekly mileage for years and decades.

First, if you're strong, you are better able to preserve good running technique even as you fatigue. If you have trained only for endurance and are deficient in muscular strength, you will hit the wall at around mile 20 of a marathon and start doing your shuffle. Whatever energy you can muster from your strong heart and resilient brain is squandered because of your blown-out hip flexors, quads, and hamstrings. But if you instead include squats, dead lifts, leg extensions, hamstring extensions, leg presses, calf raises, and other gym exercises in your workouts on a regular basis, your muscles can better respond to the demands of getting to the finish line.

Second, strength training provides an excellent stimulus to oxidative fast-twitch fibers (type 2a), which play a significant role in endurance performance. Oxidative fast-twitch fibers are especially important after your well-trained slow-twitch (type 1) fibers become fatigued from performing at medium-to-difficult heart rates for a long time. When you recruit oxidative fast-twitch fibers by doing sets of twelve in the gym, you make them more versatile and adaptable to your endurance efforts outside the gym.

Again, if you want to live a long, healthy, active, energetic life, it's simply not enough to become an endurance machine and hit your weekly mileage for years and decades. In 2012, research was conducted on elderly cross-country skiers at the prestigious Karolinska Institute, in Solna, Sweden. These were an elite group of subjects, including former Olympic and national champions who continued to compete at a high level for decades. The athletes were all over the age of eighty at the time of the study. Not surprisingly, they had the highest VO2 max values ever recorded for their age group—world-record cardiovascular function on a par with fit subjects half their age. While their tremendous aerobic capacity certainly increased their longevity and put them in a vastly superior position to inactive seniors, their endurance-oriented training patterns did not give them impressive levels of muscle strength and power. These are critically important longevity attributes that require a devotion to strength-oriented workouts.

A widely publicized 2018 study conducted by San Francisco State University on one particular set of identical twins delivered some incredible insights along these same lines. Studies of identical twins are highly valued because identical twins share virtually identical DNA, so the effects of lifestyle behaviors can be isolated and highly scrutinized—especially when researchers can find twins who engage in disparate lifestyle behaviors. The twins in the study were fifty-two years old: one had amassed around thirty years of dedicated endurance training, while the other had remained largely sedentary in a career as a truck driver. Naturally, the athletic twin was superior in most health and longevity categories—body composition, VO2 max, aerobic capacity, blood markers, and so forth. However, a surprising insight emerged: the truck driver had larger and stronger leg muscles than the endurance twin. Researchers attributed this to the unfit twin's extra body weight, which, they theorized, had helped him build and maintain muscle. The fit twin, by contrast, had been training his muscles exclusively for endurance instead of strength. A biopsy of their quadriceps revealed that the unfit twin had a typical fifty-fifty ratio of slow-twitch to fast-twitch fibers, while the endurance twin had converted his quads through training to be more than 90 percent slow-twitch, better for endurance running and cycling.

This is certainly not an exhortation to be inactive and gain weight—or to engage in round-the-clock resistance training—but the study calls to mind another important antiaging insight: fast-twitch muscle fibers decline far more quickly with age than do slow-twitch fibers. This is because slow-twitch fibers are involved in all manner of low-intensity everyday activity, while fast-twitch fibers are recruited for brief, explosive efforts that are uncommon in routine daily life and are widely avoided by people as they age.

It's essential to maintain fast-twitch fibers for many reasons. First and foremost is to prevent sarcopenia and remain independent for as long as possible. Realize that hustling up a flight of stairs or carrying a suitcase through the airport might be no sweat for you today, but eventually these will be power moves requiring lots of resources—feel the burn, baby! Fast-twitch fibers are also more metabolically active than slow-twitch, so you get more intensive glucose sink and insulin sensitivity benefits. Fast-twitch-fiber activity also supports bone density, because of the bigger demand on bones when absorbing a resistance load or performing explosive movements. Finally, high-intensity exercise is the best stimulus for adaptive hormones such as human growth hormone and testosterone. Again, you get a crop dusting of these benefits when you walk or race the occasional 5k, but you have to push the muscles with brief, challenging sets of resistance exercises (weights, stretch cords, body-weight exercises) in order to develop strength and power.

Following are basic principles that will help you conduct safe, effective strength-training sessions.

Follow Your Personal Preference

Free weights, machines, stretch tubing, or body weight? The answer is whatever is most enjoyable and convenient for you, given that you should emphasize sweeping, full-body movements and brief, intense efforts executed with precise technique.

For novices, body-weight exercises and gym machines are much safer and less intimidating than learning the complex technique necessary to lift free weights safely. Resistance bands, tubes, and cords offer an easy, convenient, and affordable way to conduct a great strength-training session at home or when traveling. You can perform all manner of resistance exercises with less risk of muscle soreness and injury than you can by lifting heavy weights. Choose resistance loads that allow you to complete around twelve reps. More than twelve carries the potential for overload injury, while fewer than twelve is not difficult enough to develop true strength and power.

Conduct Brief, Intense Workouts

Turn off your endurance-oriented brain and focus on workouts that are short in duration and feature brief, powerful, explosive efforts performed with precise technique. These are the types of workouts that challenge major muscle groups and leave you winded at the end of a set. I recommend conducting two strength sessions per week lasting between ten and thirty minutes each. Going for longer than thirty minutes is unnecessary and potentially counterproductive. You can get very strong by conducting just one challenging session per week lasting only twelve minutes, according to Dr. Doug McGuff's book, *Body by Science.* Dr. McGuff's recommended "big five" workout consists of performing a single set of five full-body exercises that collectively challenge all the major muscle groups: seated row, chest press, lat pull-down, overhead press, and leg press.

Include Full-Body Movements

Sweeping, full-body movements that recruit numerous large muscle groups, involve numerous joints, and correspond to real-life fitness, athletic, work, and daily activities are what I recommend most often. Examples include squats, dead lifts, leg presses, box jumps, push-ups, pull-ups, overhead presses, rope climbs, kettlebell swings, and sweeping movements with machines, cables, straps, or stretch tubing. Squats and dead lifts are regarded as the best strength-training exercises because they challenge the major muscle groups of both the upper and lower body and have a strong correlation to everyday movements such as picking heavy objects up from the ground and lowering the body to the ground.

Use Correct Technique

Perform all movements deliberately and powerfully, using precise technique. Certain fundamentals apply across the spectrum of most resistance exercises, including preserving a straight and elongated spine; inflating the diaphragm and engaging the core throughout the range of motion; engaging the glutes throughout the range of motion, which protects the lower spine; and keeping the shoulders in line with the spine instead of shrugged forward. Perform your sets to the point of technical failure, which is different from complete failure. Technical failure is the point where your technique begins to falter, even if only slightly, because of fatigue. You might be able to perform more reps and proceed to complete failure using sloppy form and inappropriate leverage generated by other poorly positioned joints and muscles, but this is obviously counterproductive.

Safety First

As you do in your approach to endurance training, be sure to steer clear of chronic-cardio patterns, such as pushing yourself when your muscles are stiff, sore, or significantly less powerful than usual. Always perform a brief cardiovascular warm-up before doing resistance exercises so your heart rate, respiration, and body temperature are elevated. If you are concerned about injury, the best preparation before a strength-training set is to do the exercise with minimal resistance. This might be squatting, deadlifting with a stick or empty barbell before loading weight, or going through a shorter range of motion with your stretch tubing before you do a full range of motion.

Add Microworkouts

This microworkout concept has emerged as a popular and highly effective addition to any fitness regimen. Microworkouts are brief bursts of intense effort that you can perform throughout the day to break up prolonged periods of stillness and improve fitness without the risk of fatigue that comes from formal, full-length workouts. These might include rushing up a flight or two of stairs, busting out a set of twenty deep squats or chair dips at your desk, assuming a plank position for a minute while watching screen entertainment, strapping on a mini band and doing some monster walks down the hall, or doing a set or two with stretch cords whenever you walk past them in your home.

While we have been socialized to think that getting strong entails driving to a gym and undergoing an exhaustive, hourlong workout or group class, this flying-under-the radar approach can add to tremendous cumulative benefits over time. Think about it: if you rush up a couple of flights of stairs every day, a year later you've sprinted up the equivalent of a seven-hundred-story building. Even if you're super busy, microworkouts can get the blood flowing, turbocharge fat burning, boost cognitive function, and make you feel alert and energized in just one minute.

Sprint Once in a While

Sprinting is my Primal Blueprint Law number 5. It's the ultimate anti-aging workout, honoring the natural law of longevity—"Use it or lose it." When you occasionally push your body to perform at maximum capacity for brief bursts, you experience a host of positive hormonal, psychological, neuroendocrine, and structural effects superior to those you get from any other kind of exercise.

Sprinting is also the ultimate primal workout because humans evolved amid occasional brief life-or-death threats calling for all-out physical effort. When we hone our fight-or-flight attributes once in a while, as our genes expect us to, we stay youthful, powerful, vibrant, and self-confident. Psychologically, sprint workouts reduce your perceived exertion and extend your time-to-fatigue threshold at lower levels of intensity. Becoming competent at sprinting, like becoming competent at strength training, will improve your endurance performance by making the muscles and brain more comfortable during sustained efforts.

Sprint workouts enhance oxygen utilization and promote maximal oxygen uptake in the lungs. They also improve insulin sensitivity, the ability to store and use glycogen, and muscle buffering capacity, which means better lactate clearance and less acidosis during exercise. Even a single all-out sprint of ten to thirty seconds triggers mitochondrial biogenesis and assorted other benefits through the spiking of adenosine monophosphate–activated protein kinase, or AMPK. AMPK is an enzyme lauded for its wide-ranging beneficial functions relating to cellular energy production. Sprinting also elicits that treasured spike in adaptive antiaging hormones such as testosterone and human growth hormone, which work their magic to keep your brain neurons, mitochondria, organs, muscles, joints, and connective tissue youthful and resilient.

Sprinting is the single best activity for promoting rapid reduction of excess body fat.

Sprinting is the single best activity for promoting rapid reduction of excess body fat. Even a very brief sprint session has a profound effect on your metabolic and hormonal function for days afterward. Sprinting has been found to elevate your metabolic function up to thirty times higher than it is at resting baseline. This is a measurement known as metabolic equivalent of task (see page 91). A 30-MET workout such as a sprint sends a strong signal to your genes to shed excess body fat—a far stronger signal than those sent by jogging and easy pedaling, which have MET scores ranging from 6 to 10. If you are still stuck in the flawed and dated calories in–calories out fitness mindset, it might be hard to imagine how a brief workout that you only conduct a few times a month can have a measurable impact on your fat loss and fitness progress, but this is how genetic signaling works. Throw some 30-MET fuel into your fat-burning machine, and you turbocharge fat burning for up to forty-eight hours after the workout via excess post-exercise oxygen consumption.

Research validates the idea that the EPOC after sprinting is vastly more effective for fat reduction than accumulating many more hours of comfortably paced aerobic exercise. In the aftermath of a sprint workout, body temperature, heart rate, and respiration are elevated as the body works hard to remove waste products via the bloodstream and the lymphatic system, replenish depleted energy stores, and return to homeostasis. Sprinting prompts the release of cortisol and catecholamines such as dopamine, adrenaline, epinephrine, and norepinephrine, resulting in a sustained increase in fat metabolism.

Sprinting helps target visceral fat in particular, because the catecholamine cascade elevates beta-3 adrenergic receptors that influence lipolysis (fat burning), and beta-3 receptors are more concentrated in visceral fat than in regular body fat. The elevation of body temperature and decreased blood flow to the GI tract in the hours after sprinting also have appetite-suppressing effects.

You don't have to deeply appreciate the science to understand the basic idea of genetic signaling and that it overrides the incredibly flawed, dated, and oversimplified notion that calories burned during exercise directly result in calories burned off your fat stores. Recall the previous discussion of the fact that exhausting, depleting chronic-cardio workouts increase appetite and promote laziness: that's another example of genetic signaling—in this case for fat storage instead of fat loss.

Although the term "sprinting" typically denotes running on flat ground, we can embrace a broader definition: any type of brief, explosive, all-out effort. There are many low- or no-impact sprinting options that can trigger numerous hormonal and metabolic benefits without the risk factors associated with running on flat ground. For example, you can sprint on a stationary bike, rowing machine, stair climber, or elliptical machine. Or you can even "sprint" by performing a half dozen challenging kettlebell swings.

That said, understand that sprinting on flat ground delivers the maximum benefits for fat reduction and overall athletic competence. When one produces maximum effort against gravity with each stride, a strong signal is sent to the genes to shed excess body fat. The penalty for carrying excess nonfunctional weight—i.e., body fat—in activities that are strongly regulated by gravity is far more severe than it is in any other fitness endeavor. High-impact sprinting also strengthens connective tissue and increases bone density in an adaptive response to the impact load. Remember Wolff's law of bone health—loading a bone makes it thicker and stronger.

The genetic signaling for fat reduction is still strong when performing low- or no-impact sprints, but it's a good idea to work toward eventually sprinting on flat ground if you can do so safely. I like to amuse my lecture audiences with quips such as "Nothing gets you ripped like sprinting" and "Have you ever seen a fat sprinter? No! But we see plenty of overfat endurance athletes."

Sprinting, widely validated as the most potent and time-efficient exercise for comprehensive health and fitness benefits, has been widely neglected and misappropriated by most fitness enthusiasts. Many exercisers simply never push themselves with all-out efforts, instead concentrating too much on lower-intensity endurance training. Others focus heavily on resistance training for specific sports to the exclusion of pure sprinting, while others sprint to excess by doing too many reps for too long a duration with insufficient rest periods between them. Research is compelling: fitness enthusiasts of all levels and with all manner of fitness goals can benefit tremendously from the inclusion of authentic, properly conducted sprint workouts in a well-rounded fitness program.

It's critical to understand the distinction between true sprinting and HIIT workouts, in which efforts are longer, rest is shorter, and the desired adaptations are different. Sprinting is about generating maximum speed and explosive power for very short-duration efforts. These are not workouts in which you have to hang tough through cumulative fatigue or acid accumulation in the muscles. It's a maxim of exercise physiology that a human can only deliver an all-out effort for around seven seconds. Maximum efforts between one and seven seconds are fueled by ATP–creatine phosphate—pure ATP that's stored inside the muscle cells. You don't even need to breathe for short, all-out efforts, and you won't produce any lactic acid. ATP–creatine phosphate is what fuels a high jumper or long jumper's approach and takeoff, a single-rep maximum deadlift, or a forty-yard dash at the NFL Scouting Combine. Beyond that initial burst, energy output is no longer maximal. Indeed, even Olympic 100-meter sprinters are actually decelerating during the final stages of their nearly ten-second races.

After the ATP–creatine phosphate is quickly burned through, the anaerobic glycolysis (a.k.a. ATP-lactate) process kicks in to support maximum efforts of up to around thirty seconds. With oxygen supply limited and energy demand high, the anaerobic glycolysis pathway makes ATP quickly (one hundred times faster than when making

ATP with oxygen) but with the side effect of muscle burn that constrains your performance. The familiar "burn" is actually the result of a buildup of hydrogen ions, a by-product of lactate metabolism, causing the bloodstream to become acidic. This is commonly described as "lactic acid burn." Contrary to the common misconception, lactate is actually a useful energy source for high-intensity exercise, and lactic acid does not cause muscle soreness—it's cleared quickly from the bloodstream.

If you try to go all-out for longer than thirty seconds, you transition from purely anaerobic glucose metabolism to a blend of both anaerobic and aerobic glucose metabolism, meaning that you produce more ATP but at a slower rate. Aerobic glucose metabolism allows you to sustain a maximum effort of up to two minutes without getting overwhelmed by acid accumulation, because the aerobic system helps buffer acid. This is why anaerobic-threshold workouts are a good way to improve acid-buffering capacity.

Performing an all-out effort of up to two minutes entails dealing with high levels of acid in the bloodstream, but not debilitating levels—which would be present when you attempt to maintain the pace of an all-out effort beyond two minutes. Some of the most difficult events in athletics require the participants to deliver maximum energy output longer than they would during a pure sprint. For example, Olympic 400-meter runners (for men, the world record is forty-three seconds; for women, the world record is forty-seven seconds) and 100-meter swimmers (for men, the world record is forty-seven seconds; for women, the world record is fifty-one seconds) are maxing out the creatine phosphate and the anaerobic and aerobic glycolytic pathways as they try to generate the ATP necessary to go that fast for that long. If athletes compete for beyond two minutes, the aerobic pathway provides an increasing percentage of ATP energy. Recall, too, that an all-out effort of one minute and fifteen seconds is 50 percent aerobic, a six-minute effort is 79 percent aerobic, and an hourlong effort is 98 percent aerobic (see page 149).

Aerobic glucose metabolism takes place within a cell's mitochondria. It uses oxygen to deliver a sustained source of energy for long-duration workouts at medium to difficult intensity. The chronic-cardio "sugar burner" athlete is using this pathway to excess instead of slowing down and working on fatty-acid oxidation for the most efficient, clean-burning, and long-lasting energy. Essentially, the short-duration systems supply ATP quickly, but not much of it and not for long. The glycolytic systems supply ATP less quickly, but give you more of it for longer. Finally, the aerobic system supplies tons of ATP for a long time, but produces it very slowly. The next time you get out of breath during a cardio session, realize that your ATP demands at that pace exceed your aerobic capacity, and you are switching over to less efficient, less sustainable, but more immediate sources of ATP.

Most mainstream fitness programming in the realm of HIIT is too stressful or conducted inappropriately by most participants.

A basic understanding of energy pathways is important in helping you design high-intensity training sessions that deliver maximum fitness benefits with the least amount of cellular stress and systemic fatigue. Unfortunately, most mainstream fitness programming in the realm of HIIT is too stressful or conducted inappropriately by most participants. This often results in assorted setbacks and eventual attrition from high-intensity training caused by exhaustion and burnout. When you attempt to go all-out for longer than twenty seconds, you experience an exponential increase in cellular destruction as your body struggles valiantly to supply the necessary ATP. This is the price you pay for winning an Olympic gold medal in the 400 meters, but in order to manage exercise stress and get maximum return on investment for all your workouts, sprint sessions should be carefully regulated.

This is why the sweet spot for true sprinting is between ten and twenty seconds. You get excellent fitness benefits with minimal risk of cellular destruction, lingering system-wide fatigue, and extended recovery. Sprint for ten seconds if you are inexperienced and/or sprinting on flat ground. Twenty-second sprints are fine for low- or no-impact activities and/or for experienced sprinters. You can certainly sprint for shorter periods and derive great benefits. Research suggests that six-second sprints using the ATP–creatine phosphate pathway prompt a significant spike in testosterone, which remains elevated long after the workout.

If you're accustomed to performing HIIT-style workouts consisting of more numerous and longer-lasting work efforts coupled with shorter rest intervals, becoming a true sprinter may entail an important shift in mindset. The focus with sprinting is always on quality—feeling great at every outing, demonstrating excellent technique and explosiveness on every sprint, and executing with consistency. This contrasts sharply with a common HIIT scenario in which cumulative fatigue leads to declining performance and technique, escalating perceived degree of difficulty over the course of the workout, feeling depleted, feeling exhausted afterward, and needing extended recovery time, thanks to cellular destruction and prolonged elevation of stress hormones. You'll know you've overdone it if you incur acute muscle tightness or pain during or soon after the workout, feel dizzy or nauseated, experience bouts of unusual crash-and-burn fatigue, or are inhaling more Ben & Jerry's pints than you thought possible.

Following is a basic framework for safe, effective sprint workouts.

Safety First

For all the benefits of sprinting, there are also risks of injury and exhaustion. If you are a novice, it's essential to establish a good aerobic conditioning base and lead an active lifestyle. Being active in everyday life (especially walking!), conducting regular strength-training sessions, and sprinkling in microworkouts will set you up for success in sprinting. A weekend-warrior approach to sprinting, in which you dust off your shoes and head to the track on Saturday to crush a session, is a great way to hurt yourself.

If you are new to sprinting, start with no-impact activities such as pedaling on a stationary bike or exercising on a rowing machine or an elliptical—even if you are really fit. Accumulate a handful of good sessions, then introduce low-impact options such as hills and stairs. Progress to eventually doing wind sprints on flat ground, then full sprints. Choose a reliable, flat venue such as a running track, an athletic field, or a flat, straight pedestrian trail. Don't sprint on a treadmill because it's too difficult to mess with the controls for short efforts and can be dangerous if you lose your balance.

For high-impact sprint workouts, once every seven to ten days is plenty. You can probably handle two no- or low-impact sprint sessions a week. You must always feel 100 percent rested and energized before you conduct a sprint workout. You never want to sprint in a fatigued state, because that will actually teach your central nervous system to fire muscles more slowly and less powerfully. Realize that there are many ways to trash yourself with a flawed approach, including conducting sprint workouts too frequently and doing workouts with too many sprints and/or sprints that last too long and/or have insufficient recovery time between them.

Preparation

You should always precede your main set of sprints with extensive preparations.

- First, conduct a brief cardiovascular warm-up to elevate your heart rate, respiration, and body temperature.
- Next, do some dynamic stretches that exaggerate your range of motion. For running, this could include some marching steps, walking lunges, and leg swings.
- Next, conduct some drills that teach the muscles and nervous system to fire with explosive, precise technique. For running, this can include assorted skipping drills, high knees, heel kicks, and backwards running.
- Next, conduct some wind sprints to ensure that your muscles and joints feel fluid and powerful and that your technique is sharp. If you feel sluggish or tense during wind sprints, end the workout with a cooldown and wait to attempt sprints another day.

For no- or low-impact sprinting, the dynamic stretches and technique drills are less important, but you should still spend plenty of time preparing the body for maximum effort. It's also important to prepare the mind for the delivery of maximum effort. Perform your stretches and drills with precision, and you will boost motivation and confidence.

Main-Set Protocol

I recommend that your main set consist of *four to eight sprints lasting between ten and twenty seconds each, with a six-to-one ratio of rest to work.* This entails resting for one minute after each ten-second sprint or up to two minutes after each twenty-second sprint. Observing a six-to-one rest-to-work ratio should allow you to recover fully and maintain a high standard of performance on each individual sprint. This might seem like more than necessary rest, but it's actually a *minimum* recommendation. When in doubt, take more rest to ensure that your mind and body are primed for each sprint you do.

Consistency

Consistent quality of effort is the most important concept to embrace for a successful sprint workout. If your first sprint of fifty yards across half a football field takes eight seconds and feels like a 90 on an effort scale of 100, you want your final sprint to be of similar duration and similar effort. A tiny bit of attrition is acceptable—say, nine seconds at a 93 effort level. What you don't want is to struggle and strain on your final reps to stay at around eight seconds. Nor do you want to start coming through in ten or eleven seconds at that self-reported exertion level of 90. Once performance or effort declines significantly, your sprint workout is over. It's go hard, then go home!

Since you are only sprinting when you feel great, you will be delivering somewhere between a 90 and a 95 percent effort. You could characterize this as a near-maximum effort that can be repeated with impeccable form and no strain. After some great reps, you may notice at some point a bit more fatigue, sluggishness, or loss of focus during the recovery period. These are indications that you may be nearing the limit of your productive capacity. If you experience even minor muscular or connective tissue tweaks and twinges, increased muscle tightness, or compromised form, this is a signal to end the set and commence the cooldown.

If you're an endurance athlete accustomed to suffering through grueling workouts, sprinting will require a fundamental change in mindset. Instead of the no-pain-no-gain "hang in there" mentality, you'll want to redirect your focus to exhibiting precise technique and feeling energetic and explosive throughout the workout. It's a cool feeling to conduct a workout as if you were a real athlete instead of just a plodder, so go for it!

Cooldown

After you complete the main set, always end your workout with a brief cardiovascular cooldown of between five and ten minutes. This can comprise a mixture of walking and jogging or easy efforts on the cardio machine you used for sprinting. The objective of the cooldown is to gradually lower your heart rate, respiration, blood pressure, and body temperature back to baseline. When you feel your body temperature and your sweat rate start to normalize a bit, you can stop moving and perhaps perform a few static stretches if you feel it's warranted or if it's been prescribed for you.

By the end of your cooldown, you should be able to breathe and speak normally, feel satisfied and a bit euphoric from an optimal level of workout stress, and feel pleasantly fatigued but not trashed. You should be able to walk away from the track with a little bounce in your step and an eagerness to return soon.

Next, spend five to ten minutes relaxing before you head off to your next important responsibility of the day. Dr. Jannine Krause, host of *The Health Fix* podcast, recommends a practice she calls "positional parasympathetic breathing" to facilitate coming down off the fight-or-flight state of the workout and returning to homeostasis. Lie down, relax, elevate your feet onto a chair or bench, and focus on taking gentle but deep nasal diaphragmatic breaths. You can try this technique at your workout venue or perhaps as soon as you arrive home.

So to summarize, in order to conduct an effective sprinting workout, you should

- establish a good aerobic and active-lifestyle baseline;
- follow a safe and sensible approach, starting with no- or low-impact sprinting;
- sprint only when you are 100 percent rested and energized;
- follow the recommended progression of (1) warm-up, (2) dynamic stretching, (3) technique drills, and (4) wind sprints before performing your main set;

- do four to eight sprints of ten to twenty seconds each, with a six-to-one recovery-to-work ratio;
- deliver a consistent quality of effort on each rep; and
- allow time for a deliberate cooldown and some parasympathetic chill time afterward.

Play

Play is Primal Blueprint Law number 7. Spontaneous, unstructured outdoor play is an integral element of a healthy, happy life. Unfortunately, with our deep immersion in hectic, high-tech, hyperconnected living, we've widely neglected play and collectively adopted the belief that play is for kids. But introducing play into your daily routine will make you a more creative, productive, sensitive, balanced, and happy human being.

Humans have a hardwired genetic need for play that stems from the fact that we evolved under constant life-and-death selection pressure. It's clear from anthropological and archaeological evidence that play was a vital component of our primal ancestors' lives for hundreds of thousands of years. From the magnificent ball courts found in ancient settlements throughout Mesoamerica to the architectural remnants and detailed records from the ancient Greek Olympics, there is no question that today's packed stadiums and exceptional athletic competitions are no modern creation but rather the continuing legacy of our ancestors.

Play obviously provided a needed escape from the hazards and harshness of primal life, but it also offered ancestral humans numerous other benefits. It contributed to communal living and social cohesion, nurtured creative energies, and strengthened problem-solving skills—as it still does today. Play necessitates mental modeling, critical thinking, and creative innovation, through which we develop behavioral, intellectual, and emotional creativity and flexibility. Play has been scientifically proved to increase work productivity, improve stress management, and enhance self-esteem and social competency.

Psychiatrist Stuart Brown is the founder of the National Institute for Play and author of *Play: How It Shapes the Brain, Opens the Imagination, and Invigorates the Soul*. In this book, Brown calls play a "profound biological process" and explains that play, across the span of a lifetime, wires our brains, forming new connections, creating new circuits, and organizing existing connections. The free-flowing, risk-free nature of play allows us to test skills and scenarios that prepare us for real-life challenges. Play has further allure as a stress reliever, not only from the life-and-death rigors of primal life but also from the unrelenting stress and tight structure of modern life.

The free-flowing, risk-free nature of play allows us to test skills and scenarios that prepare us for real-life challenges.

When humans are deprived of play, they can suffer from numerous symptoms of dysfunction, including lack of curiosity, diminished social competency, and uncontrollable emotions. The net result is a narrowing of social, emotional, and cognitive intelligence. This also happens to be a reliable marker of accelerated aging. Play also promotes the development and maintenance of what Dr. Brown calls a "cognitively fluid mind," characterized by abstract thinking and sophisticated problem solving. While cognitive fluidity helps us navigate the complexities of modern life, anthropologists believe it triggered one of the most significant breakthroughs on the human evolutionary timeline around sixty thousand years ago. By using play to process what-if scenarios without life-and-death consequences, our ancestors were able to increase the sophistication of their hunter-gatherer operations, further their culture, increase their population, and successfully settle the entire globe with continually advancing societies.

While play can mean anything from a tennis match to wastebasket hoops at the office to video gaming all night, let's concentrate on play, ideally in nature, that is spontaneous and unstructured, eschews tangible measurements of accomplishment, and gets you out of the focused, rational mindset that you exist in for most of the day. Find something that gets you completely absorbed in the moment and the pure joy of the experience. Such activities will deliver the best balance to our lives of stillness, predictability, and hyperconnectivity.

The integration of play into a well-rounded fitness program can be particularly beneficial for novices or people intimidated by formal workout environments. Even for highly accomplished and motivated fitness enthusiasts, play can reawaken the athletic spirit, provide a jolt of motivation and excitement, and bring a sense of newness to one's fitness experience. What's more, when one is chasing a Frisbee, trying to navigate an obstacle course, or otherwise engaged in unstructured and unfamiliar challenges, the exertion may be perceived as less stressful and less difficult than when one is hoisting weights for a certain number of reps in a gym or trying to complete a race course in a certain time.

Reflecting on my past as a marathoner, I find it amusing and poignant to realize that I have not run longer than one continuous mile in more than thirty years. Why should I? Don't get me wrong—I routinely cover perhaps five miles during epic two-hour Ultimate Frisbee battles, and I hiked more than six hundred miles during a two-month vacation in France (truth be told, I was testing my prototype Peluva shoes, so I couldn't be stopped!). I love breaking out into a jog or even a brief sprint when I'm out for urban walks or nature hikes, but I can't be bothered to set out on a structured, dogmatic, pavement-based, slightly-too-strenuous steady-state endurance run—no way.

You might think I ended my endurance training obsession because I'm cranky and worn out from the excesses of my past—fair enough. But I want you to reflect for a moment on the broken relationship we have today with spontaneous physical activity and how easy it is to drift into an overly stressful, overly regimented to approach to fitness—and the predictable and often mind-numbing routines of daily life. It's time to honor the legacy of your bold and adventurous ancestors and go for the thrill. This does not entail taking foolish, dangerous risks, like zigzagging your motorcycle down the freeway at a hundred miles an hour. Rather, this means seeking out calculated, well-managed challenges that will nevertheless deliver an emotional charge similar to that enjoyed by the foolish motorcyclist.

To access the exalted "flow" state, take on a challenge that lies just slightly outside your comfort zone—not too dangerous to paralyze you with fear but not so routine that it fails to generate an adrenaline buzz. For example, downhill skiing is not without the danger of falling and other accidents, but recreational skiers can enjoy the exhilaration of schussing down a mountain at good speed if the risk is managed appropriately. Strive to land in that "sweet spot" where exciting, intense challenges are balanced with acceptable levels of risk.

WAYS TO PLAY

There are as many ways to play as there are fish in the sea. If you've never tried them, how about having a go at the following? Don't keep score—that's a bore!

- Mountain biking
- Rock climbing
- Surfing
- Stand-up paddling
- Waterskiing
- Wakeboarding
- Wakesurfing (yep, without a rope)
- Cross-country skiing
- Ice skating
- Snowshoeing

These activities all entail synchronizing your physical efforts with forces in nature—going with the flow. Moving within a naturally varied environment, such as water, virtually demands that you transition out of an analytical state into a flowlike state.

Consider the opportunities you miss every day by staying in spectator mode. How about getting up off your folding chair and helping out at your kid's soccer practice? Or jumping into that pick-up basketball game the next time you're at the gym?

How about venturing beyond your primary competitive outlets? If you're a runner, try a mini triathlon. If you're a triathlete, try an obstacle course race. You'll toe the start line feeling buoyant and excited in a different way from the pressurized feeling you get on the start line of your important races.

Group activities are a great way to combine play with social connection. When we play with friends and family members, we infuse these intimate relationships with humor, lightheartedness, vulnerability, and a strong sense of connection. At numerous PrimalCon health and fitness retreats I hosted, we balanced educational presentations with unusual activities designed to bring out the playful spirit in everyone. These fun interludes turned out to be a highlight for many participants: a sunset ocean plunge followed by a sprint to the resort Jacuzzi; a challenging hike culminating in a jump off a fifteen-foot granite cliff into a mountain lake; and a *Survivor*-style team challenge—a blend of scavenger hunt, brain-teaser puzzles, and team-oriented physical and logistical challenges. Plan a play outing and rally your favorite group!

EPILOGUE
Expanding Your Horizons

I KNOW MANY OF YOU WILL remain enamored of endurance training despite my gentle and not-so-gentle counterarguments, so I propose that you vary your approach and evolve your perspective about what it means to be fit and how to get there. When it comes to steady-state cardio, realize that it's marketing hype, not science, that says we need it to burn calories, lose fat, and prepare for the overhyped, overly stressful races revered by the endurance community.

You can still get an A-plus in cardio by walking extensively (à la Hannes Kolehmainen, who walked and high-intensity-interval-trained his way to Olympic gold), logging 80 percent of your weekly mileage in zone 1 (à la Eliud Kipchoge), and engaging in sprinting, strength training, yoga, pickleball, team sports, and playing of all kinds. Remember the Copenhagen City Heart Study and the research conducted by Dr. James O'Keefe and many others showing that optimal cardiovascular health can be yours with as few as one to two and a half hours a week—and as many as five to eight hours a week—of comfortably paced exercise. After that, the benefits level off and even decline when exercise is taken to extremes.

If you insist upon pursuing endurance goals, I suggest that you emphasize breakthrough workouts, cross-training, and recovery and deemphasize steady-state chronic cardio. For example, if you enjoy racing, how about heading out two or three days a month for a brisk 10k? Schedule recovery workouts before and after these breakthrough workouts to ensure that you can "nail" them when race day arrives.

Emphasize zone 1 heart rates for the rest of your endurance session: don't give in to the common tendency to routinely peg your heart rate at your zone 2 maximum—and allow it to drift above the zone 2 limit here and there to boot. If you package these race-simulation workouts with a general commitment to frequent everyday movement, flexibility and mobility exercises, resistance training, and some occasional sprinting, I virtually guarantee that you will perform as well or better than you did in your chronic-cardio-fueled endeavors. You'll also have more fun and avoid the embarrassing overuse injuries so common in recreational runners.

If you're terrified that your performance will decline when you reduce your weekly mileage, think about the long-validated benefits of tapering, which means reducing your training load in advance of competition to ensure that you are fully rested and primed for a peak performance. The acknowledged pioneer in this department is Dr. David Costill, long regarded as one of the world's leading exercise physiologists. Dr. Costill is a former collegiate swimming and running coach, the holder of numerous world and American records in Masters Swimming, and professor emeritus of exercise science and director of the Human Performance Laboratory at Ball State University. He was also the first scientist to publish major research on the performance impact of tapering, and it has revolutionized the world of endurance sports.

A widely publicized study conducted by Dr. Costill in 1985 revealed that swimmers who reduced their training volume by 67 percent for fifteen days were able to achieve a 4 percent improvement in performance and a 25 percent increase in arm strength; they also had lower lactate levels while racing. Ensuing research conducted by scientists at McMaster University, in Hamilton, Ontario, revealed that highly trained runners (averaging fifty miles a week) benefited greatly from tapering. One group reduced its mileage by 64 percent, to eighteen miles a week, and achieved a 6 percent improvement in competitive performance, while another group cut its mileage by 88 percent and improved performance by a stunning 22 percent! Essentially, this group ran only short, fast intervals on a track for a week, accumulating a total of six miles. Further research in this realm has led to the widespread conclusion that the best way to taper is to dramatically reduce volume but maintain intensity.

I also encourage you to at least dabble in the workouts suggested in the appendix—jogging 2.0, walkabouts, fartlek workouts, homespun hybrid challenges, and perhaps even speedgolf. These will lead you into an empowering new phase in which you no longer have to struggle, suffer, and endure in ways that compromise your health. Instead, you can strive for excellence and personal growth in every challenge you take on.

That said, I know what it's like to feel pumped about taking a new direction in life and then find yourself gradually sliding back into old habits. This goes for everything from relationship communication skills ("Dispense all feedback with loving-kindness!") to productivity tips ("Avoid distraction—batch your emails!") and safe driving habits ("Go hands-free—no texting!"). This means that even if you are completely sold on fat max training, occasions will arrive when you are compelled to push the pace with lively training partners or otherwise bust loose from the confines of that darn heart-rate monitor. But remember: opening up the throttle once in a while is perfectly fine. A well-trained, well-rested body will respond beautifully when you ask for a peak performance effort. What I want you to avoid is the downward spiral of chronic cardio, drifting beyond harmonious passion into unhealthy obsession, and increasing reliance on cushioned shoes for dysfunctional feet.

The next time you drift into a chronic pattern or unhealthful mindset, I want you to call upon the knowledge you have gained in this book so that it can stack up proudly against the entrenched habits, flawed cultural programming, peer pressure, and ego demands that compel us to suffer and struggle instead of thrive. Remember the precepts of the running boom we shattered in chapter 1? Remember that the standard marathon distance is based not on an epic physical feat by a heroic soldier but on a whimsical 1879 poem that distorted Greek history? We might as well choose an arbitrary distance such as ten miles and call it a marathon. We'd all be better off and get to enjoy brunch sooner after the big race.

As we marvel at the unparalleled domination of East African long-distance runners on the world stage, we must acknowledge that the most prominent driving forces in their success are the massive economic incentives in elite running (combined with a dearth of other career opportunities) as well as favorable genetic attributes and a low-tech, high-altitude lifestyle. Indeed, 80 percent of the top marathon times ever recorded, and 90 percent of world records in long-distance events, are held by runners of East African descent—mainly from a single ethnic group called the Kalenjin. This is the single most impressive example of domination by people from a small geographic area ever observed in any sport. Those in your local running community who grab the podium spots and enjoy long careers on the roads and trails? They've been endowed with the genetic gifts of light frames, injury resilience, outsize competitive intensity, and a willingness to suffer that can often be at odds with a life of happiness and contentment. Deep immersion in endurance running legitimately falls into the "don't try this at home" category.

There is no "born to run" mandate but rather a genetic mandate to move frequently, lift heavy things, sprint once in a while, and play.

Remember from the section called "Professor Sisson's Evolutionary Anthropology 2.0" that there is no "born to run" mandate but rather a genetic mandate to move frequently, lift heavy things, sprint once in a while, and play. This aligns nicely with my suggestion in chapter 9 that training sessions should comprise walking interspersed with

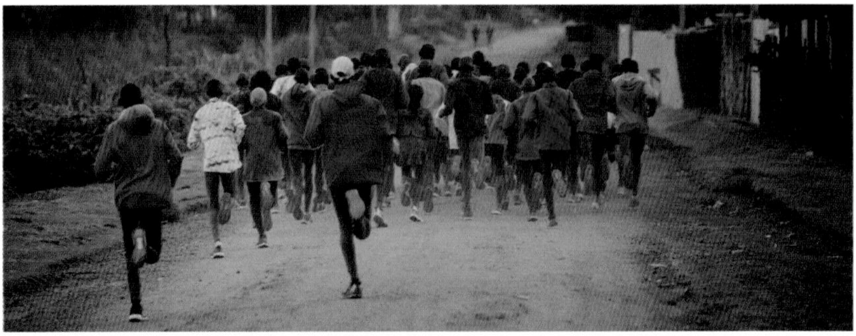

The Great Rift Valley, in Africa, is home to the most of the world's greatest endurance runners.

brief running stints—executed with a midfoot strike—and followed by walking before you blow out your heart rate. Slowing down helps you go faster because it strengthens the aerobic system, even when you walk. In fact, when you slow down, you are training in the same manner as the world's top endurance athletes.

Remember from the chapter called "The Broken Promise of Weight Loss" that body composition is mostly about dietary choices, not calories burned at workouts. Reference the scientifically validated constrained model of energy expenditure (page 208) and compensation theory (page 27). Exhausting exercise leads to increased appetite, reduced baseline activity, and genetic signaling for fat storage and muscle loss. Realize that health-destructive visceral fat accumulates as a result of activities that cause overproduction of stress hormones, including burning too many calories at workouts that are too strenuous and too frequent. Please own this important and empowering axiom: "It's not about the calories; it's about the movement." I'm concerned that the flawed, dated, and oversimplified calories in–calories out model of weight loss could be one of the deep-seated subconscious motivations leading you to push your body too hard—to run instead of walk.

Now, the calories burned when you walk are a different story. They might not be a big number on the internet calculator, but each time you get up and walk—whether for a few minutes away from your desk, a leisurely stroll in the evening, or a grand weekend outing—you are sending genetic signals for efficient fat metabolism, inflammatory balance, and stabilized appetite and satiety hormones.

"If you can't run barefoot, you probably shouldn't be running." —Graham Tuttle

Remember from the chapter called "The Broken Promise of Cushioned Shoes" that the imperative to run is driven by the use of elevated, cushioned shoes that destroy proprioception and enable the shuffling, heel-striking, overstriding, hip-drop form that almost certainly leads to recurring overuse injuries. Graham Tuttle, a.k.a. the Barefoot Sprinter—seen on YouTube and Instagram—offered a pithy insight over a video of him striding barefoot down a sidewalk: "If you can't run barefoot, you probably shouldn't be running."

You may contend that's extreme, but it's an assertion validated by research conducted by Daniel Lieberman and others. At the very least, learn to midfoot strike and perhaps try introducing a bit of running in minimalist shoes. As you muster the courage to wean yourself off a desperate reliance on your beloved cushioned footwear, acknowledge the truth that running shoes weaken and create dysfunction in your feet and lower extremities and absolutely do not protect you from injury. Nor do they lessen impact or control pronation. Your long-neglected bare feet are vastly superior to any shoe for impact absorption, balancing moving body weight, and generating propulsion. It's time to make gradual, sensible inroads toward barefoot competency.

From the chapter titled "The Catastrophe of Chronic Cardio," remember that it's easy to derive aerobic conditioning benefits from just a few hours a week of comfortably paced movement and that it's very possible to exceed your stress capacity when you combine your endurance training with all the other forms of stress in life. The fight-or-flight response is identical regardless of the stimulus. Knowing that going to extremes can mess with your heart, mitochondria, digestion, and immunity, see if you can behave in alignment with your knowledge, beliefs, and best interests and honor that heart-monitor alarm.

From the chapter called "The Ordeal of the Obligate Runner," realize that there is no mandate to endure inappropriate suffering just because we are immersed in comfort, convenience, luxury, and indulgence. No matter what baggage and issues you struggle with, you don't have to self-flagellate to cope or try to feel whole or deserving. We can still appreciate Sir Roger Bannister's observation that effort and struggle are deeply satisfying when you're pursuing peak performance goals with honor and maintaining constant vigilance over your mental and physical health.

If you continue to be influenced by fellow runners posting their workout reports on social media, reflect on the powerful pull of instant-gratification dopamine triggers. Hey, running's great if recreational drugs and all-night binges on porn and video games ain't your thing, but an addictive approach to fitness also floods the dopamine pathways and can lead to depression, anxiety, and withdrawal symptoms. Strive to detox from the obsessive pursuit of the runner's high and appreciate the rich and meaningful pleasures of exercising at a comfortable (perhaps walking!) pace and connecting with nature, with other people, and with yourself. Use exercise to manage your overall stress levels rather than heap more stress on your plate. Get over yourself!

As you say goodbye to the tailspin of chronic cardio, strive to increase all forms of general everyday movement, especially walking as much as possible in minimalist shoes. With extra precision and focus in your training, you'll be diligent about improving foot functionality instead of taking your feet for granted. Make barefoot your default at home and walk as much as possible in minimalist shoes that allow for toe splay, toe articulation, and groundfeel.

Finally, understand that broad-based full-body fitness is the key to general health, vitality, and longevity. Endurance competency is a small sliver of the big picture, and it often comes at the expense of other important pillars of fitness because you only have so much time and energy to exercise. As you gain energy and recalibrate your stress-rest balance, you can integrate regular resistance exercise, occasional all-out sprints—starting with low- or no-impact activities and working up to sprinting on flat ground—and play into your workout routines. Yes, you deserve it—play is not just for kids!

I wish you enjoyment, contentment, and fulfillment on your journey and look forward to connecting with you via BornToWalkBook.com.

APPENDIX
Fun and Challenging Non-Steady-State Workouts

I have urged you repeatedly in this book to reject the flawed dogma of steady-state cardio. So it's only fair that I suggest some alternatives. Therefore, I hereby present you with some really cool, fun, and highly effective *non*-steady-state workouts. Remember: you develop your aerobic system at all levels of exercise intensity, from walking to sprinting to stop-and-start activities and strength-training sessions in the gym. What I want you to extricate yourself from are chronic, overly stressful training patterns, which are not only ineffective but also destroy your health. Believe it or not, you can still deliver extremely impressive endurance results with a sensible, time-efficient, broad-based fitness approach.

I've been amused to witness the rise in popularity of so-called hybrid athletes on the internet. These folks try to outdo one another in endurance and strength by performing crazy self-styled challenges requiring incredibly disparate skills. YouTube is full of videos showing enthusiasts lifting massive amounts of weight and then completing extreme endurance efforts. One day in 2021, Scotsman Fergus Crawley put up an elite-level powerlifting total of 1,322 pounds (squat of 485 pounds, bench press of 308 pounds, and deadlift of 529 pounds), then ran thirty-seven miles in less than six hours. Another day, in 2023, he squatted five hundred pounds, ran a 4:58 mile, and finished the day with a sub-five-hour marathon.

One of the ultimate ambitions in the hybrid game is to deadlift five hundred pounds and run a mile in less than five minutes. A handful of hybrid athletes have achieved both feats in the same day, but in 2020, Michael Miraglia of San Diego became the only athlete to accomplish the feat on the same clock—that is, he started a stopwatch, then hoisted a weighted bar located at the track starting line, then completed four laps in a total elapsed time of 4:49. For perspective, if you were to go looking for the nearest human capable of lifting five hundred pounds off the ground, you'd find a huge waddling gym bro weighing half as much as the bar or more. Strength-training experts estimate that it takes ten years of consistent training to work up to a five-hundred-pound deadlift. In addition, running aficionados estimate that anyone who can run a sub-five-minute mile is a one-in-five-hundred specimen in his prime years (between the ages of eighteen and thirty-four) who is serious about training. It's safe to say that Miraglia is the only human ever to perform this combination feat, and I mean *ever*.

A couple of other high-profile hybrid athletes you might have seen in action are YouTube personality Nick Symmonds, a two-time US Olympic 800-meter runner and world championship bronze medalist, and Ryan Hall, the retired American record holder in the marathon (2:04) and a two-time Olympian. Symmonds produces viral videos of zany athletic challenges, often competing against young athletes or passersby in the community. He has taken videos of himself running a mile every hour, on the hour, for twenty-four consecutive hours (tougher than it sounds); chronicling his loss of ten pounds in a twenty-four-hour period; challenging an elite female hybrid athlete to a game of H-O-R-S-E using gym exercises; setting a "world record" for the fastest 400 meters run in Crocs, and so forth. Symmonds has also deadlifted four hundred pounds and run 400 meters in a combined elapsed time of fifty-six seconds.

Ryan Hall has famously transformed his body since his retirement as an elite marathoner. From toeing the line at an elfin five feet ten and 127 pounds in his heyday, he is now two hundred pounds of solid muscle. He's achieved a respectable powerlifting total of 1,340 pounds (squat 480 pounds, bench 330 pounds, deadlift 530 pounds). He, too, tackles creative hybrid challenges. Yep, he's tried and fallen short on the five-hundred-pound–sub-five-minute-mile combo, but he's expected to bag it someday—what better candidate? In 2022, Hall split a cord of wood (enough to fill two pickup trucks), ran to the bottom of the Grand Canyon, then hiked five thousand vertical feet back to the rim while carrying two jugs of water weighing sixty-two pounds each. The feat took five hours, with stops every forty-five seconds to rest the jugs on the ground. Hall was forced to retire early from elite running in 2016, at age thirty-three, because of health challenges—specifically, chronic fatigue and low testosterone. But his exploits have made him both a sad example of the ravages of extreme endurance training and the poster boy for the health-transformation potential of getting stronger and more muscular. As he mentioned to a reporter from *Men's Journal*, "I was in a bad spot when I retired. I was weak, small, and had low testosterone levels. I was tired all the time." Hall, now in his forties, claims to feel better and fitter than ever.

The exploits of Crawley, Miraglia, Symmonds, Hall, and CrossFit legends such as Rich Froning (four-time champion) and Mat Fraser (five-time champion) are awe-inspiring and help shift the paradigm about what it means to be truly fit for life. The endurance world has long been guilty of a myopic perspective in which "hybrid athlete" might have been defined as someone who could run fast over a variety of distances, from the 5k up to the marathon. But sorry—that's not going to cut it these days. Unless you are an elite athlete training for Olympics, broad-based fitness competence is the key to longevity, injury prevention, and having fun in your daily endeavors, both competitive and recreational. The following workouts have an endurance bent, but they contain exciting, challenging new elements that will keep things fresh and help you develop a variety of fitness skills.

Jogging 2.0

Instead of a humdrum steady-state training session, you can make jogging the baseline form of locomotion for your workout and sprinkle in some brief periods of medium- to high-intensity running-technique drills, dynamic stretches, jumping drills, balance and agility drills, and/or core- or leg-strengthening movements. Visit the Peluva YouTube channel for instructional videos of basic, intermediate, and advanced running-technique drills, including the popular skipping drills and many variations performed by track-and-field athletes. Skipping drills emphasize certain segments of the running stride, thus reinforcing correct technique, extending your typical range of motion, and improving your mobility and force production. Most of them are low-impact and easy to learn, even for people without racing experience.

After a five- to ten-minute warm-up jog, you can initiate your first set of drills. Focus on executing perfect form and being crisp and explosive. After fifteen seconds, stop and walk for thirty to sixty seconds, then do a few more sets of drills lasting fifteen seconds each. Walk for a couple of minutes to recover, resume jogging for a few minutes, and throw in additional sets of drills or challenges as desired over the course of the workout.

If you encounter a suitable fitness challenge en route, perhaps you'll pause for a set of step-ups or vertical jumps onto a bench or an elevated platform. You could also hit the deck for some push-ups or tackle established par course stations on your route. Search YouTube for "Brad Kearns Jogging 2.0" for inspiration. Don't worry—you'll still get your cardio "points" doing workouts like these, but you'll also develop more broad-based fitness competence, improve your resilience against injury, and stimulate some fast-twitch muscle fibers, enabling you to become more explosive. Although tradition has long mandated tightly structured workouts in distinct heart-rate zones, there is tremendous value in conducting workouts that have more variation in pace, heart rate, and muscular demand. This concept is detailed in Steve Magness's book *The Science of Running*.

Walkabouts

Instead of staying on the beaten trail or path, do some off-roading to purposely negotiate rough, varied, and/or uneven terrain. Even the most urban-dense environments offer opportunities for brief detours onto varied terrain. The idea here is to purposely challenge your proprioception and foot functionality by walking on a rock bed or natural debris, up or down steep slopes, diagonally across a steep incline, or any other variation. Even if you're confined to an urban setting, you can find ways to do this. For example, try walking a few strides with one foot on the sidewalk and another at street level before returning to a level surface. Hop onto a bus-stop bench, jump back down, and resume your walk. Grab on to a sign pole and conduct one set of single-leg straight-leg deadlifts (also known as Romanian deadlifts, or RDLs) before resuming your walk.

Mix things up! Our brains and lower extremities desperately need these challenges and variations to function optimally and maintain all-important balance skills throughout life. Unfortunately, we've been programmed to avoid attempting anything unusual in the name of safety and injury prevention. This is a ludicrous notion: when you insist upon sanitizing your exercise sessions, you steadily lose your ability to do anything as simple as hike on a rugged trail.

Benchmark Workouts

My college girlfriend used to go to the gym once a month. She did the same workout every time—a punishing sequence of high-intensity interval cardio, a single set to failure on numerous strength machines, and calisthenics and body-weight challenges. This template workout had numerous specific performance standards, including those for calorie burning, rep counts, and weight settings. If she was able to complete it, she declared herself fit and wouldn't return to the gym for another month. Whenever I tell this story, I often get knee-jerk scoffing, but the lesson here is profound. Think about it: she maintained an impressive fitness level by leading a generally active lifestyle of walking and cavorting around campus and doing one peak-performance session every month like clockwork. No risk of overtraining, injury, or burnout. There was tremendous consistency, and the workout was pretty time-efficient. While this is an extreme example, I think we can emulate it to our great benefit, especially when it comes to endurance running goals.

Unless you are intently training for a lofty standard such as a three-hour marathon, you can excel in running with vastly less weekly mileage than you think. You just have to spend sufficient time on your feet as part of a walking-inspired lifestyle, nurture broad-based functional fitness through strength training and sprinting, and conduct an occasional challenging workout that proves to your mind and your body that you've still got it—that you measure up to your desired fitness standard. In my 1989 book, *Training and Racing Biathlons*, I presented an overarching training philosophy in which workouts are categorized as *breakthrough*, *break even*, or *recovery*. A breakthrough workout is one that's difficult and challenging enough to stimulate an improvement in your fitness level. A break-even workout is a typical session conducted strictly for fitness maintenance, and a recovery workout is easy enough to be restorative. Today, runners will consider a long-distance run or high-intensity interval session a breakthrough workout, especially if the degree of difficulty and performance standards are increased over previous workouts.

Let me ask you this: Can you run a seven-minute mile right now, all-out? Can you run an eight-minute mile? Can you complete an entire boot-camp class without stopping for rest breaks? Establish whatever performance standards you wish as benchmarks, then take a crack at one every month or so. If you've been struggling with overstress and overtraining patterns, experiment with a significant or extreme reduction in your typical exercise output for a month, then attempt a benchmark workout. If you reallocate your fitness time wisely, I'll bet that you can easily attain the benchmark and perhaps surprise yourself with an improvement.

The Walk-Jog-Walk-Jog Fax Max Workout

To optimally develop your aerobic system while minimizing the risk of burnout and injury, you must honor your fat max heart rate for the vast majority of your training time. The longer the duration of your workout, the slower your average pace must be in order to remain at or below fat max. This is because cumulative fatigue causes the heart rate to drift higher when you attempt to maintain a steady pace. If you run your first mile in eleven minutes at a heart rate of 140, running your fifth mile in eleven minutes will require a higher heart rate. To run your fifth mile at a heart rate of 140, you must slow to perhaps twelve or twelve and a half minutes. There is no way to "hack" the process of aerobic development. You might have a tendency to be impatient, impulsive, highly driven, and competitive, but you can't rush your way to endurance excellence. Ask Eliud Kipchoge or Hans Kolehmainen.

If you feel frustrated with the idea that your typical run must become a walk to respect fat max, let's acknowledge that there is no rule that you need to engage in steady-state cardio to become fit or prepare for endurance events. In fact, varying the pace of your workouts can deliver excellent fitness benefits with minimal risk of overstress. Remember: our genetic expectations for health include lots of varied, low-intensity movement throughout the day, regular resistance exercise, and occasional all-out sprints. This essentially describes the hunter-gatherer lifestyle of our ancestors.

Instead of pegging your heart rate at fat max for the duration of your aerobic workouts, consider starting out at your typical jogging pace, then slowing to a walk when your heart rate reaches fat max. After you walk for a few minutes, your heart rate should drop significantly, and you can break into a jog once again. Repeat the cycle, always slowing when your heart rate reaches fat max.

The Fartlek Workout, a.k.a. the Persistence Hunt

Fartlek is a Swedish word that means "speed play." Developed by Swedish Olympic decathlete Gösta Holmér in the 1930s, when he coached distance runners, it's characterized by unstructured alterations in running pace, typically over varied terrain. Fartlek workouts are a great way to prepare for cross-country racing, in which undulating courses and the unpredictable tactics of your opponents demand a more diversified pace and effort level than what is typically seen at track events. For decades, fartlek sessions have been very popular among endurance runners seeking variety and novelty, a break from the typical rigid structure of interval workouts on the track or hill repeats. Gee, that seems pretty similar to an ancestral persistence hunt, doesn't it?

Anything goes during fartlek workouts: you are not worried about staying below fat max during such sessions. The leader of a pack of runners can set whatever pace he likes for however long he likes before ceding the lead to another runner. Or a fartlek run might entail charging up a hill encountered on the route but jogging on flats and downhills. As noted in the textbook *Exercise Physiology for Health, Fitness, and Performance*, "When properly applied, this method overloads one or all of the energy systems," and "although it lacks the systematic and quantified approaches of interval and continuous training, it also adds freedom and variety to workouts."

When I was road-testing prototype Peluva shoes during an extended summer stay in Europe, I would walk for several miles every single day. For fun and variety, I would launch into very short sprints—uphill, flat, downhill, whatever—sometimes for five seconds, sometimes for twenty seconds. Other times, I might switch from walking to jogging if I encountered a smooth stretch of road or trail. After each sprint or jogging stint, I would walk slowly for a minute or two, then resume my typical walking pace until my next spontaneous acceleration.

Walking with Purpose

In the old days, die-hard runners would scoff at the sight of earnest walkers with exaggerated arm swings and overly aggressive strides. Alas, those walkers were on to something—a safe and highly effective gait pattern. I call it walking with purpose. Essentially, you are walking as fast as you can before having to break into a jog. The hurried cadence and extra arm pumps elevate your heart rate, maximize calorie burning, and deliver excellent aerobic conditioning benefits without the impact trauma of jogging. If you feel like changing your walking pace, go for it. After all, this book is titled *Born to Walk*, not *Born to Walk Slowly*!

I find myself often walking with purpose when I'm doing local errands on foot; it's an ideal technique for those occasions when I need to return home by a certain time. Walking with purpose also offers a better opportunity for social connection than jogging or bicycling. When you're walking, you can establish a pace that's doable for all parties, which you can't do while jogging. You can converse without getting winded, and you don't have to be as vigilant about looking for safe footfalls. Cycling outdoors with a buddy, on the other hand, is best done in single file for safety, so in that situation you shouldn't be conversing at all.

Rucking

Rucking is a hot new fitness trend that entails walking or hiking with specially designed backpacks to which you can incrementally add efficiently distributed weights. The pack could be as light as fifteen pounds or as heavy as fifty pounds. "Hot new" fitness trend? Well, as author Michael Easter (*The Comfort Crisis*) explains, "Rucking has been the main fitness tool that the US military and militaries around the world have used for training for centuries." It dates back to the seventh century BCE, when the Assyrian king Sargon II outfitted his army in iron, forcing them to carry sixty or more pounds of weight as they marched. Ruck is short for rucksack, the term used in the military to describe a durable backpack carrying provisions. It's derived from the German word for back: *rück*.

Prior to World War I, soldiers typically toted their provisions around in a bindle tied to a stick—Huckleberry Finn–style—so modern rucksacks and backpacks were a great innovation. Today, US Army rangers in basic training must carry a thirty-five-pound rucksack twelve miles at a pace faster than fifteen minutes per mile. Tough! Rucking is also billed as a way to honor the persistence hunt of our ancestors, who would often be tasked with carrying their bounty back to home base. Celebrities such as Beyoncé, Justin Timberlake, Ryan Reynolds, Kylie Jenner, and Guy Fieri have all touted the weight loss and aerobic-conditioning benefits of rucking.

At first I wondered about the rationale and allure of lugging extra weight around, but like many early skeptics, I've come to appreciate the benefits, especially when the weight is distributed safely and gracefully with the assistance of proper rucking gear. I've detailed the many benefits offered by walking, but upper-body muscular strengthening is not one of them. By rucking, however, you can condition the upper body and improve aerobic fitness without the impact trauma of running. Rucking can be especially beneficial for seniors trying to ward off sarcopenia, because they lack the musculoskeletal resilience to perform medium- or high-impact exercise.

Rucking is also a great way to neutralize differences in pace and fitness among hikers. Imagine you and your partners being able to maintain similar heart rates for the duration of a hike by implementing a weight-handicap strategy instead of having to move too slowly or too fast in order to accommodate the others in the group. If you're worried about strapping up and getting some funny looks on the paths or trails in your community, fear not, because you are more likely to encounter fellow ruckers than snickerers.

Ideally, try carrying a rucking-specific backpack, but weighted fitness vests are also great. The key is to strap the weight securely to you body so you don't have the potential hazard of its bouncing around and throwing you off balance. Experts recommend starting with a weight of around 10 percent of your body weight. Hard-core enthusiasts can carry up to 40 percent of their body weight. You don't have to immediately invest in a sophisticated vest or backpack, though: you can simply load an ordinary backpack with extra water bottles or weight plates—just do the best you can to secure the pack tightly to your body. Leave some extra room for nutrition and hydration, because rucking burns more calories than you'd expect! Perhaps you'll soon become an enthusiast and be ready to invest in proper rucking gear from GoRuck.com or RogueFitness.com. As you would when starting any new workout protocol, proceed gradually. One or two sessions a week are plenty, because you'll want sufficient recovery time for your muscles and connective tissue.

Uphill Backward Walking

One of my favorite gym exercises is to walk backward on an incline treadmill. I also do this outside when I have good hills available, and I often use my rucking vest for additional resistance. Weighted backward uphill walking delivers an excellent strengthening effect to the arches, calves, quads, and glutes in a way that forward walking does not. The quads in particular get loaded much more so than they do when you're walking forward. This exercise is also great for improving balance and proprioception. It's important to wear minimalist shoes (or just socks, on a treadmill) to get full muscle activation without interference from an elevated heel. I will typically walk for three to five minutes, take a short break for forward walking, and then repeat for a few sets.

Golf

Golf is on a short list of sports with few fitness benefits and gets a deserved bit of ridicule because of it. But it doesn't have to be that way. Today's norm of riding around the course in a motorized cart is a wholly modern practice driven by laziness and a preference for convenience—not to mention the additional revenue generated for the course and the flawed notion that carts speed up play, which they don't. Of course accessibility matters: some people really need a cart to play golf. But most people who use one don't need to.

Why don't golf carts make the game go faster? First of all, you have to take a highly indirect route through the course to steer clear of tees and greens and stay on paths. You also have to alternately navigate to each player's shots in a two-person cart, creating difficult, time-consuming logistics. A USGA study revealed that carts also don't speed play because of poor cart management—for example, when players make extra back-and-forth trips from cart to ball to get a different club. The USGA study noted that "the extra time needed to walk from the cart to a golf ball is significant and creates an unpleasant golf experience for many." Furthermore, cart golf is a bastardization of the original game invented by Scottish shepherds in the 1200s, the purpose of which was to navigate a natural setting on foot while whacking a ball into a series of holes. As Mark Twain supposedly opined, and as golf journalist John Feinstein memorialized in the title of his 1995 book, "Golf is a good walk spoiled."

Golf can be one of the most fun and stimulating ways to get in some walking when you simply opt out of the option to take a cart. If lugging a heavy bag is not appealing or doable, you can use a pull cart, or consider getting a youth bag and carrying fewer clubs. A bag containing fourteen clubs is another tradition worth reconsidering for all but the most competitive players, especially given an exciting equipment innovation called the Q (visit Q.golf). This is a high-quality club engineered with an adjustable clubface. With a simple pull and twist, you can create a putter, a driving hybrid, irons of all numbers, and a few different wedge options. Who needs a bag? Or a cart?

If your walking opportunities are constrained because of the preferences of your playing partners or the rules at your course, try to minimize your reliance on the cart by grabbing extra clubs and walking from your approach shot to the green and/or from the green to the next tee. Surprisingly, a walking player won't slow down a cart player, because the walking player takes the most direct line and eliminates back-and-forth trips. Furthermore, walking the entire course helps your brain stay connected and focused on playing your best. The burden of having to navigate a motorized vehicle around the property instead of following your ball from tee to green is not to be discounted. With the incessant distractions associated with cart golf (navigating the route, servicing both your own shots and your cart partner's, and accessing beverages, snacks, music, and even a mobile phone buzzing with text messages), your focus is diverted from getting your ball along the throughline of the tee to the green—the object of the game.

The obligation to shut out distractions and refocus before every shot is tremendously draining and inefficient. This back-and-forth taxes short-term memory and disconnects us from the potential to access the state known as flow. Perhaps no other sport rewards the flow state, or punishes a distracted state, more than golf. When you walk, I'll bet you anything that you have a much more precise memory of the course layout, the decisions you've made, and the shots you've hit than when you take a cart.

Speedgolf

The sport of speedgolf takes golf-for-fitness to a whole new level. In speedgolf, you add your total number of strokes to the number of minutes it takes you to play the course to obtain your final score. As in regular tournament golf, the lowest score wins. Top players will run through the course at high speed, carrying only a handful of clubs in a youth bag, and still shoot excellent scores. You can understand why a blend of strategy, cardiovascular fitness, and Zen-like concentration is required to excel in a speedgolf tournament. But for players at all levels, it is an exhilarating way to break free from the stodgy conventions of what devoted speedgolfers like to call slow golf.

Another key benefit is you can enjoy a nine- or eighteen-hole round in a fraction of the time it typically takes to play regular golf—and get a great workout to boot. Virtually all who try the sport are able to play as well as they do when they play for four-plus hours, carry a full bag of clubs, and let their overly analytical minds get in the way of their natural athletic abilities and intuitive decision-making on the course. In speedgolf, you don't have time to fill your head with tension, uncertainty, analysis, or frustration over a poor shot. Hit the ball, for better or worse, then take off running to your next shot.

Search YouTube for "Christopher Smith Bandon Dunes" to see one of the greatest golf rounds ever played, period. Smith, a speedgolf founding father, Guinness World Record holder, and veteran PGA teaching pro, completed the highly regarded Bandon Dunes course, in Oregon, in fifty-three minutes while shooting a four-under-par 68! That's a speed-golf score of 121, achieved under the pressure of having a full CBS film crew following him around for a promotional video. While elite speedgolf professionals are something to marvel at, you can dabble in the sport the next time you're hanging around the course at twilight—perhaps after you've played a proper round and had some refreshments and social time in the clubhouse. Just head out with a few clubs in your hand (long iron, short iron, wedge, and putter to start) and tee off. Depending on your fitness level, you can walk briskly or jog between shots. Forget about practice swings, precise yardage calculations, and reading every nuance of your breaking putt. Just let loose and go with the flow: you'll likely find yourself getting *into* the flow. In 2018, my coauthor, Brad Kearns, set a Guinness World Record for the fastest single hole of golf ever played (search YouTube for "Brad Kearns Speedgolf Guinness World Record"). With just a 3-wood, he hit what he describes as four perfect shots to score a birdie and complete a 503-yard par 5 in one minute and thirty-eight seconds!

Hybrid Challenges

You've read about the signature challenges of elite hybrid athletes: deadlift a massive amount of weight, then run a mile; rack up a big powerlifting series total, then head out for an ironman; carry 124 pounds of water out of the Grand Canyon. How about taking some inspiration from them and creating a set of your own hybrid challenges? Dr. Peter Attia has developed a concept called the centenarian Olympics, a detailed list of fitness tasks he wants to accomplish after he turns one hundred. These include hoisting himself out of a swimming pool onto the deck, doing a deep squat while carrying a kettlebell that weighs as much as a great-grandchild, and much more.

I've been cooking up a list of personally meaningful fitness tasks that I'd love to be able to do ten, twenty, and thirty years from now. So inspired, I make my workout choices today essentially in order to train for the peak performances of my future self.

My workout schedule itself is essentially a hybrid challenge. I visit the gym twice a week for heavy lifting and an assortment of flexibility and mobility exercises. One such exercise is simply hanging from a bar. From a modest start, I can now hang for two minutes. I feel a tremendous improvement in grip strength while I'm doing everyday tasks. I also set a benchmark of being able to deadlift double my body weight, around 350 pounds. I've been able to do it for decades, and I'm still hanging on—barely!

Another day of the week is dedicated to a hot, challenging fat-tire bike ride on Miami Beach of up to ninety minutes in duration. When you're traveling over packed sand, it's a leisurely cruise. But when you hit the many brief patches of soft sand, you essentially have to "sprint" (while moving just a couple of miles an hour) to fight through the sand without toppling over. It's fun to invite friends along for what seems like an innocent beach cruise and see them shocked at the degree of difficulty. If you fall off in the soft sand and have to walk the bike to the edge of the quagmire, you still get out of breath! Another perk of this ride: no helmet necessary. Even the most epic wipeout is just a soft tumble into the sand.

ACKNOWLEDGMENTS

Publishing a book is a monumental project, a labor of love, and an incredible team effort requiring many peak performers sweating every detail to optimize your reading experience. My longtime writing partner, Brad Kearns, and I are incredibly grateful for the support of family, friends, and trusted confidantes who let us use them as sounding boards for ideas before we rolled up our sleeves and got to work.

We chose the best editor in the business, Barbara Clark, to dive deeply into the manuscript and refine the message to be the best it can be. Tim Tate is our trusted proofreader and indexer. The masterly illustration and graphic-design talents of Caroline De Vita are seen on the cover design, interior layout, and the great charts and drawings throughout the book. Thanks also to Ben Gambuzza for his endnote writing and research.

Oh, yeah—thanks to Brad and his trusty iPhone 15 for the cover photo. We equipped him with a $6,000 Sony digital camera for the session, and the big guy came up empty, but Brad shot a few "back-ups" with the iPhone for the heck of it. Taken in the hills above Pacific Palisades in Los Angeles, the photo shows the stunning colors of sunset over the Pacific. This is the kind of beauty that's easy to miss when you're huffing and puffing through grueling training runs instead of enjoying the seamless connection with nature afforded by walking.

We appreciate your feedback; please use the contact form at BornToWalkBook.com.

GLOSSARY

anaerobic threshold (AT): The point at which your body produces lactate faster than you are able to remove its waste products from the bloodstream. Trained athletes can maintain an anaerobic threshold effort for around one hour. AT effort is generally correlated with a blood lactate concentration of 4 mmol/mL. To achieve precision in workouts and improve anaerobic threshold performance, blood lactate can be measured in a laboratory or with portable lactate meters.

aromatase: An enzyme that converts androgen hormones (testosterone and its precursors) into estradiol (estrogen). The presence of visceral fat can prompt the aromatization of testosterone, creating the "slippery slope" of belly fat begetting more belly fat and diminished hormone status in both men and women.

CAC (coronary artery calcium) score: Measures the amount of calcified plaque in your coronary arteries via a CT scan. Your CAC score can help determine your risk of heart disease. A CAC score of over 300 puts you at very high risk for heart disease; a score of over 100 signals elevated risk; a score below 50 is considered safe, and a score of 0 indicates no calcification. Some longtime endurance athletes can have a high CAC score because of chronic scarring and inflammation of the cardiovascular system from extreme exercise. However, their heart disease risk can be lower than that of unfit people with a similarly high score because athletes' calcium deposits seem to be mostly the kind that are stable and less likely to rupture than the noncalcified plaque deposits that are implicated in heart attacks and are more common in metabolically unhealthy people.

calcaneus: The large bone that forms the heel. It's designed to support your body weight when you're standing and absorb impact during the walking gait (but not the running gait). It articulates with other bones to form joints and is the attachment point for several tendons, including the Achilles.

center of gravity/center of mass: During the running stride, the center of gravity (COG) is located in the lower pelvis in the front of the body (because the body leans slightly forward). Runners strive to land under a balanced COG instead of overstriding and causing a braking effect by landing in front of the COG. Actually, optimal landing is *slightly* in front of COG so the foot and leg can absorb impact, move through the stride pattern, and release rotational kinetic energy for takeoff.

chondromalacia: Also known as runner's knee or patellofemoral syndrome, chondromalacia occurs when cartilage in a joint softens and breaks down, allowing the ends of bones to rub together. In runners, it can be caused by overuse, poor technique, excess and inappropriate impact trauma, and muscle weakness and imbalance. It is characterized by a generalized pain and discomfort on and around the kneecap, especially during exercise requiring repeated bending of the knee.

chronic cardio: A pattern of steady-state cardiovascular workouts that are slightly to significantly too stressful, with insufficient rest between them, resulting in lingering fatigue, overuse injuries, and hormonal and metabolic problems associated with chronic overstimulation of the fight-or-flight response. In runners, chronic cardio patterns occur when fat max heart rate is routinely exceeded during workouts, putting too many workouts into the medium-to-difficult category. These workouts emphasize glucose burning instead of fat burning, hindering aerobic development and fat reduction and overstressing the body over time.

compensation theory: Overly stressful exercise patterns generate compensatory responses in the body, including increased appetite, a reduction in general everyday movement, a reduction in resting metabolic rate, and the hormone-directed shedding of lean muscle mass and hoarding of body fat. These are all genetically programmed survival responses intended to conserve energy, and store more energy, in response to chronic stress. Chronic cardio makes you soft and lazy!

cortisol: The preeminent stress hormone and fundamental driver of the fight-or-flight response. Cortisol is regulated by the pituitary gland and released into the bloodstream by the adrenal glands. It increases blood glucose levels, heart rate, blood pressure, metabolism, cognitive focus, mood, motivation, and fear and down-regulates nonemergency functions such as immune response and digestion. This is all in preparation for what is perceived by the primitive brain as a life-or-death situation. This might mean a challenging workout, a presentation in a conference room, or an argument with a loved one.

Cortisol is often discussed in a negative context, because chronically excessive cortisol production can set the stage for a number of health problems. However, healthy cortisol balance is essential for sleep-wake cycles, inflammation control (cortisol suppresses inflammation in the short term but at a potential cost of long-term inflammatory balance), blood glucose control, and many other critical bodily functions. For example, cortisol spikes naturally (and desirably) in the morning when you awaken, increasing alertness.

cytokine proteins: Inflammatory agents such as interleukin-6, TNF-alpha, and MCP-1 that are secreted by visceral fat. These proteins can interfere with normal glucose and fatty acid metabolism, suppress sex hormone levels, and drive systemic inflammation, oxidative stress, mitochondrial dysfunction, and broad-scale hormonal and metabolic dysregulation.

deadlift: A popular strength-training exercise that entails bending at the waist and lifting a weighted barbell or hexagonal bar off the ground and up to waist level as you stand up to your full height. The deadlift recruits many major muscle groups of the upper and lower body, making it widely touted as the single best full-body functional fitness exercise. It has excellent real-life application to the routine act of lifting heavy objects off the ground.

dorsiflexion: The backward bending and contracting of the foot at the ankle during walking, running, squatting, and lunging, resulting in the angle of the ankle becoming more acute.

elastic energy: Energy stored as a result of applying force, such as the compressing of a spring. When the foot lands on the ground, the bending of the knee, dorsiflexion of the toes and ankle, and the lengthening and tightening of the arch and the Achilles tendon all serve to harness elastic energy that is released upon takeoff.

endorphins: Literally "endogenous morphine," endorphins are hormones and neurotransmitters produced in the brain and released by the pituitary gland and hypothalamus in response to the pain or stress generated by activities such as a strenuous endurance workout. Endorphins block pain signals between the brain and body, creating a sense of euphoria. This is a genetically programmed survival mechanism that allows one to persevere through pain and suffering in order to survive or to make one's imminent death less painful. The endorphin response is a highly touted "benefit" of endurance running, but the pursuit of the runner's high can easily be abused and become addictive. Chasing the endorphin high too frequently can lead to exhaustion of the fight-or-flight response and diminished overall health status.

endotoxin: An internally manufactured toxin—namely, lipopolysaccharide (LPL)—that is released when the body consumes chemical-laden, nutrient-deficient processed foods. Endotoxin down-regulates fat metabolism, promotes leaky gut and systemic inflammation, interferes with the efficient burning of stored body fat, and can drive nonalcoholic fatty liver disease.

EPOC (excess post-exercise oxygen consumption): Elevated oxygen consumption and calorie burning in the hours following a high-intensity workout, also known as the afterburn effect. Your metabolic rate increases for up to forty-eight hours after a strenuous workout to facilitate returning body temperature to normal, removing lactic acid and other waste products from the bloodstream, repairing damaged muscle tissue, replenishing ATP and muscle glycogen, and restoring normal cellular oxygen levels. EPOC is the reason why even a brief, high-intensity workout that doesn't burn a large number of calories can nevertheless promote fat reduction by turbocharging fat burning around the clock.

extreme endurance exercise hypothesis: An area of research suggesting that the longer and/or more extreme one's endurance training is, the greater the risk of hormonal, immune, musculoskeletal, metabolic, and cardiovascular damage and disease. The hypothesis can be represented by an inverted U-shaped curve showing the dose-response of energy expenditure to health outcomes. Going from inactive to active brings a quick and prominent improvement in health and physical fitness. Soon a sweet spot is reached for optimal health, fitness, and protection from cardiovascular disease. But those who take exercise to the extreme and put in years and decades of big mileage at paces beyond fat max heart rate actually increase their risk of disease and accelerate the aging process. See chart on page 81.

fat max heart rate: The exercise intensity level at which the maximum number of fat calories per minute are burned. It's also known as the maximum aerobic heart rate (not to be confused with the absolute maximum heart rate), the aerobic threshold (not to be confused with the anaerobic threshold), and constitutes the upper limit of your zone 2 heart rate. Your fat max heart rate can be identified in a performance laboratory, or you can use Dr. Phil Maffetone's popular "180 minus your age" in beats per minute formula. When you increase your effort and pace beyond fat max heart rate, you of course burn more total calories per minute, but your fat-burning rate declines while your glucose burning increases sharply. Generally, the fat max heart rate pace feels very comfortable—you have more than enough oxygen to converse freely while exercising. Consequently, it's easy for exercisers to routinely exceed fat max and compromise the intended metabolic benefits (i.e., improved fat burning) of the workout. Wearing a wireless heart-rate monitor and setting a beeper alarm at fat max is the best way to ensure a productive aerobic workout with minimal anaerobic stimulation.

gene expression: The activation or deactivation of genes. This happens via a series of chemical reactions that allow cells to communicate with one another and perform various functions. The science of epigenetics studies how behaviors and environmental influences affect gene expression.

genetic signaling/genetic expectations for health: Contrary to the narrow layperson's understanding of genes as fixed heritable traits, our genes switch on and off, or are "expressed," according to signals they receive from the environment. This is the science of epigenetics. Lift weights, and you send the signal to your genes to build muscle. Watch an enjoyable movie or have a pleasant social experience, and you signal a cascade of mood-elevating hormones to enter the bloodstream. Hence genetic expectations for health are environmental influences that trigger health-promoting genetic expression. Through the life-or-death environmental selection pressure of human evolution, our genes have come to expect things like extensive everyday general movement; brief, intense exercise; and adequate sleep and sun exposure to achieve optimal gene expression.

gluconeogenesis: The conversion of amino acids, either ingested or drawn from lean muscle tissue, into glucose. This is a prominent attribute of the fight-or-flight response and serves to elevate blood glucose levels for peak performance and perceived life-or-death situations. While gluconeogenesis occurs routinely to help stabilize blood glucose, chronic fight-or-flight overstimulation can result in an excessive triggering of gluconeogenesis. This can hamper fat burning and catabolize hard-earned lean muscle tissue.

glycogen: The stored form of carbohydrate in the muscles and liver. The average person can store around 15 grams of glycogen per kilogram of body weight, but training can increase glycogen storage potential to up to 25 grams per kilogram of body weight. The liver can typically store around 100 grams (400 calories), while muscle tissue can store between 350 (1,400 calories) and 500 grams (2,000 calories), depending on body size and trainability.

heart-rate variability (HRV): A score on a scale of 1 to 100 that represents the degree of variation in beat-to-beat intervals of the heart. One's HRV score is seen as an indicator of overall cardiovascular health and the state of recovery and readiness to train. For example, a resting heart rate of sixty beats per minutes corresponds to an average of one second per heartbeat, but an HRV test might show a string of beat-to-beat intervals such as .89, 1.03, 1.06, .98, .90, and so on that average out to a heart rate of sixty beats per minute. These are known as RR intervals (R-wave peak to R-wave peak), and they are revealed on a typical EKG test by the familiar spikes off of baseline (recall that "flatline" means dead). The degree of variation in RR intervals is translated into an HRV score on a scale of 1 to 100 for user convenience only. A high HRV (i.e., a high variation in beat-to-beat intervals) is indicative of a harmonious balance between the parasympathetic and sympathetic nervous systems and a strong, athletic cardiovascular system. A low HRV score, revealing a more metronomic heartbeat, is indicative of a weak cardiovascular system or the condition of being overstressed or insufficiently recovered.

HRV readings are taken first thing in the morning, when you're in a rested state. HRV scores are highly individual, so you should establish an average HRV range over time and compare it only to your own baseline, not to those of others, whether fitter or less fit. By noticing how your daily readings compare to your personal baseline range, you can make informed training and lifestyle decisions and optimize training, recovery, and overall cardiovascular health. For example, if your typical HRV values are between 65 and 75, and a score of 60 appears, this can suggest a state of overstress and need for recovery on that particular day. If you measure your HRV over many months and see an increase in average values (e.g., going from an average of 70 to an average of 74 over time), this can suggest improved cardiovascular conditioning and/or stress management. HRV scores are not applicable to people with arrhythmia conditions such as atrial fibrillation and premature ventricular contractions (PVCs), which will cause an abnormally high HRV resulting from extra beats or skipped beats.

HIIT (high-intensity interval training): Short bursts of intense effort interspersed with recovery intervals during a workout. Literally, the word "interval" refers to the rest interval between work efforts, but it is often used to describe the duration of the work effort and/or both the work effort and the rest period. For example, a workout might be characterized as "five thirty-second bike intervals with two-minute rest intervals." HIIT workouts can consist of cardiovascular exercises (running, cycling, rowing, gym machines) or strength exercises (kettlebell, rope climbing, sled pushing), but the key feature is the rest intervals interspersed between high-intensity work efforts.

HIIT has risen in popularity, buoyed by research suggesting that it delivers fitness and weight-loss benefits superior to those of steady-state cardio. Indeed, HIIT provides a more significant and intense fitness stimulation than slower-paced, steady-state workouts, which can prompt quick improvements in physical condition and performance capability. However, a pattern of frequent HIIT workouts that are overly stressful can lead to burnout and fitness regression. The most effective HIIT workouts are challenging but not exhausting. This entails a thoughtful design of the variables—number of work efforts, intensity of work efforts, duration of work efforts, and duration of rest intervals.

hyperinsulinemia: Chronic overproduction of insulin leading to the disease state of insulin resistance and metabolic syndrome. Insulin resistance occurs when cells in specific areas of the body respond poorly to the signaling of insulin—attempts by insulin molecules to enter the cells and deliver nutrients—because of chronically elevated insulin levels. Metabolic syndrome is the term for the following five disease risk factors: high blood pressure, high triglycerides, high glucose, low

HDL cholesterol, and excess waistline measurement, indicative of the accumulation of health-destructive visceral fat. Having three of the five markers results in a diagnosis of metabolic syndrome. Many health and diet experts contend that hyperinsulinemia is the most problematic public health crisis in the developed world.

industrial seed oils: Refined oils high in polyunsaturates, also known as vegetable oils. These are highly processed oils extracted from the seeds of various plants such as corn, soybeans, rapeseed (the source of canola oil), cotton, and safflower. They are processed using high temperatures and chemical solvents that are required to extract oil from plants that don't naturally yield lots of oil. By contrast, consider the olive, coconut, and avocado plants, which are high in fat and yield healthful oils with a simple cold-pressing technique. The heavy processing of industrial oils results in oxidative damage to the end product, making them toxic to consume.

These oils are highly unstable and sensitive to further oxidative damage from exposure to light, oxygen, and heat. Hence when they are heated during cooking, they become further oxidized. When ingested (in fried, deep-fried, frozen, and packaged foods made with seed oils), they prompt an immediate and sustained disturbance to healthy cardiovascular function and interfere with healthy fat burning over time. While experts have long considered excess carbohydrate intake to be the driving factor in the development of insulin resistance and obesity, evidence is now suggesting that seed oils could be the primary culprit. Hampered fat burning from habitual seed-oil consumption (an estimated 20–32 percent of the total daily calories in the standard American diet come from seed oils) forces carbohydrates to become the main energy source, resulting in overeating, chronically excessive insulin production, and, eventually, insulin resistance, diabetes, and metabolic syndrome.

kinetic chain: A series of interactions between muscles, joints, and connective tissue that enables movements such as bending, extending, and jumping. There are an assortment of distinct kinetic chains involving groups of muscles and joints and the ways in which they connect to the spine. The five major kinetic chains in the body are intrinsic (inner core and respiratory muscles), deep longitudinal (lower legs, sacrum, hamstrings, and spinal erectors), lateral (TMJs, shoulders, sacroiliac, hips, knees, ankles, and feet), posterior (glutes, hamstrings, lumbar spine, and calves), and anterior (quads, core, and pectorals).

MET (metabolic equivalent of task): A measurement of the energy expenditure required to complete a specific physical activity. Resting in bed is 1 MET; brisk walking is 5 MET; running a ten-minute mile is 10 MET; running a 7:30 mile is 13.5 MET; sprinting is 30 MET. Extreme endurance athletes such as marathon racers (who can complete the race in three hours or less), ultrarunners, and ironman triathletes typically accumulate 200–300 MET in a week. Emerging research suggests that this elevated level of MET can increase the risk of cardiovascular problems and other health disturbances.

metabolic set point: A popular theory holding that individuals have a genetically influenced natural weight range that they tend to maintain or return to despite their efforts to gain or lose body mass. People who have "thrifty" genes—i.e., a genetic predisposition to store fat—can experience more difficulty losing excess weight and keeping it off than those who have "skinny" genes.

metatarsals: A group of five long bones in the midfoot located between the toe bones (tarsals) and the ankle bones (phalanges).

midfoot strike: A running technique in which the ball of the foot, or midfoot, makes contact with the ground first, followed by the outside edge of the middle of the foot and finally the heel. At landing, the foot is almost parallel to the ground, the lower leg is almost perpendicular to the ground, and weight is evenly distributed between the hips, knees, and ankles. A midfoot strike over a (nearly) vertical tibia and a balanced center of gravity is a feature of the correct human running gait and results in the most efficient impact absorption, harnessing of elastic energy, and forward propulsion.

midsole: The material between a shoe's inner sole (what the foot rests on inside the shoe) and outer sole (the tread). Midsoles are typically made with cushioned material called EVA (ethylene vinyl acetate) foam.

motion-control shoes: Running shoes that are built with rigid support features such as hard plastic and are said to increase stability and support, limit pronation, and reduce injury risk. No study has ever validated the idea that motion-control shoes work as promised, and many studies suggest that they interfere with natural foot functionality, promote atrophy, and increase injury risk.

NAFLD (nonalcoholic fatty liver disease): The accumulation of excess fat in the liver as a result of adverse dietary and lifestyle practices but not directly as a result of chronically excessive alcohol consumption. The name of this condition came about when nondrinkers began developing liver dysfunction similar to that which had previously been seen only in people who had consumed alcohol in excess for years.

organ reserve: The capacity of organs to perform beyond baseline levels, such as when you increase heart rate and respiration during a workout. Organs, like muscles, adhere to the natural law of "use it or lose it." When you engage your muscles to lift heavy weights, sprint, or hike long distances, your heart, lungs, liver, kidneys, skin, and other organs are called into action above and beyond baseline metabolism. Your organs help burn calories, deliver blood and oxygen to working muscles, and work hard during the period of excess postexercise oxygen consumption. By contrast, when your physical activity diminishes, as it typically does when you age, muscles and organs can atrophy in tandem. For example, an unfit person has less lung capacity (the quantity of air you exchange on each breath) and less stroke volume (the amount of blood your heart pumps with each beat) than a fit person. Since we are only as resilient as our weakest link, poor organ reserve can spell trouble when an unfit elderly person has to undergo surgery, recover from pneumonia, or confront other challenges to baseline metabolic and hormonal function.

overfat: A term popularized by Dr. Phil Maffetone in his book *The Overfat Pandemic*. Overfat is distinct from overweight because it describes someone who may be of normal total body weight but has an excessive percentage of body fat, particularly visceral fat. Dr. Maffetone estimates that 76 percent of the global population can be categorized as overfat. You are classified as overfat if you have a waist circumference of more than half your height—e.g., a thirty-four-inch waist on a sixty-seven-inch-tall (five feet, seven inches) person. The overfat benchmark is considered to be more useful than the typical body mass index (BMI) metric, which classifies obesity by the relationship of height to weight. For example, a five-foot-ten NFL running back who weighs two hundred pounds and has 6 percent body fat would be categorized as obese in a BMI table. BMI also fails to account for people with large amounts of healthy muscle mass or extra-heavy bone structure and fails to distinguish between quantities of health-destructive visceral fat and less offensive subcutaneous fat.

overstriding: Landing too far in front of one's center of gravity during running, generating a braking effect with each stride. Overstriding is often characterized by a heel-first foot strike but is more accurately identified by the angle of the tibia upon landing. If the tibia forms an acute angle to the ground, short of the desired near-ninety-degree angle, it will generate a braking effect. It's possible to heel-strike with a correct landing over a balanced center of gravity, but usually heel-striking and overstriding go hand in hand, particularly in novice runners.

oxytocin: A hormone produced in the hypothalamus and released by the pituitary gland. Oxytocin is nicknamed the love hormone because it promotes feelings of social bonding and is associated with sexual pleasure, maternal behavior, lactation, trust, romantic attachment, childbirth, and mother-infant bonding.

persistence hunting: The quintessential Homo sapiens method of hunting. Also known as endurance hunting, it involves tracking game animals over long distances for long periods of time until they become exhausted. The human genetic attributes for endurance that enable persistence hunting were a key driver of human evolution. In particular, humans' upright stature, bipedal locomotion, and ability to dissipate heat gave them an advantage over their prey, especially in hot temperatures. Our ability to access food from nutrient-dense game animals supported the complex brain development that allowed humans to rise to the top of the food chain.

These days, our genetic endurance attributes are often misinterpreted and misappropriated as evidence that humans were born to run and that endurance training delivers health and longevity benefits. Alas, our brains were by far our best competitive advantage in persistence hunting, and we did not routinely run long distances day after day in search of prey, as do today's endurance runners. It's more accurate from an evolutionary biology standpoint to acknowledge that humans have the genetic attributes to perform occasional extreme endurance feats under life-or-death selection pressure and are genetically adapted to move frequently at a slow pace throughout the day, primarily by walking and other low-level efforts. Furthermore, our genetic attributes for endurance exercise have largely been suppressed in modern times by inactivity.

plantar fascia: A band of thick tissue that connects the heel bone to the base of the toes. The plantar fascia supports the arch of the foot and absorbs shock by flattening and tightening during the walking and running strides. This flattening and tightening of the fascia to absorb shock and harness elastic energy is called the windlass mechanism—a sailing term used to describe the tightening of a rope or cable. When the plantar fascia grows weak and atrophied from a lifetime of wearing modern elevated, cushioned shoes with a rigid sole, it can become inflamed, torn, and deteriorated, causing the conditions of plantar fasciitis (inflammation) and plantar fasciosis (degeneration of tissue).

pronation: A natural side-to-side rolling motion of the foot during the landing segment of the running and walking gait characterized by the arch flattening and the foot caving inward. Pronation occurs as a combination of three simultaneous motions: subtalar eversion, ankle dorsiflexion, and forefoot abduction. The running-shoe industry has highlighted overpronation as an injury risk in the marketing of shoes said to "control" or limit pronation. Over time, the layperson has come to perceive pronation itself as negative, something to limit through the use of rigid shoes with artificial arch support. Interestingly, no study has ever shown that shoes, even the most rigid and highly arched models, can control pronation—the foot pronates anyway inside the shoe—or that pronation is a risk factor for injury. Videos and photos of some of the world's greatest long-distance runners, including Eliud Kipchoge (1:59 marathoner) and Joshua Cheptegei (world record holder at 5,000 and 10,000 meters), reveal what would be universally regarded as extreme overpronation. In fact, pronation is a key element of impact absorption and the harnessing of elastic energy for takeoff.

proprioception: The awareness of your body moving through space; your sense of position, movement, and force. Proprioception is also known as kinesthetic awareness or kinesthesia. It is your body's largely unconscious natural ability to process input from your limbs and nerve endings, especially from the bottom of your feet, and achieve feats such as walking in the dark, walking over rough terrain, swinging on parallel bars, somersaulting off a diving board, hitting a golf ball, and lifting a heavy weight off the ground. Since the majority of complex kinetic-chain activity starts from your feet, and since the soles of your feet are one of the most nerve-dense areas of the body, shoes can greatly compromise proprioception. Running in elevated, cushioned shoes enables a pattern of heel-striking, jarring, braking, and overstriding as well as the accompanying inappropriate dispersion of impact trauma through the lower extremities and a diminished sensitivity to this impact trauma.

rotational energy: The conversion of elastic (stored) energy into kinetic (active) energy. In running, elastic energy is harnessed by the temporary compression and/or dorsiflexion of various muscles and joints in the lower body upon impact, including the toes, metatarsals, longitudinal arch, Achilles, calf muscles, and even glutes. Rotational energy occurs at takeoff, helping you achieve forward propulsion. Once airborne, the ankle and toes will quickly return to a dorsiflexed position in preparation for the next foot strike and the production of more rotational energy. When you throw a ball, for example, elastic energy is harnessed by the coiling of the feet, legs, hips, and torso as well as the shoulder, elbow, hand, and fingers. Releasing the ball entails a synchronized uncoiling of the lower and upper body, generating rotational energy for a high-velocity release.

running economy (RE): The metabolic, cardiorespiratory, biomechanical, and neuromuscular efficiency of a runner at any given pace. Running economy is similar to VO2 max, because both are measured by oxygen consumption in milliliters per minute per kilogram of body weight. However, running economy applies to steady-state submaximal oxygen consumption, whereas VO2 max measures maximum oxygen consumption.

sagittal, frontal, and transverse planes: The three anatomical planes of the body. The sagittal, a.k.a. longitudinal, plane divides the body into left and right sides. Forward and backward movements—e.g., bicep curls and forward or backward lunges—along this plane involve flexion, extension, dorsiflexion, and plantar flexion. Movements along the frontal, a.k.a. coronal, plane—e.g., jumping jacks, cartwheels, and raising and lowering the arms and legs sideways—involve inversion, eversion, abduction, and adduction and proceed from side to side. The transverse, a.k.a. axial or transaxial, plane divides the body into upper and lower sections that are perpendicular to the sagittal and frontal planes and parallel to the ground. Movements along this plane—e.g., chopping wood—involve rotation, horizontal abduction, and horizontal adduction.

shoe drop: A measurement of the difference between the elevation off the ground of the heel of a shoe and its midfoot and toes. Virtually all dress shoes, work shoes, and athletic shoes are higher off the ground in the heel than in the midfoot or the toes. Hence a shoe described as having a fifteen-millimeter drop puts the heel fifteen millimeters higher off the ground than the midfoot and toes. A zero-drop shoe has a sole that's completely flat—there is no change in elevation between the heel and the toe.

spine—cervical, thoracic, and lumbar: The three sections of the vertebrae comprising the spine. The cervical is the upper section of the spinal column (the neck), consisting of the first seven vertebrae, C1 through C7. It extends from just below the skull to just above the thoracic spine and has a backward C-shaped curve. The thoracic spine starts at the base of your neck and ends at the bottom of your ribs. It consists of twelve vertebrae: T1 through T5 contain nerves that affect the upper chest, midback, abdominal muscles, and breathing muscles, and vertebrae T6 through T12 contain nerves that affect the back and abdominal muscles. The thoracic spine is very stable, supporting balance and posture. The lumbar spine is the lower part of the spine, between the ribs and sacrum. Vertebrae L1 through L5 are larger than the thoracic or cervical vertebrae. The lumbar spine typically has a slight inward curve of thirty to fifty degrees called lordosis. The lumbar spine facilitates flexion-extension movements and supports posture.

steady state: A term that describes a cardiovascular workout in which either the heart rate or the pace is kept consistent throughout—for example, running five miles at a pace of ten minutes per mile. Note that steady-state *pace* is different from steady-state *heart rate*. A steady-state pace workout, in which you attempting to maintain a pace of, for example, ten minutes per mile, will result in a gradual increase in heart rate over the course of the run because of cumulative fatigue. An aerobic-emphasis, fat max zone 2 steady-state heart-rate workout, by contrast, entails staying at or below fat max heart rate for the duration of the workout, regardless of pace. This allows for variation in terrain, temperature, and other factors and for a gradual slowing of the pace as you continue.

While steady-state workouts (both of the pace and heart-rate kind) have long been a fundamental principle of endurance training, scientific evidence as well as the training habits of elite athletes suggest that adding variation of both pace and heart rate will recruit several energy systems and prompt wide-ranging fitness adaptations. This can potentially generate better competitive preparation and avoid stagnation and regression.

subcutaneous fat: Body fat that accumulates underneath the skin, typically in the hips, thighs, rear end, and/or belly. This type of fat is less metabolically active than the health-destructive visceral fat, which accumulates around the abdominal organs. Subcutaneous fat is soft and squishy, while visceral fat is firm because it gathers deep within the abdomen in the spaces surrounding the organs. Visceral fat accumulation typically results in a firm, protruding belly, while subcutaneous fat accumulation is typically jiggly.

tib/fib; tibiofibular joints: Joints that connect the tibia and fibula at three junctions: the superior (proximal) tibiofibular joint, between the superior ends of tibia and fibula; the inferior (distal) tibiofibular joint, between their inferior ends; and the interosseous membrane of leg (middle tibiofibular joint), connecting their shafts.

toe spring: A design feature in running shoes in which the sole has a distinct upward curvature (typically around fifteen degrees), starting around the midfoot and heading toward the toes. This is also known as rocker geometry. A toe spring is apparent when a shoe rests on the ground and the toe box is slightly elevated off the surface. Toe spring is believed to improve performance for fast runners by preloading the toes into a dorsiflexed, energy-coiled position. This supposedly relieves the foot from having to work through a full range of motion, improving running economy accordingly. However, toe spring is also believed to cause atrophy, overburden the plantar fascia by continually stretching it, and disperse impact forces inappropriately to the knees and hips.

visceral fat: Body fat that accumulates around the abdominal organs as well as the heart. Visceral fat is also known as belly fat, hidden fat, intra-abdominal fat, visceral adipose tissue, and beer belly. It is metabolically active and secretes hormones and other substances directly into the bloodstream, including health-destructive inflammatory cytokine proteins. Visceral fat typically accumulates when the body's metabolic system, hormonal system, and subcutaneous fat-storage capacity become overwhelmed. Excess consumption of processed foods and alcohol can easily overtax these systems. Males have a greater tendency to accumulate visceral fat than females because they store less subcutaneous fat—i.e., their fat-storage systems are more easily overwhelmed. The condition of "skinny fat" occurs when someone who is not genetically predisposed to store much subcutaneous fat nevertheless accumulates visceral fat as a result of adverse lifestyle practices and poor metabolic health.

VO2 max: A measurement of the maximum volume of oxygen (in milliliters) one can consume per minute per kilogram of body weight (e.g., 53 mL/min/kg). Most cardiologists and respected resources such as the Mayo Clinic consider VO2 max a health marker superior to anything found in blood work, EKGs, and other routine screenings. For decades, serious endurance athletes have tracked VO2 max as a way to predict competitive potential. A VO2 max test is conducted by exercising to exhaustion on a stationary bike or treadmill while breathing into a mask connected to a device that measures oxygen consumption. As effort escalates, oxygen consumption will increase until a maximum is reached.

NOTES

Chapter 1

runners have gone from: S. Robert Lathan, "A History of Jogging and Running—the Boom of the 1970s," *Baylor University Medical Center Proceedings* 36, no. 6 (2023): 775–77, https://doi.org/10.1080/08998280.2023.2256058.

the biggest public health problem: "The Top 10 Causes of Death," World Health Organization, August 7, 2024, https://www.who.int/news-room/fact-sheets/detail/the-top-10-causes-of-death.

what experts are calling energy toxicity: Huberman Lab, "Dr. Layne Norton: The Science of Eating for Health, Fat Loss & Lean Muscle," November 6, 2022, https://www.hubermanlab.com/episode/dr-layne-norton-the-science-of-eating-for-health-fat-loss-and-lean-muscle.

"the valiant drama of a single lone runner": Dean Karnazes, *The Road to Sparta: Reliving the Ancient Battle and Epic Run That Inspired the World's Greatest Footrace* (Rodale Books, 2016), 15.

The level of obesity in America, and globally, has more than tripled: "U.S. Obesity Rates Have Tripled Over the Last 60 Years," USAFacts, last modified March 21, 2023, https://usafacts.org/articles/obesity-rate-nearly-triples-united-states-over-last-50-years/; World Health Organization, "One in Eight People Are Now Living with Obesity," news release, March 1, 2024, https://www.who.int/news/item/01-03-2024-one-in-eight-people-are-now-living-with-obesity.

only 280,000 (2 percent) have finished in under three hours: "Breaking Three Hours: Trailblazing African-American Women Marathoners," National Black Marathoners Association, accessed September 10, 2024, https://blackmarathoners.org/breaking-three-hours.shtml.

the average marathon time: Vania Nikolova, "Compare Running Finish Times [Calculator]—5K, 10K, Half Marathon, Marathon," RunRepeat, March 1, 2024, https://runrepeat.com/how-do-you-masure-up-the-runners-percentile-calculator.

the average elite sumo wrestler: Gavin Blair, "Sumo Wrestlers Present a Weighty Problem for Japan Airlines," *The Times* (London), October 16, 2023, https://www.thetimes.com/

world/asia/article/sumo-wrestlers-present-a-weighty-problem-for-japan-airlines-50xk6tznw; Jonathan Shipley, "Please Sir, I Want Sumo: How Sumo Wrestlers Fuel Up for Fights," Fed, March 10, 2022, https://www.fedfedfed.com/sliced/please-sir-i-want-sumo-how-sumo-wrestlers-fuel-up-for-fights.

"Shave one ounce off a track spike": Phil Knight, *Shoe Dog: A Memoir by the Creator of Nike* (Scribner, 2016).

"shoe company was in the position to be the touchstone": P. Ranganath Nayak and John M. Ketteringham, *Breakthroughs!* (Rawson Associates, 1986), 253.

"A Time magazine piece": "Swift Profits," *Time*, June 30, 1980, https://time.com/vault/issue/1980-06-30/page/66/.

Chapter 2

"It looks like exercise makes fat more fit": Gretchen Reynolds, "Why Exercise Is More Important Than Weight Loss for a Longer Life," *New York Times*, September 29, 2021, https://www.nytimes.com/2021/09/29/well/move/exercise-weight-loss-longer-life.html.

"[Noakes] was a marathoner": Bill Gifford, "The Silencing of Tim Noakes," *Outside*, December 9, 2016, https://www.outsideonline.com/health/nutrition/silencing-low-carb-rebel/.

the highly regarded 2015 University of Connecticut FASTER study: Jeff S. Volek et al., "Metabolic Characteristics of Keto-Adapted Ultra-Endurance Runners," *Metabolism* 65, no. 3 (2016): 100–110, https://doi.org/10.1016/j.metabol.2015.10.028.

An article on the Asics website: "How to Lose Belly Fat by Running," ASICS Advice, December 12, 2021, https://www.asics.com/gb/en-gb/running-advice/how-to-lose-belly-fat-by-running/.

who comprise an estimated 20 to 25 percent: "Everything You Need to Know About the Boston Marathon," *Runner's World*, March 15, 2022, https://www.runnersworld.com/races-places/a19605700/boston-marathon-faq/.

You experience a boost in metabolism: Wesley J. Tucker et al., "Excess Postexercise Oxygen Consumption after High-Intensity and Sprint Interval Exercise, and Continuous Steady-State Exercise," *Journal of Strength and Conditioning Research* 30, no. 11 (2016): 3090–97, https://doi.org/10.1519/JSC.0000000000001399.

he asserts that 76 percent: Philip Maffetone, *The Overfat Pandemic: Exposing the Problem and Its Simple Solution for Everyone Who Needs to Eliminate Excess Body Fat* (Skyhorse Publishing, 2017), 2.

Researchers call him TOFI: Patricia Yárnoz-Esquiroz et al., "'Obesities': Position Statement on a Complex Disease Entity with Multifaceted Drivers," *European Journal of Clinical Investigation* 52, no. 7 (2022), https://doi.org/10.1111/eci.13811.

Visceral fat accounts for around 10 percent: "Visceral Fat," Cleveland Clinic, accessed September 11, 2024, https://my.clevelandclinic.org/health/diseases/24147-visceral-fat; Matthew Solan, "An Inside Look at Body Fat," Harvard Health, October 1, 2023, https://www.health.harvard.edu/mens-health/an-inside-look-at-body-fat.

One UK study revealed: Jane E. Brody, "The Dangers of Belly Fat," *New York Times*, June 11, 2018, https://www.nytimes.com/2018/06/11/well/live/belly-fat-health-visceral-fat-waist-cancer.html.

Research from India revealed: Brody, "The Dangers of Belly Fat."

A thirty-six-year study in California: Brody, "The Dangers of Belly Fat."

A study of 350,000 European males and females: Brody, "The Dangers of Belly Fat."

Public health and medical experts contend: Jamal Hossain et al., "Diabetes Mellitus, the Fastest Growing Global Public Health Concern: Early Detection Should Be Focused," *Health Science Reports* 7, no. 3 (2024), https://doi.org/10.1002/hsr2.2004.

"liquidating your assets": Brad Kearns, *Get Over Yourself*, episode 54, "Deconstructing Tommy, Part 1," March 1, 2019, 6:36, https://bradkearns.com/2019/03/01/tommyb1-2/.

a survey published: Beate Pfeiffer et al., "Nutritional Intake and Gastrointestinal Problems During Competitive Endurance Events," *Medicine & Science in Sports & Exercise* 44, no. 2 (2012): 344–51, https://pubmed.ncbi.nlm.nih.gov/21775906/.

"Exercise not only delays actual death": Ben Court, "Get Stronger, Live Longer!," *Men's Health*, March 10, 2023, https://www.menshealth.com/fitness/a43137717/peter-attia-outlive-exercise-longevity/.

"F45 Training merges": "Why F45 Works," F45 Training, accessed September 11, 2024, https://f45training.com/.

exercise physiology research validates: "High-Intensity Workouts Can Help You Get Fit Fast, but Preparation Is Key," *Cultivating Health*, UC Davis Health, September 28, 2022, https://health.ucdavis.edu/blog/cultivating-health/high-intensity-workouts-can-help-you-get-fit-fast-but-preparation-is-key/2022/09.

"literally no different from consuming radiation in a bottle": Brad Kearns, *Get Over Yourself*, episode 264, "Carnivore Insights Inspired by Dr. Paul Saladino," March 26, 2021, https://bradkearns.com/2021/03/26/carnivore-insights-inspired-by-dr-paul-saladino/.

Chapter 3

A 1997 study: Shawn Robbins and Edward Waked, "Hazard of Deceptive Advertising of Athletic Footwear," *British Journal of Sports Medicine* 31, no. 4 (1998): 299–303, https://doi.org/10.1136/bjsm.31.4.299.

A 2022 Chinese study: Masen Zhang et al., "The Effect of Heel-to-Toe Drop of Running Shoes on Patellofemoral Joint Stress During Running," *Gait Posture* 93 (2022): 230–34, https://doi.org/10.1016/j.gaitpost.2022.02.008.

Our technology ensures enhanced stability: "Men's Stability Running Shoes," Saucony, accessed September 11, 2024, https://www.saucony.com/en/mens-stability-running-shoes/.

a heavily scientifically referenced article: Steve Magness, "Why Running Shoes Do Not Work: Looking at Pronation, Cushioning, Motion Control and Barefoot Running," *Science of Running*, January 25, 2010, https://www.scienceofrunning.com/2010/01/why-running-shoes-do-not-work-looking.html?v=47e5dceea252.

"Running shoes are built upon two central premises": Magness, "Why Running Shoes Do Not Work."

Magness cites three studies: Dennis Y. Wen et al., "Lower Extremity Alignment and Risk of Overuse Injuries in Runners," *Medicine & Science in Sports & Exercise* 29, no. 10 (1997): 1291–98, https://doi.org/10.1097/00005768-199710000-00003; Dennis Y. Wen et al., "Injuries in Runners: A Prospective Study of Alignment," *Clinical Journal of Sports Medicine* 8, no. 3 (1998): 187–94, https://doi.org/10.1097/00042752-199807000-00005; Alex Stacoff et al., "Effects of Foot Orthoses on Skeletal Motion During Running," *Clinical Biomechanics* 15, no. 1 (2000): 54–64, https://doi.org/10.1016/s0268-0033(99)00028-5; Alex Stacoff, "Effects of Shoe Sole Construction on Skeletal Motion During Running," *Medicine & Science in Sports & Exercise* 33, no. 2 (2001): 311–19, https://doi.org/10.1097/00005768-200102000-00022.

"The foot no longer gets the proprioceptive cues": Magness, "Why Running Shoes Do Not Work," quoted in Golden Harper, *Golden: Run Better*, May 1, 2017, https://goldenharper.net/.

"half of recreational runners are still injured every year": "Running Injuries," Yale Medicine, accessed September 11, 2024, https://www.yalemedicine.org/conditions/running-injury.

"Running shoes are based on a kind of cult idea": Adam Weiner, "Will Running Barefoot Cure What Ails Us?," *Popular Science*, May 13, 2009, https://www.popsci.com/entertainment-amp-gaming/article/2009-05/running-barefoot/.

"because it's largely their fault": Christopher McDougall, *Born to Run: A Hidden Tribe, Superathletes, and the Greatest Race the World Has Never Seen* (Vintage Books, 2011), 179.

"Just placing a little wedge under our foundation": Katy Bowman, *Every Woman's Guide to Foot Pain Relief: The New Science of Healthy Feet* (BenBella Books, 2011), 62.

the primary evolutionary adaptation: William Irvin Sellers et al., "Evolutionary Robotic Approaches in Primate Gait Analysis," *International Journal of Primatology* 31, no. 2 (2010): 321–38, https://doi.org/10.1007/s10764-010-9396-4.

increasing our oxygen uptake: Amelie Werkhausen et al., "Technologically Advanced Running Shoes Reduce Oxygen Cost and Cumulative Tibial Loading per Kilometer in Recreational Female and Male Runners," *Scientific Reports* 14 (2024), https://doi.org/10.1038/s41598-024-62263-0.

the streamlined toe box: Sabrina Imbler, "Why Were Medieval Europeans So Obsessed with Long, Pointy Shoes?," *Atlas Obscura*, May 22, 2019, https://www.atlasobscura.com/articles/medieval-europeans-pointy-shoes.

research suggests that this is one of the key reasons: Alecsa Stewart, "Are Super Shoes So Super?," *Slate*, December 16, 2023, https://slate.com/technology/2023/12/nike-super-shoes-fast-injury-carbon-plate-worth-it.html.

Over time, this can cause atrophy: Freddy Sichting et al., "Effect of the Upward Curvature of Toe Springs on Walking Biomechanics in Humans," *Scientific Reports* 10, no. 1 (2020), https://doi.org/10.1038/s41598-020-71247-9.

Toe spring is also believed to: Matthew Klein, "What Is Toe Spring in Running Shoes?," *Runner's World*, March 4, 2021, https://www.runnersworld.com/gear/a35713264/toe-spring-running-shoes/.

A 2018 study: Christopher Bramah et al., "Is There a Pathological Gait Associated with Common Soft Tissue Running Injuries?," *American Journal of Sports Medicine* 46, no. 12 (2018): 3023–31, https://doi.org/10.1177/0363546518793657.

heel-striking, overstriding inefficiency: Daniel E. Lieberman et al., "Foot Strike Patterns and Collision Forces in Habitually Barefoot Versus Shod Runners," *Nature* 463 (January 2010): 531–35, https://www.nature.com/articles/nature08723.

a complex mathematical calculation: "Impact Force," ShoeSense, accessed September 11, 2024, https://shoesenserunning.com/pages/impact-force.

There has to be energy storage: Steve Magness, "Why We Land in Front of Our Center of Gravity," *Science of Running*, August 23, 2010, https://www.scienceofrunning.com/2010/08/why-we-land-in-front-of-our-center-of.html.

"The tendons fool you": Brad Kearns (@bradkearns1), "It felt good to run some wind sprints on the track for the first time in nearly 4 months, but I am exerting great discipline to ease back into the game," Instagram, March 23, 2023, https://www.instagram.com/p/CqJwW7ovWJw/.

The National Institutes of Health reports: Tatiana Munhoz da Rocha lemos Costa et al., "Stress Fractures," *Archives of Endocrinology and Metabolism* 66, no. 5 (November 2022): 765–73, https://doi.org/10.20945%2F2359-3997000000562.

sales grew to $160 million: "Vibram FiveFingers Sees Slower Growth Ahead . . .," SGB Media, March 19, 2012, https://sgbonline.com/vibram-fivefingers-sees-slower-growth-ahead/.

but only to the $20–$25 million range: Ashwin Rodrigues, "'Barefoot' Sneakers Are Extending Their Grip on the Sneaker World. Here's Why," *Fast Company*, July 16, 2023, https://www.fastcompany.com/90920435/barefoot-sneakers-nike-five-fingers-vivobarefoot.

numerous highly respected research studies: Cindy Kuzma, "What You Do (and Don't) Need in a Running Shoe," *New York Times*, March 30, 2023, https://www.nytimes.com/2023/03/30/well/move/running-shoes.html; Gretchen Reynolds, "Super Cushioned Running Shoes Are All the Rage, but Aren't Foolproof," *New York Times*, February 19, 2020, https://www.nytimes.com/2020/02/19/well/move/super-cushioned-running-shoes-maximal-ist-pronation-injuries.html.

Exercise physiology studies reveal: Wouter Hoogkamer et al., "A Comparison of the Energetic Cost of Running in Marathon Racing Shoes," *Sports Medicine* 48, no. 4 (April 2018): 1009–19, https://pubmed.ncbi.nlm.nih.gov/29143929/.

the top fifty male marathoners in the world: Jonathan Taylor, "Super Shoes: Explaining Athletics' New Technological Arms Race," *The Conversation*, March 2, 2021, https://theconversation.com/super-shoes-explaining-athletics-new-technological-arms-race-156265#:~:-text.

50–70 percent of the kinetic energy: Jonathan Beverly, "The Truth About Energy Return in Your Shoes," *Runner's World*, October 15, 2015, https://www.runnersworld.com/gear/a20855198/the-truth-about-energy-return-in-your-shoes/.

return more than 85 percent of the energy: Claire Maldarelli, "Nike Put Its Energy-Returning Foam into a Shoe You Can Train In," *Popular Science*, July 13, 2018, https://www.popsci.com/nike-pegasus-turbo-review-faster-training-runs/.

"teeter-totter" theory: Benno M. Nigg et al., "Teeter-Totter Effect: A New Mechanism to Understand Shoe-Related Improvements in Long-Distance Running," *British Journal of Sports Medicine* 55, no. 9 (May 2021): 462–63, https://doi.org/10.1136/bjsports-2020-102550.

Researchers at the University of Colorado: Hoogkamer et al., "A Comparison of the Energetic Cost of Running in Marathon Racing Shoes."

scientists at St. Edward's University: Dustin P. Joubert et al., "Effects of Highly Cushioned and Resilient Racing Shoes on Running Economy at Slower Running Speeds," *International Journal of Sports Physiology and Performance* 18, no. 2 (January 2023): 164–70, https://doi.org/10.1123/ijspp.2022-0227.

A 2023 study: Adam Tenforde et al., "Bone Stress Injuries in Runners Using Carbon Fiber Plate Footwear," *Sports Medicine* 53, no. 8 (February 2023): 1499–1505, https://doi.org/10.1007%2Fs40279-023-01818-z.

Chapter 4

suggests that running two to five days per week: James O'Keefe, "Run for Your Life! At a Comfortable Pace, and Not Too Far: James O'Keefe at TEDx UMKC," TEDx talk, Kansas City, Missouri, November 27, 2012, https://www.youtube.com/watch?v=Y6U728AZnV0.

The highly regarded Copenhagen City Heart Study: Yasmine Aguib and Jassim Al Suwaidi, "The Copenhagen City Heart Study (Østerbroundersøgelsen)," *Global Cardiology Science & Practice* 2015, no. 3 (October 2015): 33, https://doi.org/10.5339%2Fgcsp.2015.33.

continue to accrue with an exercise regimen: Christie Aschwanden, "Can Exercising Too Hard and Too Long Cause Heart Problems?," *Washington Post*, June 13, 2020, https://www.washingtonpost.com/health/can-exercising-too-hard-and-too-long-cause-heart-problems/2020/06/12/8b85b43c-a5c6-11ea-b473-04905b1af82b_story.html.

"you're not training for health": Aschwanden, "Can Exercising Too Hard and Too Long Cause Heart Problems?"

conducted another landmark study in 2019: Alex Hutchinson, "There's Finally Heart Health Data on Extreme Exercise," *Outside*, November 25, 2019, https://www.outsideonline.com/health/training-performance/extreme-exercise-heart-health-study/.

"effortful but not exhaustive": Laura F. De Fina et al., "The Association Between Midlife Cardiorespiratory Fitness and Later Life Chronic Kidney Disease: The Cooper Center Longitudinal Study," *Preventive Medicine* 89 (August 2016): 178–83, https://doi.org/10.1016/j.ypmed.2016.05.030.

published a review: Kim Blond et al., "Association of High Amounts of Physical Activity with Mortality Risk: A Systematic Review and Meta-Analysis," *British Journal of Sports Medicine* 54, no. 20 (August 2019): 1195–1202, https://doi.org/10.1136/bjsports-2018-100393.

Medical experts are now referring: Justin E. Trivax and Peter A. McCullough, "Phidippides [sic] Cardiomyopathy: A Review and Case Illustration," *Clinical Cardiology* 35, no. 2 (February 2012): 69–73, https://doi.org/10.1002%2Fclc.20994.

A study of longtime marathoners: "The Agony of Long-Distance Runners: Coronary Plaque," ABC News, March 18, 2010, https://abcnews.go.com/Health/HeartDisease/coronary-plaque-plague-long-distance-runners/story?id=10140233.

Dr. O'Keefe cites research: Aschwanden, "Can Exercising Too Hard and Too Long Cause Heart Problems?"

"I've been an exercise addict": Aschwanden, "Can Exercising Too Hard and Too Long Cause Heart Problems?"

He reports that 12 percent: Konrad Marshall, "Heart Attacks of the Mega-Fit: How Safe Is Extreme Sport?," *Sydney Morning Herald*, March 30, 2018, https://www.smh.com.au/sport/heart-attacks-of-the-mega-fit-how-safe-is-extreme-sport-20180328-p4z6m7.html.

"We can't ignore that": Marshall, "Heart Attacks of the Mega-Fit."

The fitness patterns for conferring longevity: O'Keefe, "Run for Your Life!"

According to a study: Harshal R. Patil et al., "Cardiovascular Damage Resulting from Chronic Excessive Endurance Exercise," *Missouri Medicine* 109, no. 4 (July-August 2012): 312–21, https://pubmed.ncbi.nlm.nih.gov/22953596.

The MET scale ranks activities: Don Hall, "MET: Levels of Common Recreational Activities," Wellsource, 2008, https://media.hypersites.com/clients/1235/filemanager/MHC/METs.pdf.

"Humans are not genetically adapted": Patil et al., "Cardiovascular Damage Resulting from Chronic Excessive Endurance Exercise," 314.

published an analysis: Sergej M. Ostojic, "Exercise-Induced Mitochondrial Dysfunction: A Myth or Reality?," *Clinical Science* 130, no. 16 (August 2016): 1407–16, https://doi.org/10.1042/CS20160200.

describes what happens in the cells: Peter Attia, *The Drive* episode 66, "Vamsi Mootha, M.D.: Aging, Type 2 Diabetes, Cancer, Alzheimer's Disease, and Parkinson's Disease—Do All Roads Lead to Mitochondria?," August 12, 2019, https://peterattiamd.com/vamsimootha/.

"bravado and beer": John Branch, "The Enduring Fight over the First Ironman Triathlon," *New York Times*, January 25, 2019, https://www.nytimes.com/2019/01/25/sports/iron-man-original-lawsuit.html.

you would have the same lab results: Beatriz Lara et al., "Elevation of Cardiac Troponins After Endurance Running Competitions," *Circulation* 139, no. 5 (December 2018): 709–11, https://doi.org/10.1161/CIRCULATIONAHA.118.034655.

A study published in the *American Journal of Kidney Diseases*: Sherry G. Mansour et al., "Kidney Injury and Repair Biomarkers in Marathon Runners," *American Journal of Kidney Diseases* 70, no. 2 (August 2017): 252–61, https://doi.org/10.1053/j.ajkd.2017.01.045.

inspired to conduct a study: David C. Nieman et al., "Infectious Episodes in Runners Before and After the Los Angeles Marathon," *Journal of Sports Medicine and Physical Fitness* 30, no. 3 (September 1990): 316–28, https://pubmed.ncbi.nlm.nih.gov/2266764/.

helps promote the formation: Vincenzo Monda et al., "Exercise Modifies the Gut Microbiota with Positive Health Effects," *Oxidative Medicine and Cellular Longevity* 2017, no. 3831972 (March 2017), https://doi.org/10.1155/2017/3831972.

A 2017 Italian study: Monda et al., "Exercise Modifies the Gut Microbiota with Positive Health Effects."

Australian researcher Ricardo Costa, PhD, explains: Ricardo J. S. Costa, "Gut-Training: The Impact of Two Weeks Repetitive Gut-Challenge During Exercise on Gastrointestinal Status, Glucose Availability, Fuel Kinetics, and Running Performance," *Applied Physiology, Nutrition, and Metabolism* 42, no. 5 (March 2017): 547–57, https://doi.org/10.1139/apnm-2016-0453.

Dr. Robert Lustig cites research: Olivia Grady, "Dr. Robert Lustig Offers Insights into Connection Between Food Choices and Chronic Disease," *Today at Elon*, Elon University, September 22, 2023, https://www.elon.edu/u/news/2023/09/22/dr-robert-lustig-offers-insights-into-connection-between-food-choices-and-chronic-disease/.

a study of sixty amateur finishers: Lisa Rosenbaum, "Extreme Exercise and the Heart," *The New Yorker*, July 15, 2014, https://www.newyorker.com/tech/annals-of-technology/extreme-exercise-and-the-heart.

"If even the healthiest hearts": Rosenbaum, "Extreme Exercise and the Heart."

"100 percent immunity": David Crossen, "Marathon's Benefit to Heart Is Debated," *New York Times*, October 16, 1979, https://www.nytimes.com/1979/10/16/archives/marathons-benefit-to-heart-is-debated-marathons-benefit-to-the.html.

recounted the conversation: "Did Nathan Pritikin Foretell Jim Fixx's Death?," *Fanatic Cook*, November 24, 2014, https://fanaticcook.com/2014/11/24/did-nathan-pritikin-foretell-jim-fixxs-death/.

"He was not a health nut": John L. Parker Jr., *Once a Runner: A Novel* (Scribner, 2009), 122.

"Exercise is king": Andrew Siegel, *Finding Your Own Fountain of Youth: The Essential Guide to Maximizing Health, Wellness, Fitness & Longevity* (Paul Mould Publishing, 2008), 191.

Hutchinson cites research: Alex Hutchinson, "There's New Evidence on Heart Health in Endurance Athletes," *Outside*, August 7, 2021, https://www.outsideonline.com/health/training-performance/endurance-athletes-heart-health-research-2021/.

According to Dr. Brian Olshansky: Rosenbaum, "Extreme Exercise and the Heart."

Consider a study: "Cardiac Risks Appear Low for Elite Athletes with Diagnosed, Treated Genetic Heart Disease," American College of Cardiology news release, March 6, 2023, https://www.acc.org/About-ACC/Press-Releases/2023/03/06/14/02/Cardiac-Risks-Appear-Low-for-Elite-Athletes.

16 percent of global deaths: "The Top 10 Causes of Death," World Health Organization, August 7, 2024, https://www.who.int/news-room/fact-sheets/detail/the-top-10-causes-of-death.

Chapter 5

"most of us find effort and struggle deeply satisfying": Roger Bannister, *The Four-Minute Mile* (Lyons Press, 2004), vii.

coined the term "obligate runner": Richard M. Restak, "The Jim Fixx Neurosis: Running Yourself to Death," *Washington Post*, July 28, 1984, https://www.washingtonpost.com/archive/opinions/1984/07/29/the-jim-fixx-neurosis-running-yourself-to-death/681bd977-8295-4d4a-802c-bbfd54684be5/.

surveyed nearly five hundred runners: Restak, "The Jim Fixx Neurosis."

The researchers observed: Restak, "The Jim Fixx Neurosis."

A 1983 study: Alayne Yates et al., "Running—An Analogue of Anorexia?," *New England Journal of Medicine* 308, no. 5 (February 1983): 251–55, https://doi.org/10.1056/nejm198302033080504.

A 2015 Italian study: Fabio Lucidi et al., "Running Away from Stress: How Regulatory Modes Prospectively Affect Athletes' Stress Through Passion," *Scandinavian Journal of Medicine & Science in Sports* 26, no. 6 (June 2016): 703–11, https://doi.org/10.1111/sms.12496.

As Muir says: Sophie Parsons, "Is Olympic 1500m Athlete Laura Muir a Practicing Vet?," August 5, 2021, *The Herald* (Scotland), https://www.heraldscotland.com/news/19492990.olympic-1500m-athlete-laura-muir-practicing-vet/.

Brené Brown believes: Brené Brown, "Shame vs. Guilt," BrenéBrown.com, January 15, 2013, https://brenebrown.com/articles/2013/01/15/shame-v-guilt/.

broke world records: Neil Shuttleworth, "Ron Hill Obituary," *The Guardian*, May 23, 2021, https://www.theguardian.com/sport/2021/may/23/ron-hill-obituary.

when he reported that: Jason Daley, "World's Largest Running Streak Comes to an End," *Smithsonian Magazine*, January 31, 2017, https://www.smithsonianmag.com/smart-news/worlds-longest-running-streak-comes-end-180961985/.

every day for forty-eight years: Heather Mayer Irvine, "For 48 Years, Robert 'Raven' Kraft Ran the Same Eight Miles. Every Single Day.," *Runner's World*, November 9, 2023, https://www.runnersworld.com/runners-stories/a45765996/robert-raven-kraft-ends-8-mile-run-streak/.

magazine profile titled: Sarah Barker, "The Minds and Habits of Master Streakers," *Outside*, July 6, 2021, https://run.outsideonline.com/people/the-minds-and-habits-of-master-streakers/.

In an ESPN.com article: Doug Williams, "Sutherland Keeps on Running, Rocking," ESPN.com, October 16, 2013, https://www.espn.com/sports/endurance/story/_/id/9834548/endurance-sports-44-years-jon-sutherland-running-streak-going-strong.

Saremi offers a few suggestions: Allie Burdick, "5 Signs You're Obsessed with Running," *Women's Running*, October 11, 2018, https://www.womensrunning.com/health/5-signs-running-unhealthy-obsession/.

"You are in danger of living a life": David Goggins, *Can't Hurt Me: Master Your Mind and Defy the Odds* (Lioncrest Publishing, 2018), 9.

"It's a lot more than mind over matter": Goggins, *Can't Hurt Me*, 163.

"A lot of my injuries": *Joe Rogan Experience* episode 1212, "David Goggins," December 5, 2018, https://www.youtube.com/watch?v=BvWB7B8tXK8&ab_channel=PowerfulJRE.

40 percent rule: Chris Myers, "The 40% Rule: The Simple Secret to Success," *Forbes*, October 6, 2017, https://www.forbes.com/sites/chrismyers/2017/10/06/the-40-rule-the-simple-secret-to-success/.

"The whole team loved her": Phil Richards, "She's an Inspiration to Many," *Indianapolis News*, June 4, 1996.

a newspaper interview related: Richards, "She's an Inspiration to Many."

As she said about the incident: Richards, "She's an Inspiration to Many."

Her father shared a similar sentiment: Richard Demak, "'And Then She Just Disappeared,'" *Sports Illustrated*, June 15, 1986, https://vault.si.com/vault/1986/06/16/and-then-she-just-disappeared.

described the sentiments: Mark Heisler, "The Ormsby Ordeal: Problem Is, Kathy Wasn't the First Runner to Consider Jumping," *Los Angeles Times*, June 29, 1986, https://www.latimes.com/archives/la-xpm-1986-06-29-sp-117-story.html.

As Dr. Lustig says: Robert Lustig, "Eat Real Food," RobertLustig.com, accessed September 13, 2024, https://robertlustig.com/real-food/.

Dr. Lustig puts it even more bluntly: "Book Dr. Robert Lustig to Speak," RobertLustig.com, accessed September 13, 2024, https://robertlustig.com/speaking/.

"people often bypass admiring you": Morgan Housel, *The Psychology of Money: Timeless Lessons on Wealth, Greed, and Happiness* (Harriman House, 2020), 95, https://ia800402.us.archive.org/18/items/the-psychology-of-money-morgan-housel/The%20Psychology%20of%20Money%20%28Morgan%20Housel%29.pdf.

eighteen to thirty-three times more potent: H. H. Loh et al., "Beta-Endorphin Is a Potent Analgesic Agent," *Proceedings of the National Academy of Sciences of the United States of America* 73, no. 8 (August 1976), 2895–98, https://doi.org/10.1073%2Fpnas.73.8.2895.

"Modern life leaves our minds restless": Arthur De Vany, "Evolutionary Fitness," *Evolutionarily*, December 11, 2000, https://evolutionarily.com/wp-content/uploads/2018/10/Arthur-De-Vany-Evolutionary-Fitness.pdf.

David Brooks wrote: David Brooks, "The Moral Bucket List," *New York Times,* April 11, 2015, https://www.nytimes.com/2015/04/12/opinion/sunday/david-brooks-the-moral-bucket-list.html.

"focus on process": Ashley Merryman, "Forget Trophies, Let Kids Know It's O.K. to Lose," *New York Times*, October 6, 2016, https://www.nytimes.com/roomfordebate/2016/10/06/should-every-young-athlete-get-a-trophy/forget-trophies-let-kids-know-its-ok-to-lose.

"Is this working": Brad Kearns, *Get Over Yourself*, "Ashley Merryman," March 12, 2019, https://bradkearns.com/2019/03/12/merryman/.

obligate runner research suggests: Restak, "The Jim Fixx Neurosis."

Craig Virgin is one of the greatest: "Craig Virgin," Athlete Overview, World Athletics, accessed September 13, 2024, https://worldathletics.org/athletes/united-states/craig-virgin-14346700.

some choice comments: "Illinois' Homegrown Champion," NBC Chicago, December 15, 2011, https://www.nbcchicago.com/news/local/illinoiss-homegrown-champion/1917459/.

"In the early stages of addiction": Caleb Daniloff, "Why Running Could Be the Answer to Beating Addiction," *Runner's World*, June 9, 2017, https://www.runnersworld.com/uk/health/mental-health/a775765/why-running-could-be-the-answer-to-beating-addiction/.

Chapter 6

Research published by Dr. Paul Gastin: Paul B. Gastin, "Energy System Interaction and Relative Contribution During Maximal Exercise," *Sports Medicine* 31, no. 10 (August 2001): 725–41, https://doi.org/10.2165/00007256-200131100-00003.

A healthy person will typically have: Tripthi M. Mathew and Sandeep Sharma, "High Altitude Oxygenation," StatPearls, last modified April 10, 2023, https://www.ncbi.nlm.nih.gov/books/NBK539701/.

"We think there's a psychological tripwire": Roy M. Wallack, *Bike for Life: How to Ride to 100—and Beyond* (Hachette Books, 2015), 37.

As Eliud Kipchoge said: Eliud Kipchoge, "Eliud Kipchoge & David Bedford | Full Address and Q&A | Oxford Union," January 5, 2018, https://www.youtube.com/watch?v=Tc00m-DtzIJU&ab_channel=OxfordUnion.

Extensive anecdotal research: Phil Maffetone, "Is My Ideal Marathon Pace Always 15 Seconds Per Mile Faster Than My MAF Pace?," MAF Fitness, last modified May 18, 2018, https://burnfat.philmaffetone.com/article/97-is-my-ideal-marathon-pace-always-15-seconds-per-mile-faster-than-my-maf-pace.

"Kipchoge pace on treadmill": "Runners Attempt Eliud Kipchoge's World Record Marathon Pace," October 15, 2018, https://www.youtube.com/watch?v=SRYtn0j5ccA&ab_channel=Runner%27sWorld.

April 1–7: 108 kilometers: From Tim Noakes, MD, *Lore of Running* (Human Kinetics, 2003), 379.

He revealed that he trains: Evelyn Watta, "Eliud Kipchoge's Revolutionary Training Methods: How the Olympic Champion's Slow Runs Have Made Him the Fastest," Olympics.com, February 15, 2023, https://olympics.com/en/news/eliud-kipchoge-marathon-revolutionary-training-methods.

offers further support: "Polarized Training Pathway," Fast Talk Laboratories, accessed September 13, 2024, https://www.fasttalklabs.com/pathways/polarized-training/.

five zones, ranked from easy to hard: "Heart Rate Zones Explained," Cleveland Clinic, December 12, 2023, https://health.clevelandclinic.org/exercise-heart-rate-zones-explained.

also reminds us that: Ross Tucker and Sarah Gearhart, "How to Train Like Eliud Kipchoge," *Runner's World*, last modified June 20, 2023, https://www.runnersworld.com/uk/training/marathon/a42722004/eliud-kipchoge-training/.

"fittest man in history": Tris Dixon, "Mat Fraser on Life After Being the Fittest Man on Earth (Five Times)," British *GQ*, April 7, 2021, https://www.gq-magazine.co.uk/lifestyle/article/mat-fraser-on-life-after-being-the-fittest-man-on-earth. TK Consider changing to "fittest man on Earth."

Here's how Hinshaw describes: "My 12 Weeks with Rich Froning," Aerobic Capacity, accessed September 13, 2024, https://www.aerobiccapacity.com/my12weeks.

A study of sixty-six thousand participants: Ron Winslow, "To Double the Odds of Seeing 85: Get a Move On," *Wall Street Journal*, March 9, 2010, https://www.wsj.com/articles/SB10001424052748703954904575109673558885594.

says about the study data: Winslow, "To Double the Odds of Seeing 85."

Booth asserts that: Wes Judd, "To Look and Feel Younger, Running Is the Real Miracle Drug," *Runner's World*, February 9, 2018, https://www.runnersworld.com/news/a20865704/to-look-and-feel-younger-running-is-the-real-miracle-drug/.

American Heart Association states: Trisha D. Scribbans et al., "The Effect of Training Intensity on VO_2max in Young Healthy Adults: A Meta-Regression and Meta-Analysis," *International Journal of Exercise Science* 9, no. 2 (April 2016): 230–47, https://pubmed.ncbi.nlm.nih.gov/27182424.

one's VO2 max is hugely influenced: Ada N. Nordeidet et al., "Exploring Shared Genetics Between Maximal Oxygen Uptake and Disease: The HUNT Study," *Physiological Genomics* 55, no. 10 (September 2023): 440–51, https://doi.org/10.1152/physiolgenomics.00026.2023.

Here's a reminder: Arthur Lydiard and Garth Gilmour, *Running with Lydiard* (Meyer & Meyer Sport, 2000), 25.

Chapter 7

BDNF has been shown to help: Camille S. Wang et al., "BDNF Signaling in Context: From Synaptic Regulation to Psychiatric Disorders," *Cell* 185, no. 1 (January 2022): 62–76, https://doi.org/10.1016/j.cell.2021.12.003.

"Miracle-Gro for the brain": John J. Ratey, *Spark: The Revolutionary New Science of Exercise and the Brain* (Little, Brown, 2008), 19.

widely publicized 2017 study: Zaldy S. Tan et al., "Physical Activity, Brain Volume, and Dementia Risk: The Framingham Study," *Journals of Gerontology* 72, no. 6 (June 2017): 789–95, https://doi.org/10.1093/gerona/glw130.

prominent Stanford University study: Marily Oppezzo and Daniel L. Schwartz, "Give Your Ideas Some Legs: The Positive Effect of Walking on Creative Thinking," *Journal of Experimental Psychology: Learning, Memory, and Cognition* 40, no. 4 (2014): 1142–52, https://doi.org/10.1037/a0036577.

Researchers speculate that walking: Oppezzo and Schwartz, "Give Your Ideas Some Legs."

A three-phase study: Jeffrey Conrath Miller and Zlatan Krizan, "Walking Facilitates Positive Affect (Even When Expecting the Opposite)," *Emotion* 16, no. 5 (2016): 775–85, https://doi.org/10.1037/a0040270.

A Harvard University study revealed: "5 Surprising Benefits of Walking," Harvard Health, December 7, 2023, https://www.health.harvard.edu/staying-healthy/5-surprising-benefits-of-walking.

Studies conducted at the University of Exeter: Hwajung Oh and Adrian H. Taylor, "A Brisk Walk, Compared with Being Sedentary, Reduces Attentional Bias and Chocolate Cravings Among Regular Chocolate Eaters with Different Body Mass," *Appetite* 71 (2013): 144–49, https://doi.org/10.1016/j.appet.2013.07.015.

One study of a thousand subjects: "5 Surprising Benefits of Walking."

the leading cause of injury and death: "About Older Adult Fall Prevention," Centers for Disease Control and Prevention, May 16, 2024, https://www.cdc.gov/falls/about/index.html.

As author Rebecca Solnit writes: Rebecca Solnit, *Wanderlust: A History of Walking* (Penguin, 2001), 250.

Americans take only half that number: David R. Bassett Jr. et al., "Pedometer-Measured Physical Activity and Health Behaviors in U.S. Adults," *Medicine & Science in Sports & Exercise* 42, no. 10 (October 2010): 1819–25, https://doi.org/10.1249%2FMSS.0b013e3181dc2e54.

"Even just going up the stairs": Mark Sisson, *Keto for Life: Reset Your Biological Clock in 21 Days and Optimize Your Diet for Longevity* (Harmony Books, 2019), 40.

"the closest thing we have to a wonder drug": "5 Surprising Benefits of Walking."

A 2022 Finnish study: Vahid Farrahi et al., "Joint Profiles of Sedentary Time and Physical Activity in Adults and Their Associations with Cardiometabolic Health," *Medicine and Science in Sports & Exercise* 54, no. 12 (December 2022): 2118–28, https://doi.org/10.1249%2FMSS.0000000000003008.

2018 Nielsen Total Audience Report: "Time Flies: U.S. Adults Now Spend Nearly Half a Day Interacting with Media," Nielsen Media Research, July 2018, https://www.nielsen.com/insights/2018/time-flies-us-adults-now-spend-nearly-half-a-day-interacting-with-media/.

Kaiser Family Foundation reported: "Generation M2: Media in the Lives of 8- to 18-Year-Olds," Kaiser Family Foundation news release, January 20, 2010, https://www.kff.org/other/event/generation-m2-media-in-the-lives-of/.

considered a "master hormone": Vanessa Rae Romero, "A Lesson on Leptin," *Healthy Living How To*, August 2, 2012, https://healthylivinghowto.com/guest-post-a-lesson-on-leptin/.

Research on the concept of sustained attention: A. C. Shilton, "How to Tell If Your Brain Needs a Break," *New York Times*, February 3, 2023, https://www.nytimes.com/2023/02/03/well/mind/brain-break-focus-productivity.html.

This is validated by research: Herman Pontzer et al., "Hunter-Gatherer Energetics and Human Obesity," *PLOS One* 7, no. 7 (July 2012), https://doi.org/10.1371/journal.pone.0040503.

advanced in Dr. Pontzer's book: Herman Pontzer, "The Exercise Paradox," *Scientific American*, February 1, 2017, https://www.scientificamerican.com/article/the-exercise-paradox/.

groundbreaking 2017 research: David A. Raichlen et al., "Physical Activity Patterns and Biomarkers of Cardiovascular Disease Risk in Hunter-Gatherers," *American Journal of Human Biology* 29, no. 2 (March-April 2017), https://doi.org/10.1002/ajhb.22919.

who famously walked the talk: Henry David Thoreau, "Walking," *Atlantic Monthly* 9, no. 56 (June 1862): 657–74, https://cdn.theatlantic.com/media/archives/1862/06/9-56/131953850.pdf.

Dr. James Levine cites research: Ryan Fiorenzi, "Sitting Is the New Smoking," Start Standing, July 12, 2023, https://www.startstanding.org/sitting-new-smoking/.

A 2022 meta-analysis: Aidan J. Buffey et al., "The Acute Effects of Interrupting Prolonged Sitting Time in Adults with Standing and Light-Intensity Walking on Biomarkers of

Cardiometabolic Health in Adults: A Systematic Review and Meta-Analysis," *Sports Medicine* 52 (2022): 1765-1787, https://doi.org/10.1007/s40279-022-01649-4.

Hong Kong residents have: Roger Yat-Nork Chung and Sir Michael Marmot, "People in Hong Kong Have the Longest Life Expectancy in the World: Some Possible Explanations," *NAM Perspectives*, January 21, 2020, https://doi.org/10.31478%2F202001d.

that they describe as: Dan Buettner, *The Blue Zones: Lessons for Living Longer from the People Who've Lived the Longest* (National Geographic, 2008), 3; Buettner, *The Blue Zones of Happiness: Lessons from the World's Happiest People* (National Geographic, 2017), 24.

validated the importance of walking: Pedro F. Saint-Maurice et al., "Association of Daily Step Count and Step Intensity with Mortality Among US Adults," *Journal of the American Medical Association* 323, no. 12 (March 2020): 1151–60, https://doi.org/10.1001/jama.2020.1382.

unwittingly offers support: Dylan Tweney, "To Run Better, Start by Ditching Your Nikes," *Wired*, July 10, 2009, https://www.wired.com/2009/07/barefoot/.

McDougall also points out: Tara Parker-Pope, "The Human Body Is Built for Distance," *New York Times*, October 26, 2009, https://www.nytimes.com/2009/10/27/health/27well.html.

305 people have died: Alan Arnette, "Everest 2022: Welcome to Everest 2022 Coverage," AlanArnette.com, March 1, 2022, https://www.alanarnette.com/blog/2022/03/01/everest-2022-welcome-to-everest-2022-coverage/.

As Ed Viesturs noted: Bonnie Berkowitz and Weiyi Cai, "What It's Like to Climb Mount Everest Without Oxygen," *The Independent*, May 23, 2016, https://www.independent.co.uk/news/world/asia/mount-everest-what-it-s-like-to-climb-without-oxygen-a7044021.html.

paved the way for many more: Willa Frej, "Arianna: Office Nap Rooms Will Soon Be As Common As Conference Rooms," *HuffPost*, April 4, 2016, https://www.huffpost.com/entry/arianna-huffington-office-nap-rooms-conference-rooms_n_57025cbfe4b0a06d58060ff1.

researchers in New Zealand suggest: "Short Walks After Meals May Prove Important Tool in Managing Diabetes," University of Otago news release, October 18, 2016, https://www.otago.ac.nz/news/newsroom/short-walks-after-meals-may-prove-important-tool-in-managing-diabetes.

Chapter 8

American Podiatric Medical Association reports: "Down at Their Heels: Heel Pain Tops American's List of Persistent Foot Ailments," American Podiatric Medical Association news release, January 23, 2009, https://www.apma.org/files/FileDownloads/APMAFootAilmentsSurveyNewsWorthyAnalysis012309.pdf.

This research revealed: Daniel E. Lieberman et al., "Foot Strike Patterns and Collision Forces in Habitually Barefoot Versus Shod Runners," *Nature* 463 (January 2010): 531–35, https://doi.org/10.1038/nature08723.

Numerous studies suggest: Stephen J. Slade et al., "Somatosensory Perception of Running Shoe Mass," *Ergonomics* 57, no. 6 (March 2014): 912–20, https://doi.org/10.1080/00140139.2014.904009; "No Surprise—Heavier Running Shoes Can Slow You Down," *Women's*

Running, accessed September 15, 2024, https://www.womensrunning.com/training/heavier-running-shoes-slow-down/.

Keeping the arms nearly straight: Andrew K. Yegian et al., :Straight Arm Walking, Bent Arm Running: Gait-Specific Elbow Angles," *Journal of Experimental Biology* 222, no. 13 (July 2019), https://journals.biologists.com/jeb/article/222/13/jeb197228/2704/Straight-arm-walking-bent-arm-running-gait.

Notice how Bolt's legs strike: "100m Usain Bolt Slow Motion Art of Sprinting Fastest Man," September 20, 2012, https://www.youtube.com/watch?v=4fjC1Oim0UQ&ab_channel=OleEejkeEe.

Then watch a video of Eliud Kipchoge: Eliud Kipchoge, "#Londonmarathon #Slowmotion #Running Eluid [sic] Kipchoge Slow Motion Cámara Lenta Técnica de Carrera," April 30, 2019, https://www.youtube.com/watch?v=9p7NT_elwk4&ab_channel=BuyinredTiendaonline.

A study of three hundred finishers: Aravind Ajad Yarra, "Power Your Running with Big Stride," Geeks on Feet, September 4, 2020, https://geeksonfeet.com/run/stride/.

Search YouTube for "Nike—Just Do It (1988)": "Nike – Just Do It (1998) – Very First Commercial," August 30, 2017, https://www.youtube.com/watch?v=0yO7xLAGugQ&ab_channel=tvcommercials.

Daniel Lieberman asserts: Rebecca Hersher, "Barefoot Running Easier on Feet Than Running Shoes," *Harvard Gazette*, January 27, 2010, https://news.harvard.edu/gazette/story/2010/01/barefoot-running-easier-on-feet-than-running-shoes/.

One study of more than six hundred: James R. Barrett et al., "High- Versus Low-Top Shoes for the Prevention of Ankle Sprains in Basketball Players: A Prospective Randomized Study," *American Journal of Sports Medicine* 21, no. 4 (July 1993): 582–85, https://doi.org/10.1177/036354659302100416.

emerging research suggests: Kate Sawkins et al., "The Placebo Effect of Ankle Taping in Ankle Instability," *Medicine & Science in Sports & Exercise* 39, no. 5 (May 2007): 781–87, https://doi.org/10.1249/mss.0b013e3180337371.

Chapter 9

Emerging science is validating: Gabrielle Doré, "Muscle Is the Cornerstone of Longevity," Yahoo! Finance, March 8, 2023, https://finance.yahoo.com/news/muscle-cornerstone-longevity-140025059.html.

Our skeletal muscles make up: "Skeletal Muscle," Cleveland Clinic, last modified September 9, 2021, https://my.clevelandclinic.org/health/body/21787-skeletal-muscle.

cites as the number one cause: "About Older Adult Fall Prevention," Centers for Disease Control and Prevention, May 16, 2024, https://www.cdc.gov/falls/about/index.html.

a study of six thousand Japanese participants: Taina Rantanen et al., "Midlife Grip Strength as a Predictor of Old Age Disability," *Journal of the American Medical Association* 281, no. 6 (February1999): 558–60, https://doi.org/10.1001/jama.281.6.55; "Honolulu Heart Program (HHP)," National Heart, Lung, and Blood Institute, last updated October 23, 2023, https://biolincc.nhlbi.nih.gov/studies/hhp/.

In a 1999 study in Brazil: "Ability to Sit and Rise from the Floor Is Closely Correlated with All-Cause Mortality Risk," European Society of Cardiology news release, December 13, 2012, https://www.escardio.org/The-ESC/Press-Office/Press-releases/Ability-to-sit-and-rise-from-the-floor-is-closely-correlated-with-all-cause-mort.

A British study of 324 identical twins: Claire J. Steves et al., "Kicking Back Cognitive Ageing: Leg Power Predicts Cognitive Ageing after Ten Years in Older Female Twins," *Gerontology* 62, no. 2 (February 2016): 138–49, https://doi.org/10.1159%2F000441029.

Dr. Claire Steves, said: "Strong Legs Contribute to a Healthier Brain in Old Age, Study Finds," *The Guardian*, November 9, 2015, https://www.theguardian.com/uk-news/2015/nov/09/strong-legs-healthier-brain-in-old-age.

Primal Fitness Expert Certification course: "Primal Health Coach Certification," Primal Health Coach Institute, accessed September 15, 2024, https://www.primalhealthcoach.com/primal-health-coach-certification/.

In 2012, research was conducted: Scott Trappe et al., "New Records in Aerobic Power Among Octogenarian Lifelong Endurance Athletes," *Journal of Applied Physiology* 114, no. 1 (January 2013): 3–10, https://doi.org/10.1152%2Fjapplphysiol.01107.2012.

A widely publicized 2018 study: Lisa Owens Viani, "SF State Study Compares Athlete and Truck Driver, Identical Twins," San Francisco State University news release, July 20, 2018, https://news.sfsu.edu/archive/news-story/sf-state-study-compares-athlete-and-truck-driver-identical-twins.html.

Sprinting has been found: "Regular Sprints Boost Metabolism," *ScienceDaily*, January 30, 2009, https://www.sciencedaily.com/releases/2009/01/090127190344.htm.

Research validates the idea: Beau Kjerulf Greer et al., "EPOC Comparison Between Resistance Training and High-Intensity Interval Training in Aerobically Fit Women," *International Journal of Exercise Science* 14, no. 2 (August 2021): 1027–35, https://pubmed.ncbi.nlm.nih.gov/34567357.

Research is compelling: Michael Venutolo-Mantovani, "The Fastest Way to Boost Your Fitness," *New York Times*, April 23, 2024, https://www.nytimes.com/2024/04/23/well/move/sprints-running-workout.html.

It's a maxim of exercise physiology: Angela Harter Alger, "Phosphagen System (ATP-CP System)," in *Nutrition and Physical Fitness* (Pressbooks, 2022), https://pressbooks.calstate.edu/nutritionandfitness/chapter/8-2-phosphagen-system-atp-cp-system/.

Play has been scientifically proved: Lawrence Robinson et al., "The Benefits of Play for Adults," HelpGuide, June 4, 2024, https://www.helpguide.org/mental-health/wellbeing/benefits-of-play-for-adults.

IMAGE CREDITS

Page viii: Photo courtesy of Peluva

Page 13: Bob Daemmrich/Alamy Stock Photo

Page 16: Thames Hare & Hounds

Page 17: Harry Trask/Boston Herald

Page 73: xMarshall/Shutterstock.com

Page 74: iStock.com/davidf

Page 149: Photo by Bernd Dittrich/Unsplash

Page 165: Smith Archive/Alamy Stock Photo

Page 168: Maxisport/Shutterstock.com

Page 227: iStock.com/Suraj Pokhrel

Page 240: The Picture Art Collection/Alamy Stock Photo

Page 243: adike/Shutterstock.com

Page 286: kovop/Shutterstock.com

INDEX

italic page numbers indicate images

B

C

F

G

H

N

T

U

V

W

Y

Z